Secondary Headaches

Editor

RANDOLPH W. EVANS

NEUROLOGIC CLINICS

www.neurologic.theclinics.com

Consulting Editor
RANDOLPH W. EVANS

May 2024 • Volume 42 • Number 2

ELSEVIER

1600 John F. Kennedy Boulevard • Suite 1800 • Philadelphia, Pennsylvania, 19103-2899

http://www.theclinics.com

NEUROLOGIC CLINICS Volume 42, Number 2
May 2024 ISSN 0733-8619, ISBN-13: 978-0-443-18360-7

Editor: Stacy Eastman
Developmental Editor: Varun Gopal

Neurologic Clinics (ISSN 0733-8619) is published quarterly by Elsevier Inc., 360 Park Avenue South, New York, NY 10010–1710. Months of issue are February, May, August, and November. Periodicals postage paid at New York, NY, and additional mailing offices. Subscription prices are $360.00 per year for US individuals, $100.00 per year for US students, $445.00 per year for Canadian individuals, $504.00 per year for international individuals, $210.00 for foreign students/residents, and $100.00 for Canadian students/residents. For institutional access pricing please contact Customer Service via the contact information below. To receive student/resident rate, orders must be accompanied by name of affiliated institution, date of term, and the *signature* of program/residency coordinator on institution letterhead. Orders will be billed at individual rate until proof of status is received. Foreign air speed delivery is included in all *Clinics* subscription prices. All prices are subject to change without notice. **POSTMASTER:** Send address changes to *Neurologic Clinics*, Elsevier Health Sciences Division, Subscription Customer Service, 3251 Riverport Lane, Maryland Heights, MO 63043. **Customer Service: Telephone: 1-800-654-2452 (U.S. and Canada); 314-447-8871 (outside U.S. and Canada). Fax: 314-447-8029. E-mail: journalscustomerservice-usa@elsevier.com (for print support); journalsonlinesupport-usa@elsevier.com (for online support).**

Reprints. For copies of 100 or more of articles in this publication, please contact the Commercial Reprints Department, Elsevier Inc., 360 Park Avenue South, New York, New York, 10010-1710; Tel.: +1-212-633-3874; Fax: +1-212-633-3820, and E-mail: reprints@elsevier.com.

Neurologic Clinics is also published in Spanish by Nueva Editorial Interamericana S.A., Mexico City, Mexico.

Neurologic Clinics is covered in *Current Contents/Clinical Medicine*, *MEDLINE/PubMed (Index Medicus)*, *EMBASE/Excerpta Medica*, and *PsycINFO*, and *ISI/BIOMED*.

Contributors

CONSULTING EDITOR

RANDOLPH W. EVANS, MD
Clinical Professor, Department of Neurology, Baylor College of Medicine, Houston, Texas, USA

EDITOR

RANDOLPH W. EVANS, MD
Clinical Professor, Department of Neurology, Baylor College of Medicine, Houston, Texas, USA

AUTHORS

OSAMA AL DEYABAT, MD
Physician, Department of Ophthalmology, Blanton Eye Institute, Houston Methodist Hospital, Houston, Texas, USA

ANTHONY K. ALLAM, BBA
Department of Neurosurgery, Baylor College of Medicine, Houston, Texas, USA

JAMES R. ALLISON, BDS (Hons), MFDS RCSEng/RCPS (Glasg), MDTFEd, FHEA
Clinical Research Fellow, School of Dental Sciences, Faculty of Medical Sciences, Newcastle University, Newcastle Upon Tyne Hospitals NHS Foundation Trust, Newcastle Upon Tyne, United Kingdom

SAIF ALDEEN ALRYALAT, MD
Physician, Department of Ophthalmology, University of Jordan, Amman, Jordan; Department of Ophthalmology, Blanton Eye Institute, Houston Methodist Hospital, Houston, Texas, USA

JENNIFER P. BASSIUR, DDS
Associate Professor, Center for Oral, Facial and Head Pain, College of Dental Medicine, Columbia University Medical Center, Division of Oral and Maxillofacial Surgery, New York, New York, USA

EMMA V. BEECROFT, BDS, MFDS RCS (Ed & Eng)
PG Dip Con Sed, Associate Clinical Lecturer, School of Dental Sciences, Faculty of Medical Sciences, Newcastle University, Newcastle Upon Tyne Hospitals NHS Foundation Trust, Newcastle Upon Tyne, United Kingdom

SOOMI CHO, MD
Clinical Fellow, Department of Neurology, Yonsei University College of Medicine, Seoul, South Korea

MIN KYUNG CHU, MD, PhD
Professor, Department of Neurology, Yonsei University College of Medicine, Seoul, South Korea

FRED MICHAEL CUTRER, MD
Neurologist, Professor, Chair, Headache Division, Mayo Clinic, Rochester, Minnesota, USA

EVERTON EDMONDSON, MD
Professor, Department of Neurology, Baylor College of Medicine, Houston, Texas, USA

DAVID EDWARDS, BDS (Hons), MRes, MSc, MFDTEd, MFDS RCS (Ed), PGDip Con Sed, PGDip Rest Dent RCS (Eng), PGCert MEd Ed, FHEA
Dentist, School of Dental Sciences, Faculty of Medical Sciences, Newcastle University, Newcastle Upon Tyne Hospitals NHS Foundation Trust, Newcastle Upon Tyne, United Kingdom

RANDOLPH W. EVANS, MD
Clinical Professor, Department of Neurology, Baylor College of Medicine, Houston, Texas, USA

DEBORAH I. FRIEDMAN, MD, MPH
Neurologist, Yellow Rose Headache and Neuro-Ophthalmology, Dallas, Texas, USA

JONATHAN GLADSTONE, MD, FRCPC
Headache Neurology Consultant, Department of Pediatrics, Division of Neurology, The Hospital for Sick Children, University of Toronto, Toronto, Ontario, Canada; Headache Neurology Consultant, Gladstone Headache Clinic, North York, Ontario, Canada

JAMES IM, MD
PGY5, Adult Neurology Resident, Department of Medicine, Division of Adult Neurology, St. Michael's Hospital, University of Toronto, Toronto, Ontario, Canada

ZAZA KATSARAVA, MD, PhD, MSc
Professor, Department of Neurology, University of Duisburg-Essen, Essen, Germany; Evangelical Hospital Unna, Unna, Germany; EVEX Medical Corporation, Tbilisi, Georgia

DORIS KUNG, DO
Associate Professor, Department of Neurology, Baylor College of Medicine, Houston, Texas, USA

ANA MARISSA LAGMAN-BARTOLOME, MD, FRCPC, FAHS
Department of Pediatrics, Division of Neurology, Children's Hospital, London Health Sciences Center, Schulich School of Medicine & Dentistry, University of Western Ontario, London, Ontario, Canada; Department of Pediatrics, Division of Neurology, The Hospital for Sick Children, University of Toronto, Toronto, Ontario, Canada

M. BENJAMIN LARKIN, MD, PharmD
Resident Physician, Department of Neurosurgery, Baylor College of Medicine, Houston, Texas, USA

ANDREW G. LEE, MD
Chair, Department of Ophthalmology, Blanton Eye Institute, Houston Methodist Hospital, Houston, Texas, USA; Sam Houston State, Conroe, Texas, USA; Department of Ophthalmology, Cullen Eye Institute, Baylor College of Medicine, Houston, Texas, USA; Departments of Ophthalmology, Neurology, and Neurosurgery, Weill Cornell Medicine,

New York, New York, USA; Department of Ophthalmology, University of Texas MD Anderson Cancer Center, Houston, Texas, USA; Texas A&M College of Medicine, Bryan, Texas, USA; Department of Ophthalmology, University of Iowa Hospitals and Clinics, Iowa City, Iowa, USA

MONIQUE MONTENEGRO, MD
Neurologist, Assistant Professor, General Neurology and Headache Division, University of Minnesota Medical School, Minneapolis, Minnesota, USA

MARK OBERMANN, MD, PhD, MHBA
Head, Department of Neurology, Hospital Weser-Egge, Hoexter, Germany; Department of Neurology, University of Duisburg-Essen, Essen, Germany

AISHWARYA V. PAREEK, MD
Department of Pediatrics, Section of Neurology and Developmental Neuroscience, Baylor College of Medicine, Texas Children's Hospital, Houston, Texas, USA

MARCELA ROMERO-REYES, DDS, PhD
Clinical Professor, Director, Brotman Facial Pain Clinic, University of Maryland, School of Dentistry, Department of Neural and Pain Sciences, University of Maryland, Baltimore, School of Dentistry, Baltimore, Maryland, USA

JOHN F. ROTHROCK, MD
Professor of Neurology and Director of APC Headache Fellowship, Inova Health, University of Virginia School of Medicine, Editor in Chief, Migraineur, Fairfax, Virginia, USA

PEDRO AUGUSTO SAMPAIO ROCHA-FILHO, MD, PhD
Professor, Division of Neuropsychiatry, Centro de Ciências Médicas, Universidade Federal de Pernambuco (UFPE), Headache Clinic, Hospital Universitario Oswaldo Cruz, Universidade de Pernambuco, Recife, Brazil

HIMANSHU SHARMA, MD, PhD
Resident Physician, Department of Neurosurgery, Baylor College of Medicine, Houston, Texas, USA

ASHWIN VISWANATHAN, MD
Professor, Department of Neurosurgery, Baylor College of Medicine, Houston, Texas, USA

SHUU-JIUN WANG, MD
Neurologist, Department of Neurology, Neurological Institute, Taipei Veterans General Hospital, College of Medicine, National Yang Ming Chiao Tung University, Brain Research Center, National Yang Ming Chiao Tung University, Taipei, Taiwan

JR-WEI WU, MD
Neurologist, Department of Neurology, Neurological Institute, Taipei Veterans General Hospital, Center for Quality Management, Taipei Veterans General Hospital, Assistant Professor, College of Medicine, National Yang Ming Chiao Tung University, Taipei, Taiwan

DAVID S. YOUNGER, MD, DrPH, MPH, MS
Clinician, Department of Clinical Medicine and Neuroscience, CUNY School of Medicine, New York, New York, USA; Department of Medicine, Section of Internal Medicine and Neurology, White Plains Hospital, White Plains, New York, USA

Contents

abnormality. It is either primary (idiopathic intracranial hypertension, IIH) or secondary. A secondary cause is unlikely when adhering to the diagnostic criteria. Permanent visual loss occurs if undetected or untreated, and the associated headaches may be debilitating. Fulminant disease may result in blindness despite aggressive treatment. This chapter addresses the diagnosis and management of IIH including new insights into the pathobiology of IIH, updates in therapeutics and causes of overdiagnosis.

Spontaneous intracranial hypotension (SIH) typically presents as an acute orthostatic headache during an upright position, secondary to spinal cerebrospinal fluid leaks. New evidence indicates that a lumbar puncture may not be essential for diagnosing every patient with SIH. Spinal neuroimaging protocols used for diagnosing and localizing spinal cerebrospinal fluid leaks include brain/spinal MRI, computed tomography myelography, digital subtraction myelography, and radionuclide cisternography. Complications of SIH include subdural hematoma, cerebral venous thrombosis, and superficial siderosis. Treatment options encompass conservative management, epidural blood patches, and surgical interventions. The early application of epidural blood patches in all patients with SIH is suggested.

The prevalence of brain tumors in patients with headache is very low; however, 48% to 71% of patients with brain tumors experience headache. The clinical presentation of headache in brain tumors varies according to age; intracranial pressure; tumor location, type, and progression; headache history; and treatment. Brain tumor-associated headaches can be caused by local and distant traction on pain-sensitive cranial structures, mass effect caused by the enlarging tumor and cerebral edema, infarction, hemorrhage, hydrocephalus, and tumor secretion. This article reviews the current findings related to epidemiologic details, clinical manifestations, mechanisms, diagnostic approaches, and management of headache in association with brain tumors.

Identification of substances that may cause or trigger headache is important to start effective treatment early to prevent unnecessary suffering, deterioration in quality of life, and the development of chronic pain. Treatment in case of medication overuse and other chronic headache should be decisive and effective. Drug withdrawal and introduction of effective prophylactic medication for the underlying headache disorder should be the primary treatment strategy. Typical headache-inducing substances are nitric oxide, phosphodiesterase, cocaine, alcohol, histamine, carbon oxide, and calcitonin gene-related peptide. The withdrawal of caffeine, estrogen, and opioids is most often associated with the development of headache.

Pedro Augusto Sampaio Rocha-Filho

Headache affects around half of patients in the acute phase of COVID-19 and generally occurs at the beginning of the symptomatic phase, has an insidious onset, and is bilateral, and of moderate to severe intensity. COVID-19 may also present complications that cause acute and persistent headaches, such as cerebrovascular diseases, rhinosinusitis, meningitis, and intracranial hypertension. In 10% to 20% of patients with COVID-19, headache may persist beyond the acute phase. In general, the headache improves over time. To date, there are no clinical trials that have assessed the treatment of persistent post-COVID-19 headache.

Ana Marissa Lagman-Bartolome, James Im, and Jonathan Gladstone

Headaches attributed to disorders of homeostasis include those different headache types associated with metabolic and systemic diseases. These are headache disorders occurring in temporal relation to a disorder of homeostasis including hypoxia, high altitude, airplane travel, diving, sleep apnea, dialysis, autonomic dysreflexia, hypothyroidism, fasting, cardiac cephalalgia, hypertension and other hypertensive disorders like pheochromocytoma, hypertensive crisis, and encephalopathy, as well as preeclampsia or eclampsia. The proposed mechanism behind the causation of these headache subtypes including diagnostic criteria, evaluation, treatment, and overall management will be discussed.

Aishwarya V. Pareek, Everton Edmondson, and Doris Kung

Cervicogenic headaches are a secondary headache disorder attributable to cervical spine dysfunction resulting in head pain with or without neck pain. Diagnosis of this condition has been complicated by varied clinical presentations, causations, and differing diagnostic criteria. In this article, we aim to clarify the approach to diagnosing cervicogenic headaches by providing an overview of cervicogenic headaches, clinical case examples, and a practical diagnostic algorithm based on the most current criteria. A standardized approach will aid in confirmation of the diagnosis of cervicogenic headaches and facilitate further research into this condition.

Saif Aldeen Alryalat, Osama Al Deyabat, and Andrew G. Lee

Eye pain is a common complaint among patients presenting to the neurology clinic. It can be related to neurologic diseases, but it can also be a localized eye condition. Such disorders can be misleading, as their benign appearance might mask more grave underlying conditions, potentially leading to misdiagnoses or delayed treatment. Clinicians should be aware of the specific neurologic or systemic disorders (eg, demyelinating diseases or vascular abnormalities) that might first manifest as eye pain. Formal ophthalmic consultation is recommended for patients presenting with

NEUROLOGIC CLINICS

THE CLINICS ARE AVAILABLE ONLINE!
Access your subscription at:
www.theclinics.com

Preface

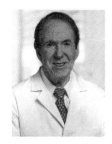

Randolph W. Evans, MD
Editor

Although an estimated 90% of headaches are of the primary type, the other 10% are secondary headache disorders, which are diverse and fascinating, at times potentially life-threatening, and sometimes challenging to diagnose. We update our well-received second issue on this topic, which appeared in May 2014.

This issue reviews 15 types and causes of secondary headache and facial pain disorders: posttraumatic headaches; headaches due to vascular disorders; headaches and vasculitis; idiopathic intracranial hypertension; spontaneous intracranial hypotension; headache in brain tumors; headaches attributed to a substance or its withdrawal; headache associated with COVID-19; metabolic headache; cervicogenic headache; ophthalmologic disorders, temporomandibular disorders, bruxism, and headache; trigeminal neuralgia and glossopharyngeal neuralgia; cough, exertional, and sex headaches; and other secondary headaches.

These headaches range from the rare to the mundane and from the well-established to the highly controversial. We're all too familiar with the tragic new entity, COVID-19 and associated headaches. I hope this issue will stimulate further interest in the subspecialty of headache medicine.

I appreciate the outstanding contributions of our distinguished contributors. I thank Stacy Eastman, Senior Editor, *Neurologic Clinics*; Varun Gopal, Content Development Specialist, *Neurologic Clinics*; and the production team at Elsevier for their great work.

Randolph W. Evans, MD
Baylor College of Medicine
1200 Binz #1370
Houston, TX 77004, USA

E-mail address:
revansmd@gmail.com

Neurol Clin 42 (2024) xiii
https://doi.org/10.1016/j.ncl.2024.02.003
0733-8619/24/© 2024 Elsevier Inc. All rights reserved.

neurologic.theclinics.com

The Postconcussion Syndrome and Posttraumatic Headaches in Civilians, Soldiers, and Athletes

Randolph W. Evans, MD

KEYWORDS

- Postconcussion syndrome • Mild traumatic brain injury • Headaches
- Posttraumatic • Occipital neuralgia • Soldiers • Athletes • Concussion

KEY POINTS

- Mild traumatic brain injuries account for about 80% of all traumatic brain injuries.
- Headache is the most common symptom of the postconcussion syndrome, which develops in 30-90% of those who are symptomatic after mild head injuries.
- Paradoxically, headache prevalence and lifetime duration is greater in those who have mild head injury compared with those who have more severe trauma.
- Tension-type-like and migraine-like are the most common phenotypes.
- There are few randomized placebo-controlled trials for treatment, which is based on the phenotype.

Headaches resulting from head trauma are one of the most common secondary headache types. Because of the medicolegal aspects, posttraumatic headaches (PTHs) have been one of the most controversial headache topics, and, for many physicians, one of their least favorite types to treat. However, in the last 25 years, there has been increasing interest in PTHs among physicians and the public because of athletes with concussion and headaches occurring in United States soldiers with blast trauma. This article reviews the postconcussion syndrome (PCS) and PTHs with a focus on adults and updates the literature from the prior review in this issue in 2014.[1]

THE POSTCONCUSSION SYNDROME

PCS refers to a large number of symptoms and signs that may occur alone or in combination, usually after a mild traumatic brain injury (mTBI).[2] Concussion, the mildest form of TBI, is a clinical syndrome of biomechanically induced alteration of

Neurology, Baylor College of Medicine, 1200 Binz #1370, Houston, TX 77004, USA
E-mail address: revansmd@gmail.com

Neurol Clin 42 (2024) 341–373
https://doi.org/10.1016/j.ncl.2023.12.001
0733-8619/24/© 2023 Elsevier Inc. All rights reserved.

brain function, typically affecting memory and orientation, which may or may not involve loss of consciousness.[3]

The patient's account of loss of consciousness and duration may not be reliable.[4] Loss of consciousness does not have to occur for PCS to develop. Although confusion or disorientation is used as a criterion for mTBI in the World Health Organization criteria,[5] these signs are not specific to mTBI and can occur as a strong emotional reaction to an unexpected event that places a person in serious danger.[6] The diagnosis of concussion may not be reliable even by an unaffiliated sideline neurotrauma expert in the National Football League (NFL; see case 3).[7]

It is controversial whether the symptoms of PCS are a specific, cohesive, and predictable syndrome because the symptoms are nonspecific, subjective, and common in the uninjured general population and among those with nonhead injuries and comorbidities such as depression, insomnia, and pain.[8,9] There is controversy over the diagnostic criteria such as the International Statistical Classification of Diseases and Related Health Problems (ICD-10) and Diagnostic and Statistical Manual of Mental Disorders.[10–12]

A high base rate level of PCS symptoms in the general population can lead to misattribution of symptoms to PCS. In one study of 104 healthy university community adults (61% women) with a mean age of 23 years, the following percentages endorsed the following symptoms from the ICD-10 criteria for PCS as present in the prior 2 weeks: fatigue, 76%; irritable, 72%; nervous or tense, 63%; poor sleep, 62%; poor concentration, 61%; sad, 61%; temper problems, 53%; headaches, 52%; memory problems, 51%; dizziness, 42%; extra sensitive to noises, 40%; nausea, 38%; and difficulty reading, 36%.[13] Several studies have compared patients with mTBI to nonhead injured controls finding a high prevalence of the same symptoms in both groups, indicating a high prevalence of base rate symptoms in the general population[14] similar to those with persistent PCS.[15]

Prevalence rates of PCS vary from 11% to 82% depending on diagnostic criteria, population, and the time of assessment.[16] The following symptoms and signs are associated with PCS: headaches, dizziness, vertigo, tinnitus, hearing loss, blurred vision, diplopia, convergence insufficiency, light and noise sensitivity, diminished taste and smell, irritability, anxiety, depression, personality change, fatigue, sleep disturbance, decreased libido, decreased appetite, posttraumatic stress disorder, memory dysfunction, impaired concentration and attention, slowing of reaction time, and slowing of information processing speed (**Box 1**).[17] In a prospective longitudinal study, the most to least common symptoms are as follows: fatigue, headaches, taking longer to think, poor memory, poor concentration, dizziness, frustrated, irritable, noise sensitivity, restlessness, sleep disturbance, light sensitivity, blurred vision, depressed, nausea, and double vision.[18]

In another study of 118 patients who sustained a mTBI, symptoms were reported 1 month following the injury in the following percentages of patients: fatigue, 91%; headaches, 78%; forgetfulness, 73%; sleep disturbance, 70%; anxiety, 63%; irritability, 62%; dizziness, 59%; noise sensitivity, 46%, and light sensitivity, 44%.[19] PCS may be subdivided into early PCS and a late or persistent PCS, which is when symptoms and signs persist for more than 6 months.[20] Among 53 patients referred to a headache clinic with chronic PTHs, about half had cognitive complaints, a quarter had psychological complaints, and 17% had an isolated complaint of headache.[21]

In a survey of headache medicine specialists, the mean response on the Likert scale (1, strongly disagree and 5, strongly agree) was 3.66 for the following statement: I like to treat PCS. Of the 7 headache types queried, only refractory migraine (3.62) and new daily persistent headache (3.52) were less liked.[22]

Box 1
Sequelae of mild head injury

Headaches
  Tension type
  Migraine with and without aura
  Medication overuse
  Trigeminal autonomic cephalalgias
  Hemicrania continua
  Occipital neuralgia
  C2–3 facet joint
  Cervicogenic
  Supraorbital and infraorbital neuralgia
  Scalp lacerations and local trauma
  Temporomandibular joint
  Subdural or epidural hematomas
  Low CSF pressure syndrome
  Hemorrhagic cortical contusions
  Carotid and vertebral artery dissections
  Cerebral venous thrombosis
  Carotid–cavernous fistula

Cranial nerve symptoms and signs
  Dizziness
  Vertigo
  Tinnitus
  Hearing loss
  Blurred vision
  Diplopia
  Convergence insufficiency
  Light and noise sensitivity
  Diminished taste and smell

Psychological and somatic complaints
  Irritability
  Anxiety
  Depression
  Personality change
  Posttraumatic stress disorder
  Fatigue
  Sleep disturbance
  Decreased libido
  Decreased appetite
  Initial nausea or vomiting

Cognitive impairment
  Memory dysfunction
  Impaired concentration and attention
  Slowing of reaction time
  Slowing of information processing speed

Rare sequelae
  Subdural and epidural hematomas
  Cerebral venous thrombosis
  Second impact syndrome
  Seizures
  Nonepileptic posttraumatic seizures
  Transient global amnesia
  Tremor
  Dystonia

From Evans RW. Post-concussion syndrome. In: Evans RW, Baskin DS, Yatsu FM, editors. Prognosis of neurological disorders. 2nd edition. New York: Oxford University Press; 2000. p. 366–80.

DIAGNOSTIC TESTING FOR MILD TRAUMATIC BRAIN INJURY
Imaging

Computerized tomography (CT) abnormalities of the brain (complicated mTBI) have been detected in up to 5% of patients with a Glasgow Coma Scale (GCS) score of 15 and as high as 30% of those with a GCS score of 13.[23] According to a meta-analysis of 23,079 patients with minor head trauma (defined as a GCS score of 13–15), the prevalence of severe intracranial injury was 7.1% and the prevalence of injuries leading to death or requiring neurosurgical intervention was 0.9%.[24] For those without loss of consciousness, the likelihood ratio was only 0.60 for intracranial injury. The Canadian CT Head Rule, the New Orleans Criteria, and the National Emergency X-ray Utilization Study provide clinical rules to identify patients with mTBI who can safely avoid undergoing CT.[23]

MRI is more sensitive than CT for the detection of axonal injury, small hemorrhages, contusions, and small extra-axial collections. In a study of 1375 patients with mTBI (79% with loss of consciousness) with negative CT findings within 24 hours of injury, MRI's of the brain were positive for acute posttraumatic changes in 27% (isolated traumatic axonal injury in 54%, isolated diffuse axonal injury in 18%, isolated contusions in 2%, pure extra-axial lesions in 12%, and mixed lesions in 15%.[25]

According to guidelines from the Radiological Society of North American,[26] for patients presenting with acute TBI, noncontrast head CT is the imaging of choice. "MRI has a higher sensitivity for detecting axonal injury among mild TBI patients; however, the routine use of brain MRI for the detection of injury in the setting of acute mild TBI is not supported at the present time. MRI may be indicated in particular instances when there are persistent neurologic, cognitive, and behavioral symptoms, such as new-onset, progressive or worsening symptoms."

According to guidelines from the American College of Radiology[21] and the Radiological Society of North America (RSNA),[27] there is insufficient evidence to support the routine clinical use of MRI of the brain with diffusion tensor imaging and single photon computerized tomography (SPECT) for the evaluation of TBI. The RSNA guideline states the following: "However, at present, there is insufficient evidence supporting the routine clinical use of these advanced neuroimaging techniques (MRI diffusion tensor imaging, functional MRI, MR spectroscopy, perfusion imaging, positron emission tomography/ single photon computerized tomography and magnetoencephalography for diagnosis and/or prognostication of TBI at the individual patient level."[21]

MRI DTI findings are nonspecific with abnormal findings present in 60% of normal controls,[28] depression, attention deficit disorder, posttraumatic stress disorder, obstructive sleep apnea, diabetes mellitus, hypertension, and alcohol use disorders.

According to the United States Department of Veteran Affairs and Department of Defense guidelines, "Currently, evidence does not support the use of laboratory imaging or physiologic testing [neuroimaging, serum biomarkers, electroencephalogram(EEG)] for diagnosing mTBI or directing the care of patients with symptoms attributed to mTBI."[29] The guidelines also have recommendations for management of postacute mTBI.

Electroencephalogram

Routine EEG and quantitative EEG (QEEG) are not indicated for diagnosis and/or prognosis of mTBI. According to the United States Department of Veteran Affairs and Department of Defense guidelines, "Unfortunately, there were no studies identified in this systematic evidence review to support the use of EEG for diagnosis and/ or prognosis in postacute mTBI."[25]

In a review of the utility of QEEG in mTBI, Nuwer and colleagues stated, "There are no clear EEG or QEEG features unique to mild traumatic brain injury. Late after head injury, the correspondence is poor between electrophysiologic findings and clinical symptoms. ... There are no proven pathognomonic signatures useful for identifying head injury as the cause of signs and symptoms, especially late after the Injury. ...Conversely, an EEG abnormality is not apt or proving an organic basis for a patient's complaints...EEG does not predict, confirm or measure PCS [postconcussion syndrome] or PPCS [persistent postconcussion syndrome], nor should mild EEG abnormality be used to substantiate an objective clinical brain injury. Nor can a normal EEG exclude an initial significant brain injury."[30]

According to the Guideline Committee of the American Clinical Neurophysiology Society, "It was found that for patients with or without symptoms of abnormal cognition or behavior, current evidence does not support the clinical use of qEEG either at the time of the injury or remote from the injury to diagnose mTBI."[31]

Neuopsychological Testing

For those with persistent cognitive symptoms, neuropsychological testing by a qualified neuropsychologist is necessary to determine the presence of neurocognitive impairment due to TBI.[11] In a prospective study of 656 patients with mTBI who presented to level 1 trauma centers within 24 hours of mTBI, poor cognitive outcome at 1 year affected 13.5% of patients versus 4.5% of controls.[32]

Computerized neuropsychological testing does not allow for direct observation or interpretation by a neuropsychologist, is a brief snapshot of limited cognitive domains, may be used incorrectly if not interpreted by a neuropsychologist, and does not substitute for formal neuropsychological testing by a neuropsychologist. "Interpretation of test scores following a neuropsychological evaluation is intricate and requires specialized knowledge about the psychometric properties of assessment (e.g., validity, reliability, normative data, base rates, and reliable change). Additional factors such as culture, preexisting (e.g., learning disorder or ADHD), or co-occurring diagnoses (e.g., mood symptoms) can influence test performance and the interpretive process of any neuropsychological assessment. Furthermore, the most recent consensus statement highlights the growing body of literature reporting that psychological factors play a significant role in symptom recovery and presentation."[33]

HISTORICAL ASPECTS OF POSTCONCUSSION SYNDROME

PCS has been controversial for more than 160 years.[34,35] Erichsen, a London surgeon, beginning with a series of lectures in 1866, opined that minor injuries to the head could result in severe disability as a result of "subacute cerebral meningitis and arachnitis."[36] Symptoms reported by these patients included headaches, memory complaints, nightmares, irritability, and light and noise sensitivity. Erichsen was defensive about these cases of cerebral concussion because many occurred after railway accidents in which litigation was involved. On the title page of his book, he quotes Montaigne, "Je raconte, je ne juge pas" (I tell, I do not judge). These injuries became known as "railway brain" and those of the spine as "railway spine." He pointed out that earlier investigators had described the same symptoms in the prerailway era. He also was concerned about misdiagnosing these cases as hysteria: "Hysteria is the disease for which I have more frequently seen concussion of the spine, followed by meningo-myelitis, mistaken, and it certainly has always appeared extraordinary to me that so great an error of diagnosis could so easily be made."

Railway spine and brain became topics of intense controversy. In 1879, Rigler[37] raised the important issue of compensation neurosis when he described the increased incidence of posttraumatic invalidism after a system of financial compensation was established for accidental injuries on the Prussian railways in 1871. In 1888, Strumpell discussed how the desire for compensation could lead to exaggeration. In 1889, Oppenheim popularized the concept of traumatic neurosis, in which a strong afferent stimulus resulted in impairment of function of the central nervous system. Charcot countered Oppenheim's work and suggested that the impairment described actually was the result of hysteria and neurasthenia.

PCS also was controversial throughout the twentieth century. In one of the first uses of the term in 1934, Strauss and Savitsky's concluded: "In our opinion, the subjective post-traumatic syndrome, characterized by headache, dizziness, inordinate fatigue on effort, intolerance to intoxicants and vasomotor instability, is organic and is dependent on a disturbance in intracranial equilibrium due directly to the blow on the head. We suggest the term "postconcussion syndrome" for this symptom complex."[38]

Miller, in 1961, summarized the viewpoint of those who believed that PCS actually was a compensation neurosis: "The most consistent clinical feature is the subject's unshakable conviction of unfitness for work."[39] In 1962, Symonds took an equally strong opposing viewpoint: "It is, I think, questionable whether the effects of concussion, however slight, are ever completely reversible."[40]

In a 2017 survey of Texas neurologists,[41] 31% of respondents agreed, "PCS is a clearly defined syndrome with a solid basis for determining prognosis." The statement, "Most physicians tend to question the authenticity of patients' reports of symptoms with PCS," was endorsed by 34.2% and the statement, "I personally tend to question the authenticity of patients' reports of symptoms with PCS" was endorsed by 10.9%. Only 10.9% of respondents agreed, "Prolonged symptoms are more likely to be psychogenic in origin than due to any true pathology for patients with PCS." There is a growing acceptance of PCS among neurologists compared with a 1992 American survey.[42]

EPIDEMIOLOGY OF TRAUMATIC BRAIN INJURY
Civilians

TBI is a cause of significant morbidity and mortality worldwide with approximately 50 to 60 million injuries annually including at least 3.5 million in the United States.[43] In the United States, the causes of TBI are approximately as follow: falls, 42%; motor vehicle accidents, 20%; sports and recreational accidents, 10%; assaults, 10% (including nonfatal gunshot wound); and occupational, 4%. Motor vehicle accidents are a more common cause of TBI in the young (almost 30% for ages 15–19 years) and falls a more common cause in the elderly (60% for ages 65 years and older). Men are injured more frequently than women, with an approximate 2:1 ratio.[44] Perhaps, 25% or more of people who have mTBI injuries do not seek treatment.[45]

About 80% of reported traumatic brain injuries are mild.[46] In a Canadian study, the annual incidence of concussion was 1.2%.[47] In a population-based United States survey with random sampling, 36.4% of respondents reported at least one mTBI in the lifetime.[48] In addition, some patients may have hidden TBI, where they develop PCS but do not make the causal connection between the injury and its consequences.[49]

United States Military

Approximately 20% of veterans of Operations Enduring Freedom (Afghanistan) and Iraqi Freedom sustained a TBI, the "signature wound" of the conflicts.[50] According to the Congressional Research Service,[51] "Of the total 253,330 TBI cases between January 1, 2000 and August 20, 2012, 194,561 have been mild, 42,083 have been moderate, 6476 have been severe or penetrating, and 10,210 have not been classifiable." Blast exposure is the most common mechanism of injury contributing to 75% of mTBI.[52,53]

Sports

In the United States, 1.6 to 3.8 million persons per year sustain sport-related mTBI with many not obtaining immediate medical attention.[54] In 2017, 2.5 million high school students reported sustaining at least one sport or activity-related concussion in the past year, and one million high school students reported sustaining more than one sport-related or activity-related concussion in the past year.[55] in a 2021 survey, 11.9% of high school students reported a concussion from playing a sport or being physically active.[56] For high school sports, football has the highest rate of concussion.[57]

The incidence of concussion among high school and college football players per 1000 games was 1.55 and 3.02, respectively.[58] Women have more concussions in high school and college basketball and soccer (highest rates) compared with men. The rates per 1000 games for soccer are as follows: high school, males 0.59, females 0.97; college, males 1.38, females 1.80. For collegiate sports, from most to least, the most common causes of concussion are men's wrestling, men's ice hockey, women's ice hockey, and football.[59] In gender-comparable sports, women have higher concussion rates.[60–62]

According to the NFL, there were 149 concussions in 271 games reported during the 2022 season compared with 126 in 2018 and the 2018 to 2020 3-year average of 130. A recent consensus statement of concussion in sports includes recommendations for return to play.[63]

Based on a meta-analysis, "More evidence is needed to support the protective effect of mouthguards, additional padding in American football helmets, appropriate helmet fit in collision sport, policy limiting contact practice in adolescent American football, head contact rule enforcement in contact sports (eg, American football, ice hockey), and training strategies targeting modifiable intrinsic risk factors."[64]

In the NFL, changes to reduce concussions include targeting rule changes, eliminating specific practice drills, and in-game blind-side blocks. Measures taken to improve concussion detection and diagnosis include introduction of a centralized clinical electronic health record, Athletic Trainer spotter program, and unaffiliated neurotrauma consultants.

Postcraniotomy

Iatrogenic trauma may also cause headaches. Moderate to severe pain has been reported in up to 60% to 90% of patients undergoing craniotomy and 30% suffer from chronic pain.[65] Possible mechanisms include damage of the nerve branches, formation of neuromas, nerve entrapment in the scar, traction of the dura, formation of adhesions (dura to bone, dura to muscle, or dura to brain), or muscle incision. In some cases, aseptic meningitis and intracranial hypotension due to a cerebrospinal fluid (CSF) leak need to be excluded. In one study of surgery for acoustic neuromas, risk factors included young age, female gender, preoperative headaches, anxiety, and depression.[66]

In a prospective study of patients for the risk of headaches after the treatment of intracranial aneurysms followed for 4 months after the procedure, the incidence of headache was 28 out of 51 cases (54.9%) after surgery compared with 12 out of 47 cases (25.5%) after embolization.[67] Less than a third had persistent headaches for more than 3 months. In another study of postcraniotomy headaches during the 6 months after craniotomy for the treatment of supratentorial intracranial aneurysms, there was an incidence of postcraniotomy headache of 40% with 30% having migrainous headaches at 6 months.[68]

In a study of patients undergoing supratentorial craniotomy for epilepsy, 11.9% had ongoing headaches 1 year after surgery with 4% medically uncontrolled.[69] In another study of 107 patients who underwent craniotomies for brain tumors or epilepsy, no patients had debilitating headaches.[70]

In a meta-analysis of 1653 patients who underwent resection of acoustic neuromas, long-term significant headaches were reported by 36% of those who underwent a retrosigmoid approach as compared with 16% and 1% of those who underwent translabyrinthine and middle fossa approaches, respectively.[71] Some patients with chronic headaches following acoustic nerve resection have occipital nerve injuries improving after excision of the greater and lesser occipital nerves.[72] In another study of 311 patients who underwent suboccipital craniotomy, headaches were present in 49%. Most cases had an onset within 7 days and disappeared within 30 days of surgery.[73]

HEADACHES

Headaches are estimated as occurring variably in 30% to 90% of persons who are symptomatic after mild head injury.[74] Head and neck injury account for approximately 15% of chronic daily headaches.[75] Paradoxically, headache prevalence and lifetime duration is greater in those who have mild head injury compared with those who have more severe trauma.[76,77] A prospective study of mTBI found no difference in acute headache frequency in those who reported loss of consciousness or posttraumatic amnesia compared to those without.[78]

According to the International Classification of Headache Disorders-3 (ICHD-3), "It is recognized that some patients develop headache following very minor trauma to the head – so minor that it does not meet criteria even for mTBI. These headaches may begin after a single trauma or following repetitive minor head impacts (e.g. in players of rugby or American football). However, headache due to very minor head trauma has not been adequately studied, so there are insufficient data."[79]

Risk factors for acute posttraumatic headache in civilians adults include younger age, female sex, fewer years of formal education, computed tomography-positive scans, alteration of consciousness, psychiatric history, and history of migraine. Risk factors for persistent posttraumatic headache include female sex, fewer years of formal education, and history of migraine.[80,81]

ICHD-3 categories for acute headache attributed to trauma or injury to the head and/or neck are in **Box 2**.[64] The criteria for acute headache attributed to traumatic injury to the head are in **Box 3**.

Persistent headache attributed to traumatic injury to the head is the presence of headache for more than 3 months. White matter hyperintensities and cerebral microbleeds are no more prevalent in those with persistent PTHs compared with controls.[82]

Box 2
Headache attributed to trauma or injury to the head and/or neck

5.1. Acute headache attributed to traumatic injury to the head
    5.1.1. Acute headache attributed to moderate or severe traumatic injury to the head
    5.1.2. Acute headache attributed to mild traumatic injury to the head

5.2. Persistent headache attributed to traumatic injury to the head
    5.2.1. Persistent headache attributed to moderate or severe traumatic injury to the head
    5.2.2. Persistent headache attributed to mild traumatic injury to the head

5.3. Acute headache attributed to whiplash

5.4. Persistent headache attributed to whiplash

5.5. Acute headache attributed to craniotomy

5.6. Persistent headache attributed to craniotomy

ICHD-3 criteria.

Box 3
Acute headache attributed to traumatic injury to the head

A. Any headache fulfilling criteria C and D

B. Traumatic injury to the head[1] has occurred

C. Headache is reported to have developed within 7 d after one of the following:
   1. The injury to the head
   2. Regaining of consciousness following the injury to the head
   3. Discontinuation of medication(s) impairing ability to sense or report headache following the injury to the head

D. Either of the following:
   1. Headache has resolved within 3 mo after its onset
   2. Headache has not yet resolved but 3 mo have not yet passed since its onset

E. Not better accounted for by another ICHD-3 diagnosis.

ICHD-3 criteria.

Time of onset

According to the ICHD-3 criteria, the onset of the headache should be less than 7 days after the injury.[66] Some argue that 3 months is a more reasonable latency for onset than 7 days[83,84] although some patients with new onset primary headaches will be misdiagnosed as having PTHs.

The less than 7-day onset is arbitrary, particularly because the cause of posttraumatic migraine is not understood. For example, posttraumatic epilepsy may have a latency of months or years. Similarly, it would not be surprising if there were a latency of weeks or months for posttraumatic migraine to develop. Conversely, because migraine is a common disorder, the longer the latency between the trauma and onset, the more likely the trauma may not have been causative. Consider the hypothetical case of a 27-year-old man who develops new-onset migraine 2 months after a mild head injury in a motor vehicle accident. The incidence of migraine in men aged younger than 30 years is 0.25% per year or, in this case, 0.042% per 2 months.[85] Was the new-onset migraine the result of the mTBI or coincidence?

So consider the increased incidence of new or worse headaches found with onset after 7 days at 3-month assessment in 3 studies. In a prospective study of 212 subjects hospitalized with mTBI for observation or other injuries, an additional 59% of subjects reported new or worse headache (compared with preinjury) at 3 months who had not previously reported headache within the first 7 days after injury (baseline assessment).[69] However, the cohort was 76% men with 58% injured in vehicle-related accidents (which are potentially compensable).

Two other studies found a high percentage of new onset headache with onset after 7 days: 23% additional headaches at the 3-month assessment in consecutive patients with moderate-to-severe TBI[86] and 19% in a retrospective cohort of United States Army soldiers.[87]

However, 2 studies found onset almost always within 7 days. Lieba-Samal and colleagues performed a study of 100 patients (66% men) with acute mild head injury presenting to the department of trauma surgery in Vienna with last assessment 90 to 100 days after trauma.[88] Among the 66% who reported acute PTHs, the onset was within 48 hours in 92%.

Langer and colleagues agree with the ICHD-3 criteria and recommend not extending the headache onset to more than 7 days, which could even be shorter to allow for greater diagnostic precision.[63] In a prospective study of 302 adults with concussion (originating from injuries that were not work related or due to motor vehicle accidents) recruited from the emergency room and seen within 1 week, 92% endorsed posttraumatic headache with 94% endorsing onset within 24 hours. During the 12 weeks of follow-up after injury, 0% endorsed a new onset acute posttraumatic headache with onset beyond 1 week of the concussion.

Langer and colleagues opine that headaches with onset after 7 days are not a direct sequela of the head injury but have other precipitants including the following: affective symptoms, acute psychosocial, financial stressors, or workplace stressors; narcotic medication use for other trauma; and sleep deprivation and interruptions.[63]

Epidemiology of Phenotypes

Civilians

In a meta-analysis[89] of 5 studies of PTHs,[21,90-93] most were of the tension type (ranging from 6.9% to 85.7%, mean = 33.6%) and the second most had migraine characteristics (ranging from 1.9% to 40.7%, mean = 28.6%). The following features were present: mild-to-moderate intensity pain, about 60%; bilateral, 72.5%; nonthrobbing, 83%; light sensitivity, 35.8%; noise sensitivity, 29.1%; and aggravation by routine physical activities, 71.1%. Analgesic overuse was reported as present in 18.8% to 45.8%. The percentage of mixed or unclassifiable headaches ranged from 4.2% to 36.5%.

In the prospective study of 302 subjects, acute headache location was not correlated with the site of injury and was described as pressure/squeezing in 60% and throbbing/pulsing in 22%.[63] The most common durations were continuous (35%), lasting 2 to 3 hours (16%), or lasting 30 minutes (14%). In those with daily headache, the pain was intermittent in 59% or continuous in 25%. Locations included the following: holocranial, 19%; temple, 50%; forehead, 49%; behind the eyes, 49%, and back of the head, 46%. Neck pain was endorsed by 34%. Visual aura was present in 12%. Associated symptoms included the following: difficulty concentrating/thinking, 75%; sensitivity to light, 74%; sensitivity to sound, 72%; fatigue, 72%, lightheadedness, 69%; and nausea, 55%; In a prospective 1-year study of 212 subjects, which included headaches with onset at any time, up to 49% of headaches met criteria for migraine and probable migraine, up to 40% met tension-type criteria, 4% were cervicogenic, and up to 16% were unclassified.[69] Of the up to 27% of subjects who reported having headaches several times per week to daily, 62% of the headache types were migraine in this highest frequency group at 1 year. Individuals aged older than 60 years were significantly more likely to report no headaches over time and at all time points.

In another prospective 1-year study (which included headaches with onset at any time) of 378 subjects who sustained moderate-to-severe traumatic brain injuries, migraine occurred in up to 38%, probable migraine in up to 25%, tension-type headache in up to 21%, cervicogenic headache in up to 10%, and unclassifiable in up to 30%.[94] Women were more likely to have preinjury migraine than men and to have migraine or probable migraine at all time points after injury.

In a prospective study of 543 patients after TBI (96.9% mild), migraine/probable migraine was reported as follows: 3 months, 70.1%; 6 months, 72.8%; and 12 months, 69.5%.[95] At 12 months, the headaches were reported as monthly in 74.4%, weekly in 20.7%, daily in 4.3%, and constant in 0% with a pain score of 1 to 4 in 65.2%, 5 to 7 in 31.1%, and 8 to 10 in 3.7%. Headaches were reported as disabling in 3.7%.

In a study of 100 people with persistent posttraumatic headache attributed to mTBI, the mean headache frequency was 25.4 ± 7.1 days per month.[96] Phenotypes were as follows: chronic migraine-like, 61%; combined episodic migraine-like and tension-type-like headaches, 29%; and chronic tension-type, 9%. The most frequent trigger factors were stress, lack of sleep, and bright lights.

United States military
The Department of Defense estimates that 394,591 service members sustained a mTBI from 2000 through the first quarter of 2023.[97] Case 1 is an example of PTH.

Migraine is the most common type of posttraumatic headache occurring in 60% to 97% of cases.[98] Blast trauma had been sustained by 77% of soldiers with chronic PTHs.[99] The onset of PTH after injury was within 1 week for nearly 40%, within 1 month for 20%, and beyond 1 month for 40%.[100]

In a retrospective study of 95 soldiers with persistent posttraumatic headache due to concussion sustained during the wars in Afghanistan and Iraq, the migraine type was diagnosed in 60%.[101] The onset was 7 days or less in 77.9% and more than 1 month in 6.3%. A continuous headache of any type was present in 75%.

Interestingly, there was a high prevalence of migraine in US Soldiers deployed to combat in Iraq without physical trauma, with 17.4% of men and 34.9% of women reporting a headache consistent with migraine during the prior year, much greater than a civilian population.[102]

Athletes
In a study of 296 student athletes aged 12 to 25 years who sustained sport-related concussions, migraines occurred in 52, headache in 176, and no headache in 68.[103] Female athletes were 2.13 times more likely than male athletes to report posttraumatic migraine characteristics. Those with migraine characteristics had prolonged symptom recovery including cognitive, neurobehavioral, and somatic symptoms. Only one patient reported migraine at 90 days. Another study of high school and college athletes found that those with posttraumatic migraines had significantly greater neurocognitive deficits when compared with those who had concussions with nonmigraine headaches and controls.[104]

A convenience sample of 50 retired NFL players with a mean age of 45.5 years found a 1-year prevalence of migraine of 92%, 56% with episodic, and 36% with chronic.[105] The onset of the migraines was as follows: 4% before playing in the NFL, 48% while playing in the NFL, and 48% after retiring with a mean age of onset of 33.0 years (range of age of onset of 12–63 years). The reason for the increased prevalence of migraine with late onset after playing is not certain. Possibilities include the following: concussions or subconcussive impacts causing brain injury causing later onset migraine; co-morbid depression and anxiety (reported by 78% and 86% of subjects); chronic nonheadache pain (reported by 88%); and medication rebound with use of opioids 8 or more days per month for nonheadache chronic pain (reported by 25%).[106]

In the survey of Texas neurologists, 68.4% of respondents disagreed or strongly disagreed with the following statement: I would support my son or grandson (or if you do not have one, relative's or friend's) playing football.[27]

Postcraniotomy
Up to 90% of cases start immediately postoperative at a median time of 4 days typically different than headaches if present before surgery.[107] Most patients have headaches on the same side and at the site of surgery with the tension-type phenotype. Allodynia at the site of the surgical scar is reported by 82%.

There is a single case report of a patient with new onset hemicrania continua 2 days after resection of a large left-sided acoustic neuroma with complete resolution of headache on indomethacin 50 mg twice daily.

Possible overdiagnosis of migraine

Tension type, cervicogenic headaches, and occipital neuralgia have the potential for being misdiagnosed as migraine because light and noise sensitivity and nausea are commonly associated with PCS.[16,70,71]

Neck injuries commonly accompany head trauma and can produce headaches such as those associated with whiplash injuries,[108] which are beyond the scope of this review. Pareek and colleagues review cervicogenic headache in this issue.[109] Although not part of PCS, headaches associated with subdural and epidural hematomas also are described.

CASES

Case 1. Migraine from Blast Trauma

This 39-year-old United States male army soldier was standing outside of his truck in Afghanistan when 3 rocket-propelled grenades hit the truck. The blast threw him 25 to 30 feet resulting in loss of consciousness for 3 to 4 minutes and confusion following. He had a mild headache immediately following, developed severe headaches 2 days later, which were initially 2 to 3 times per week, and then became daily 10 months after the trauma. He was started on amitriptyline 50 mg at bedtime and the headaches decreased to 1 to 2 times per week. He described a right-sided, especially, frontoparietal throbbing with an intensity ranging from 3 to 10 out of 10 associated with nausea, vomiting at times, light and noise sensitivity but no aura. The headache would resolve in about 40 minutes with an oral triptan but without medication could last 24 hours. Weightlifting and stomach crunches were triggers. There was no prior history of headaches. An MRI of the brain was normal. He also had posttraumatic stress disorder.

Comment

This is a typical case of posttraumatic migraine with onset within 1 week following blast trauma in a soldier associated with comorbid posttraumatic stress disorder.

Case 2. Footballer's Migraine

Late in the first quarter of Super Bowl XXXII on January 25, 1998, Terrell Davis, a 25-year-old running back for the Denver Broncos with a history of migraine with and without aura since age 7, was unintentionally kicked in the helmet by a Green Bay Packers defender.[110] A few minutes later, he went to the sidelines with a migraine visual aura. Coach Shanahan sent him back in for one more play, which was a fake where Elway kept the ball and ran into the end zone. Davis was given his usual migraine medication, dihydroergotamine nasal spray, on the sideline by the trainer. He went into the locker room and his severe headache was gone by the start of the third quarter with the benefit of the extra Super Bowl halftime minutes. When he returned for the second half, he had 20 carries for 90 yards including the winning touchdown and won the game's most valuable player award.[111] He had a Super Bowl-record 3 rushing touchdowns.

Comment

This is the most famous example of "footballer's migraine" witnessed by 800 million viewers occurring in American football rather than in soccer as originally described. Early treatment of migraine can get your patient back to school or work and even enable them to be Super Bowl MVP.

Case 3

In the game on September 25, 2022, Miami Dolphin's quarterback, 24 year-old Tua Tagovailoa, took a hit without loss of consciousness and then struggled to get to his feet and fell after a couple of steps. Four days later, he had another hit with loss of consciousness during which he displayed a fencing response (extension in one arm and flexion in the contralateral arm immediately after injury usually lasting for seconds).[112] The sideline neurotrauma expert who examined him after the September 25, 2022, episode was fired for not following the concussion protocol.[7] On October 7, 2022, the NFL and NFL Players Association announced that the step-by-step protocol was followed in his case. In response to an investigation, the league's protocol was modified by adding the diagnosis of "ataxia" to the mandatory "no-go" symptoms.[113]

He returned to play after 1 month and started 9 games. On December 25, 2022, he hit his head on the turf late in the first half. He had 3 interceptions in the second half. He had symptoms and was placed in the concussion protocol after the game.

During the offseason, Tagovailoa considered retiring but then trained in jiu-jitsu 1 day a week to learn how to fall in a safe manner.[114] He next played during the 2023 season wearing the VICIS ZERO2 MATRIX QB, the NFL's new quarterback specific helmet designed to prevent concussion.[115] For the 2023 season, he had a league-leading 4451 passing yards.

Comment

Even with up to 24 cameras at an NFL game and an unaffiliated neurotrauma physician consultant on the sideline, concussion can be difficult to diagnose. Obviously, there is no gold standard for diagnosing concussion.

Based on a meta-analysis, visible signs of concussion among professional athletes were identified in 53% to 78.9%. The visible signs with the highest specificity include the following: tonic posturing (97%), impact seizure (96%), suspected loss of consciousness (93%), ataxia/motor incoordination with difficulty getting up (81%), abnormal behavior (55%), and blank/vacant/dazed look (62%).[116]

Subconcussive impacts may also cause cognitive impairment and increase the risk of chronic traumatic encephalopathy.[117] This reminds me of Ralph Nader's 1965 book, *Unsafe at Any Speed: The Designed-In-Dangers of the American Automobile*.[118]

Based on a systemic review, "No evidence was identified to support the inclusion of any patient-specific, injury-specific or other factors (e.g., imaging findings) as absolute indications for retirement or discontinued participation in contact or collision sport following SRC (sport related concussion)."[119]

TYPES AND FEATURES OF HEADACHES
Tension-Type Headache

These headaches occur in a variety of distributions, including generalized, nuchal-occipital, bifrontal, bitemporal, cap-like, or headband. The headache, which may be constant or intermittent with variable duration, usually is described as pressure, tight, or dull aching.

Temporomandibular joint injury can be caused by either direct trauma or jarring associated with the head injury. Patients may complain of temporomandibular joint area pain with chewing and hemicranial or ipsilateral frontotemporal aching or pressure headaches although the pain may be referred anywhere in the trigeminal and cervical complex. See the Romero-Reyes and Bassiur review in this issue.[120]

Occipital Neuralgia

This term is in some ways a misnomer because the pain is not necessarily from the occipital nerve and usually does not have a neuralgic quality. Greater occipital neuralgia is a common posttraumatic headache[121] and also is seen frequently without injury. The aching, pressure, stabbing, or throbbing pain may be in a nuchal-occipital or parietal, temporal, frontal, periorbital, or retro-orbital distribution. Occasionally, a true neuralgia may be present with paroxysmal shooting-type pain. The headache may last for minutes, hours, or days and be unilateral or bilateral not fitting the ICHD-3 criteria for duration.[122]

Occasionally, referred ipsilateral facial paresthesias or subjective numbness especially in the cheek, which is a diagnosis of exclusion, may be present due to convergence of the C2 afferents, which supply the greater occipital nerve and trigeminal afferents on second-order neurons within the trigeminocervical complex.[123] Lesser occipital neuralgia similarly can occur with pain generally referred more laterally over the head with reproduction of symptoms by digital pressure over the nerve.

The headache may be the result of direct trauma to the nerve, an entrapment of the greater occipital nerve in the aponeurosis of the superior trapezius or semispinalis capitis muscle, or instead be referred pain without nerve compression from trigger points in these or other suboccipital muscles. Digital pressure over the greater occipital nerve reproduces the headache. Pain referred from the C2–3 facet joint or other upper cervical spine pathology and posterior fossa pathology, however, may produce a similar headache.

Migraine

Recurring attacks of migraine with or without aura can result from mild head injury or preexisting migraine may be exacerbated. Medication overuse for the treatment of other types of posttraumatic pain can also increase the frequency of migraine whether de novo or preexisting.

Impact also can cause acute migraine episodes in adolescents who have a family history of migraine. This originally was termed "footballer's migraine" to describe headaches in young men who played soccer who had multiple migraine with aura attacks triggered only by impact.[124] Similar attacks can be triggered by mild head injury in any sport (see case 2).

After minor head trauma, children, adolescents, and young adults can develop a variety of transient neurologic sequelae that are not always associated with migraine and are perhaps the result of vasospasm. Five clinical types can cause the following: hemiparesis; somnolence, irritability, and vomiting; a confusional state[125,126]; transient blindness, often precipitated by occipital impacts; and brainstem signs.[127]

Trigeminal Autonomic Cephalalgias and Hemicrania Continua

Cluster headaches rarely result from mild head injuries.[128] There are case reports of posttraumatic chronic paroxysmal hemicrania occurring with and without aura (3 cases),[129,130] short-lasting unilateral neuralgiform headache attacks with conjunctival injection, tearing, sweating, and rhinorrhea,[131] short-lasting unilateral headache with cranial autonomic symptoms,[132] and hemicrania continua.[133]

Cranial neuralgias[134]

Injury of the supraorbital branch of the first trigeminal division as it passes through the supraorbital foramen just inferior to the medial eyebrow can cause supraorbital neuralgia.[135] Similarly, infraorbital neuralgia can result from trauma to the inferior orbit.[136] Shooting, tingling, aching, or burning pain along with decreased or altered sensation and sometimes decreased sweating in the appropriate nerve distribution may be present. The pain can be paroxysmal or fairly constant. A dull aching or throbbing pain also may occur around the area of injury. Auriculotemporal and supratrochlear neuralgias can also occur.

Scalp Lacerations and Local Trauma

Dysesthesias over scalp lacerations occur frequently. In the presence or absence of a laceration, an aching, soreness, tingling, or shooting pain over the site of the original trauma can develop. Symptoms may persist for weeks or months but rarely for more than 1 year.

Subdural Hematomas

Tearing of the parasagittal bridging veins (which drain blood from the surface of the hemisphere into the dural venous sinuses) leads to hematoma formation within the subdural space. Even minor injuries without loss of consciousness, such as bumps on the head or riding a roller coaster[137] or motion simulator ride,[138] can result in this tearing. Falls and assaults are more likely to cause subdural hematomas than motor vehicle accidents.

Subdural hematomas usually are located over the hemispheres, although other locations, such as between the occipital lobe and tentorium cerebelli or between the temporal lobe and base of the skull, can occur. A subdural hematoma becomes subacute between 2 and 14 days after the injury when there is a mixture of clotted and fluid blood and becomes chronic when the hematoma is filled with fluid more than 14 days after the injury. Rebleeding can occur in the chronic phase. Most patients who have chronic subdural hematomas are late middle aged or elderly. Subdural hematomas can be present with a normal neurologic examination. Rarely, after mild head injury and a normal CT scan of the brain, subdural hematomas can have a delayed onset.[139,140]

In a study of 1080 patients with surgically treated chronic subdural hematoma, headache was recognized in 22.6%, nausea and vomiting in 3%, and papilledema in only 1 patient.[141] Headaches associated with subdural hematomas are nonspecific, ranging from mild to severe and paroxysmal to constant.[142] Unilateral headaches usually are the result of ipsilateral subdural hematomas. Headaches associated with chronic subdural hematomas have at least one of the following features in 75% of cases: sudden onset; severe pain; exacerbation with coughing, straining, or exercise; and vomiting and or nausea.

Epidural Hematomas

Bleeding into the epidural space from a direct blow to the head produces an epidural hematoma. The source of the bleeding is variable and can be arterial or venous or both. In the supratentorial compartment, bleeding is of the following origins: middle meningeal artery, 50%; middle meningeal veins, 33%; dural venous sinus, 10%; and other sources, including hemorrhage from a fracture line, 7%. Most epidural hematomas in the posterior fossa are the result of dural venous sinus bleeding. The locations of epidurals are as follows: temporal region (usually under a fractured squamous temporal bone), 70%; frontal convexity, 15%; parieto-occipital, 10%; and parasagittal or posterior fossa, 5%. Ninety-five percent of epidurals are unilateral.

Epidural hematomas usually occur between the ages of 10 and 40 years and much less frequently in those younger than 2 or older than 60 years. Motor vehicle accidents and falls are the most common causes. Trivial trauma without loss of consciousness can be a cause.

Forty percent of patients who have an epidural hematoma present with a GCS of 14 or 15. Less than one-third of patients have the classic lucid interval (initially unconscious, then recovery, and then unconscious again). Uncommonly, traumatic delayed epidural hematomas where the hematoma is insignificant or not present on the initial CT scan after trauma can occur.[143]

Up to 30% of epidural hematomas are of the chronic type.[144] The patient often is a child or young adult who sustains what seems to be a trivial injury often without loss of consciousness.[145] A persistent headache then develops, often associated with nausea, vomiting, and memory impairment, which might seem consistent with PCS. After the passage of days to weeks, focal findings develop. The headaches of acute and chronic epidural may be unilateral or bilateral and can be nonspecific.

Other Causes

Trauma can cause a spinal CSF leak or an anterior skull base fracture (sinus leaks more common than cribiform plate) and result in a low-CSF pressure headache.[146,147] Traumatic subarachnoid hemorrhage can cause headaches.[148] Headaches can be the only symptom of posttraumatic carotid and vertebral artery dissections.[149] Posttraumatic cerebral venous thrombosis[150] and carotid-cavernous fistulas[151] are other rare causes.

PATHOPHYSIOLOGY
Neurobiologic Factors

The pathogenesis of PTHs is poorly understood.[152,153] Mild traumatic brain injury may result in cortical contusions after coup and contre-coup injuries or diffuse axonal injury resulting from sheer and tensile strain damage.[154] Marvoudis and colleagues describe the following pathophysiologic mechanisms involved in posttraumatic headache pathogenesis: impaired descending pain modulation, neurometabolic changes, neuroinflammation, cortical spreading depression, release of calcitonin gene-related peptide (CGRP); trigeminal system activation, secondary cascade of metabolic and cellular excitotoxic and inflammatory changes, and hypersensitivity to CGRP.[155]

Neuroimaging studies, including MRI, single photon emission computerized tomography, PET, magnetic source imaging, MR diffusion tension imaging, functional MRI, and MRI spectroscopy can demonstrate structural and functional deficits.[156–158]

Nonorganic Explanations

There are many nonorganic explanations for PCS, which suggest an origin for their subjective symptoms other than TBI for some including psychogenic factors, psychosocial, sociocultural, base rate misattribution, expectation as etiology, chronic pain, nocebo effects,[159] litigation, perceived injustice and entitlement,[160] and malingering.[161]

Effects of Litigation

In a survey of Texas neurologists, only 15% agreed with the statement, "Once litigation is settled, symptoms quick resolve in patients with PCS."[27] However, some authors think that PTHs and PCS are a creation of the legal system.[162]

Patients who have litigation are similar to those who do not in the following respects: symptoms that improve with time,[163] types of headaches, cognitive test results,[138] and response to migraine medications.[164] Symptoms usually do not resolve with the settlement of litigation.[165] In a study of 44 patients with persistent PTHs in Copenhagen, Denmark, only one reported some improvement in headache following the end of litigation.[96]

Pending litigation may increase the level of stress for some claimants and may result in increased frequency of symptoms after settlement.[166] Skepticism of physicians also may accentuate the level of stress and compel some patients to exaggerate so that the doctors take them seriously.

However, studies without litigants suggest that litigation is a factor in headache prolongation. In a retrospective and prospective study in Lithuania, there was no difference in frequency one or more years after injury compared with controls.[167,168] In a prospective study in Vienna, Austria, 0% reported headaches at 90 to 100 days after injury.[73]

"If you have to prove you are ill, you can't get well."[169] Studies have also found that litigation and/or compensation is a significant factor for PCS in slower recovery[170] and persistent symptoms.[171,172]

In a study of consecutive outpatient neuropsychological evaluations performed on an average more than 1 year after injury, mTBI subjects (who had equivocal or very mild brain injury) who failed 2 symptom validity tests and may also be involved in litigation reported more symptoms (including headaches in 80%) and to a higher degree than those who had sustained moderate-to-severe TBI (headaches in 45%).[173]

Some patients may have persistent headache complaints resulting from secondary gain,[147] malingering, and psychological disorders. Potential indicators of malingering after mild head injury include the following: premorbid factors (antisocial and borderline personality traits, poor work record, and prior claims for injury); behavioral characteristics (uncooperative evasive or suspicious); neuropsychologic test performance (missing random items, giving up easily, inconsistent test profile, or stating frequently, "I don't know"); postmorbid complaints (describing events surrounding the accident in great detail or reporting an unusually large number of symptoms); and miscellaneous items (engaging in general activities not consistent with reported deficits, having significant financial stressors, resistance, and exhibiting a lack of reasonable follow-through on treatments).[174]

In a study of mild head injured litigants, Andrikopoulos compared 72 patients who had no improvement or worsening headache with 39 patients who had improving headache. Those who had no improvement or worsening performed worse on cognitive tests and had greater psychopathology on the Minnesota Multiphasic Personality Inventory-2 (MMPI-2) than those who had improving headaches, suggesting the possibility of malingering.[175]

Not surprisingly, there are many controversial topics for physicians who are involved in litigation as treating physicians or expert witnesses in mTBI cases.[176] Hubbard and Hodge review legal case studies involving PTHs, the physician as expert witness, and the controversy over whether litigation prolongs posttraumatic headache symptoms.[177]

TREATMENT OF HEADACHES
Civilians

There is a dearth of randomized placebo-controlled trials of medications for PTHs. Only a few studies, all done without controls, have been performed for the prevention of PTHs. There is a low level of evidence to support any pharmacologic treatment.[178] The International Headache Society has proposed guidelines for controlled trials of pharmacologic treatment of persistent posttraumatic headache attributed to mTBI.[179]

Three studies in civilian adults, which involved either monotherapy or combined therapy with propranolol, amitriptyline,[139,180] or valproate,[181] showed efficacy although a small study showed no benefit with amitriptyline.[182] A retrospective study performed in a sports medicine clinic with 277 child and adult subjects found no long-term improvement in those prescribed gabapentin and tricyclic antidepressants compared with those not prescribed medication.[183]

In a prospective study of 63 patients aged 18 to 65 years with persistent posttraumatic headache predominantly migraine-like, 79% reported failure of at least one preventive drug and 19% reported failure of at least 4 preventive medications.[141] Medications included antihypertensives, anticonvulsants, antidepressants, and onabotulinum toxin A (lack of efficacy in 67%).

The only prospective randomized trial of an anti-CGRP medication for the prevention of PTHs was negative (with fremanezumab).[184] In a 12-week open label study of erenumab for 100 patients aged 18 to 65 years with persistent posttraumatic headache attributed to mTBI, there was a reduction of moderate-to-severe headache days.[185] In an open label study of 15 patients with persistent PTHs, erenumab might result in an improvement in quality of life.[186]

Soldiers

There are open-label retrospective studies of chronic PTHs among United States soldiers. One found no significant benefit of treatment with low-dose tricyclic antidepressants but improvement with preventive treatment with topiramate.[99] A second found benefit from onabotulinum toxin A injections with 56% reporting more than one headache type.[187] A third found no long-term improvement in those prescribed gabapentin and tricyclic antidepressants compared with those not prescribed medication.[183] Onabotulinum toxin A may be effective in United States soldiers with the migraine phenotype[188] and with the migraine and tension-type phenotype.[189] Triptans may be effective for posttraumatic migraine.[141,155,190]

Treatment Options

Posttraumatic tension-like and migraine-like headaches are treated with the usual symptomatic and preventative medications used for nontraumatic tension-type and migraine headaches.[191] The physician should be concerned about the potential for medication overuse headaches with the frequent use of over-the-counter medications, such as acetaminophen, aspirin, and combination products containing caffeine, and prescription opioids, butalbital, and benzodiazepines. In one survey, more than 70% of those with headache during the first year after mTBI used acetaminophen or an NSAID, which was usually not effective.[192] Habituation also is a concern with opioids, butalbital, and benzodiazepines.

It is not clear whether biofeedback, cognitive behavioral therapy, physical therapy and manual therapy, acupuncture, immobilization devices, ice, and neuromodulation devices are of benefit.[10,164,193–195]

Occipital neuralgia may improve with local anesthetic nerve blocks (eg, 3 ml of 1% xylocaine). Combined with an injectable corticosteroid can be combined if patients do not respond adequately to local anesthetic alone (eg, 2.5 mL of 1% xylocaine and 3 mg of betamethasone).[96,196–198] Other blocks may be helpful for the posttraumatic migraine phenotype include lesser occipital nerve, supraorbital, supratrochlear, and auriculotemporal.[199,200]

Natsis and colleagues, based on a cadaver study, recommend injecting about 20 to 25 mm below the external occipital protuberance and about 15 mm lateral from the midline starting infiltration shortly after the injection needle has overcome the resistance of the trapezius muscle aponeurosis.[201] Others recommend injecting one-third of the way laterally along an imaginary line connecting the occipital protuberance to the mastoid process.[164,167] Before injection, the physician should aspirate to avoid inadvertent vascular injection.

Injection of corticosteroids can uncommonly cause Cushing syndrome, cutaneous atrophy, and alopecia.[202] The addition of corticosteroids to local anesthetic is probably not of additional benefit.[167]

Anecdotally, nonsteroidal anti-inflammatory drugs and muscle relaxants may also be beneficial. If there is a true occipital neuralgia with paroxysmal lancinating pain, baclofen, tizanidine, carbamazepine, gabapentin, or pregabalin may help. Physical therapy and transcutaneous nerve stimulators may help relieve some headaches. A variety of other treatments have been proposed for refractory cases including pulsed radiofrequency therapy[203,204] and occipital nerve stimulation.[205,206]

There are studies suggesting benefit from occipital nerve decompression.[207,208] There remain questions about the efficacy of decompression because of differences in definitions and diagnosis of occipital neuralgia and suggestions for a sham surgery comparison group.

Treatment of Athletes

Treatment of PTHs is problematic in athletes. There are side effects of migraine preventive medications such as amitriptyline (sedation and weight gain), beta-blockers (which may cause exercise intolerance and bradycardia), and topiramate (which may cause cognitive side effects, depression, and weight loss). Various acute and preventive treatments have been recommended.[92,209]

For collegiate and professional athletes who have returned to play, the physician should be familiar with prohibited substances.[92] Most organizations use the World Anti-Doping Agency or similar guidelines, which may prohibit the use of anabolic steroids, peptide hormones and growth factors, beta-2 agonists, hormone and metabolic modulators, diuretics and masking agents, stimulants, narcotics, cannabinoids, glucocorticoids, and β-blockers (in certain sports).[210] As an example of professional sports, the NFL has the same list of prohibited substances and a detailed policy on performance-enhancing substances.[211]

For athletes with persistent headache only, application of return to play guidelines[63] is problematic because of the lack of evidence that playing with PTH only poses any risk to the brain.

Cervicogenic and Temporomandibular Joint

Treatment of posttraumatic cervicogenic headaches and those originating from the temporomandibular joint are discussed in other articles in this issue.[93,95]

EDUCATION

One of the most important roles of the physician is education of the patient and family members, other physicians, and when appropriate, employers, attorneys, and representatives of insurance companies. There is widespread ignorance about the potential effects of mTBI because of what Evans has termed "the Hollywood head injury myth."[212] Patient complaints of chronic daily headaches of any type, especially posttraumatic, often are met with skepticism by much of the public, who cannot imagine that headaches occur with such frequency.

Most people's knowledge of the sequelae of mild head injuries largely is the result of movie magic. Some of the funniest scenes in slapstick comedies and cartoons depict the character sustaining single or multiple head injuries, looking dazed, and then recovering immediately. In cowboy movies, action, detective stories, and boxing and martial arts films, seemingly serious head trauma often is inflicted by blows from guns and heavy objects, motor vehicle accidents, falls, fists, and kicks, all without lasting consequences. Our experience is minimal compared with the thousands of simulated head injuries seen in the movies and on television.

The physician can provide education by summarizing the literature and using vivid examples from sports. The public is familiar with dementia pugilistica, or punch-drunk syndrome, of cumulative head injury in boxers. The examples of Joe Louis and Floyd Patterson are well known. Many have witnessed powerful punches resulting in dazed, disoriented boxers or knockouts. Contrary to popular belief, Mohammed Ali had young-onset Parkinson disease.[213]

There also is growing awareness of the effects of cumulative concussions in the NFL (eg, quarterbacks Steve Young, Troy Aikman, Stan Humphries, Brett Favre, Jay Cutler, and Tua Tagovailoa) and National Hockey League (eg, Pat Lafontaine and Marc Savard) and the fear of chronic traumatic encephalopathy. Reports of concussions and headaches preventing athletes from returning to play make the sports pages on a regular basis.

PROGNOSIS

Prognostic or natural history studies are difficult to compare due to the heterogeneity of study populations and differences in case definition. Prognostic studies reviewed go back to 1944.[190] These study problems are reflected in the range of patients with persistent headaches, which are incompletely understood without control groups.

The percentage of adult patients who have headaches after injury at 1 month varies from 31.3%[59] to 90%[214]; at 3 months from 23%[215] to 78%[216]; and at 1 year from 8.4%[217] to 70.2%,[218] at 3 years, 50.9%,[219] and at 4 years, 24%.[220] In a prospective study, headaches were reported by those with mTBI compared with controls, respectively, as follows: 1 year, 70.2%, 52%; and 10 years, 41.5%, 31%.[195] A few prospective studies are of interest.

In a prospective study of 100 consecutive patients with mild head injury and a normal CT of the brain in Norway and Sweden followed-up at 3 months, headaches were present in 42%, 62% reported the presence of one or more symptoms, and 40% had 3 or more PCS symptoms.[221]

In a prospective study of 543 patients with TBI (96.9% mild) in Binzhou, China, headaches were reported as follows: 3 months, 57.7%; 6 months, 53.9%; and 12 months, 49.4%.[84]

In a prospective study in the Netherlands of patients who sustained an mTBI, there were 409 respondents at 3 months with transient loss of consciousness reported by 85% (which was not a risk factor for headache).[192] Headaches were reported by 23% and 35% had not returned to work. Those with headache were less likely to have returned compared with those without headache.

A multicenter prospective cohort study of 1301 subjects with mTBI (648 with uncomplicated and 599 with complicated mTBI) was performed in Europe and Israel.[222] Complicated mTBI was defined as intracranial abnormalities present on CT scan. Headaches were reported at 3 months in about 30% of subjects at 3 and 6 months with no significant difference between those with uncomplicated and complicated mTBI. Complicated mTBI was a weak indicator for postconcussion symptoms and higher PCS rates.

In a recent prospective study of 1594 adult patients who had sustained a mTBI within 24 hours prior evaluated at level 1 trauma centers in the United States, acute PTH was reported 2 weeks following the injury in 60.4% (n = 1594).[223] Among those with PTHs, persistent headaches were present at the following times after the injury: 3 months, 52.4%; 6 months, 37.5%; and 12 months, 28.9%. The risk factors for acute PTHs included the following: younger age, female sex, fewer years of formal education, CT-positive scans, alteration of consciousness, psychiatric history, and history of migraine. The risk factors for persistent headaches included the following: female sex, fewer years of formal education, and history of migraine.

In the only population-based study, which was performed in Norway among subjects aged 30 to 44 years, the 1-year period prevalence of chronic posttraumatic headache was 0.21% and of postcraniotomy headache, 0.02%.[224] Significant improvement was present at 3-year follow-up of the subjects with chronic PTHs with a mean duration of 10 years.[225]

CLINICS CARE POINTS

- The symptoms of PCS are not specific for the effects of mTBI and are common in the general population and among those with co-morbidities.

- CT and MRI scans of the brain are usually normal after mTBI. Routine EEG and quantitative EEG and advanced neuroimaging such as MRI with diffusion tensor imaging are not indicated for diagnosis or prognosis of mTBI.

- Neuropsychological testing is indicated for those with persistent cognitive symptoms. Cognitive impairment in present after 1 year in about 15% of those who sustained a mTBI.

- PTH is treated like the primary headache phenotype.

DISCLOSURE

Speaker's Bureau: Abbvie [Migraine]; Biohaven [Migraine]; Impel [Migraine]; Teva [Migraine]. Other Financial Interest: Elsevier [Royalties]; Medscape Neurology [Royalties]; Oxford University Press [Royalties].

REFERENCES

1. Evans RW. Posttraumatic headaches in civilians, soldiers, and athletes. Neurol Clin 2014;32(2):283–303.
2. Evans RW. Postconcussion syndrome. In: UpToDate, Connor RF, editors. UpToDate. Wolters Kluwer; 2023.
3. Giza CC, Kutcher JS, Ashwal S, et al. Summary of evidence-based guideline update: Evaluation and management of concussion in sports: Report of the Guideline Development Subcommittee of the American Academy of Neurology. Neurology 2013;80:2250–7.
4. Friedland D, Swash M. Post-traumatic amnesia and confusional state: hazards of retrospective assessment. J Neurol Neurosurg Psychiatry 2016;87(10): 1068–74.
5. Carroll LJ, Cassidy JD, Holm L, et al. Methodological issues and research recommendations for mild traumatic brain injury: the WHO Collaborating Centre Task Force on Mild Traumatic Brain Injury. J Rehabil Med 2004;43(Suppl): 113–25.
6. Ruff RM, Iverson GL, Barth JT, et al. NAN Policy and Planning Committee. Recommendations for diagnosing a mild traumatic brain injury: a National Academy of Neuropsychology education paper. Arch Clin Neuropsychol 2009;24(1):3–10.
7. Belson K, Vrentas J, Morgan E. Doctor who examined Tagovailoa is Dismissed; N.F.L. Assessing concussion rules. New York Times 2022.
8. van der Vlegel M, Polinder S, Toet H, et al. Prevalence of Post-Concussion-Like Symptoms in the General Injury Population and the Association with Health-

Related Quality of Life, Health Care Use, and Return to Work. J Clin Med 2021; 10(4):806.

9. Broshek DK, Pardini JE, Herring SA. Persisting symptoms after concussion: Time for a paradigm shift. Pharm Manag PM R 2022 Dec;14(12):1509–13.

10. Dwyer B, Katz DI. Postconcussion syndrome. Handb Clin Neurol 2018;158: 163–78.

11. Cancelliere C, Verville L, Stubbs JL, et al. Post-Concussion Symptoms and Disability in Adults With Mild Traumatic Brain Injury: A Systematic Review and Meta-Analysis. J Neurotrauma 2023;40(11–12):1045–59.

12. Taylor AA, McCauley SR, Strutt AM. Postconcussional Syndrome: Clinical Diagnosis and Treatment. Neurol Clin 2023;41(1):161–76.

13. Iverson GL, Lange RT. Examination of "postconcussion-like" symptoms in a healthy sample. Appl Neuropsychol 2003;10(3):137–44.

14. Gouvier WD, Uddo-Crane M, Brown LM. Base rates of post-concussional symptoms. Arch Clin Neuropsychol 1988;3(3):273–8.

15. Dean PJ, O'Neill D, Sterr A. Post-concussion syndrome: prevalence after mild traumatic brain injury in comparison with a sample without head injury. Brain Inj 2012;26:14–26.

16. Polinder S, Cnossen MC, Real RGL, et al. A Multidimensional Approach to Post-concussion Symptoms in Mild Traumatic Brain Injury. Front Neurol 2018;9(9): 1113.

17. J Bazarian J, Wong T, Harris M. Epidemiology and predictors of post-concussive syndrome after minor head injury in an emergency population. Brain Inj 1999;13:173–89.

18. Theadom A, Parag V, Dowell T, et al, BIONIC Research Group. Persistent problems 1 year after mild traumatic brain injury: a longitudinal population study in New Zealand. Br J Gen Pract 2016;66(642):e16–23.

19. Paniak C, Reynolds S, Phillips K, et al. Patient complaints within 1 month of mild traumatic brain injury: a controlled study. Arch Clin Neuropsychol 2002;17(4): 319–34.

20. P Alexander M. Mild traumatic brain injury: pathophysiology, natural history, and clinical management. Neurology 1995;45:1253–60.

21. Baandrup L, Jensen R. Chronic post-traumatic headache–a clinical analysis in relation to the International Headache Classification 2nd Edition. Cephalalgia 2005;25(2):132–8.

22. Evans RW, Ghosh K. A Survey of Headache Medicine Physicians on the Likeability of Headaches and Their Personal Headache History. Headache 2016; 56(3):540–6.

23. Useche JN, Bermudez S. Conventional Computed Tomography and Magnetic Resonance in Brain Concussion. Neuroimaging Clin N Am 2018;28(1):15–29.

24. Easter JS, Haukoos JS, Meehan WP, et al. Will Neuroimaging Reveal a Severe Intracranial Injury in This Adult With Minor Head Trauma?: The Rational Clinical Examination Systematic Review. JAMA 2015;314(24):2672–81.

25. Yue JK, Yuh EL, Korley FK, et al. TRACK-TBI Investigators. Association between plasma GFAP concentrations and MRI abnormalities in patients with CT-negative traumatic brain injury in the TRACK-TBI cohort: a prospective multicentre study. Lancet Neurol 2019;18(10):953–61.

26. Expert Panel on Neurological Imaging. ACR Appropriateness Criteria. 2020. p 21-23. Available at: https://acsearch.acr.org/docs/69481/Narrative/). Accessed November 25, 2023.

27. Radiological Society of North America Statement on Traumatic Brain Injury (TBI) Imaging Reviewed: 4/15/2023. Available at: https://www.rsna.org/-/media/Files/RSNA/Media/Traumatic-Brain-Injury-TBI-Imaging.ashx?la=en&hash=041FB0B84B9 846BE2149368FAF9DCB1E44009B64#:~:text=Reviewed%3A%204%2F15% 2F2023,The%20Radiological%20Society&text=Traumatic%20brain%20injury %20(TBI)%20is,assaults%20and%20sports%2Drelated%20injuries.&text=Imaging %20plays%20an%20essential%20role%20in%20identifying%20TBI%20patients %20with%20intracranial%20injury. Accessed November 25, 2023.

28. Weaver LK, Wilson SH, Lindblad AS, et al, NORMAL Study Team. Comprehensive Evaluation of Healthy Volunteers Using Multi-Modality Brain Injury Assessments: An Exploratory, Observational Study. Front Neurol 2018;9:1030.

29. Department of Veterans Affairs and Department of Defense. VA/DoD clinical practice guideline for the management and rehabilitation of post-acute mild traumatic brain injury. 2021, p 27-28. Available at: https://www.healthquality.va.gov/guidelines/Rehab/mtbi/VADoDmTBICPGFinal508.pdf. Accessed November 25, 2023.

30. Nuwer MR, Hovda DA, Schrader LM, et al. Routine and quantitative EEG in mild traumatic brain injury. Clin Neurophysiol 2005;116(9):2001–25.

31. Tenney JR, Gloss D, Arya R, et al. Practice Guideline: Use of Quantitative EEG for the Diagnosis of Mild Traumatic Brain Injury: Report of the Guideline Committee of the American Clinical Neurophysiology Society. J Clin Neurophysiol 2021; 38(4):287–92.

32. Schneider ALC, Huie JR, Boscardin WJ, et al. TRACK-TBI Investigators. Cognitive Outcome 1 Year After Mild Traumatic Brain Injury: Results From the TRACK-TBI Study. Neurology 2022;98(12):e1248–61.

33. Jennings S, Collins MW, Taylor AM. Neuropsychological Assessment of Sport-Related Concussion. Clin Sports Med 2021;40(1):81–91.

34. Trimble M. Post-traumatic neurosis: from railway spine to the whiplash. Chichester (England): Wiley; 1981.

35. Evans RW. The post-concussion syndrome: 130 years of controversy. Semin Neurol 1994;14:32–9.

36. J.E Erichsen on railway and other injuries of the nervous system. Philadelphia: Henry C. Lea; 1867.

37. Rigler J. Ueber die Folgen der Verletzungen auf Eisenbahnen Insbesondere der Verletzungen des Rueckenmarks. Berlin: Druck and Verlag von G. Reimer; 1879.

38. Strauss I, Savitsky N. Head injury: Neurologic and psychiatric aspects. Arch Neurol Psychiatry 1934;31:893–955.

39. Miller H. Accident neurosis. Br Med J 1961;1:919–25, 9928.

40. Symonds C. Concussion and its sequelae. Lancet 1962;1:1–5.

41. Evans RW, Ghosh K. A Survey of Neurologists on Postconcussion Syndrome. Headache 2018;58(6):836–44.

42. Evans RW, Evans RI, Sharp M. The physician survey on the post-concussion and whiplash syndromes. Headache 1994;34:268–74.

43. Lefevre-Dognin C, Cogné M, Perdrieau V, et al. Definition and epidemiology of mild traumatic brain injury. Neurochirurgie 2021;67(3):218–21.

44. Taylor CA, Bell JM, Breiding MJ, et al. Traumatic Brain Injury–Related Emergency Department Visits, Hospitalizations, and Deaths — United States, 2007 and 2013. MMWR Surveill Summ 2017;66(No. SS-9):1–16.

45. Gordon KE. The Silent Minority: Insights into Who Fails to Present for Medical Care Following a Brain Injury. Neuroepidemiology 2020;54(3):235–42.

46. Moore M, Sandsmark DK. Clinical Updates in Mild Traumatic Brain Injury (Concussion). Neuroimaging Clin N Am 2023;33(2):271–8.
47. Langer L, Levy C, Bayley M. Increasing Incidence of Concussion: True Epidemic or Better Recognition? J Head Trauma Rehabil 2020;35(1):E60–6.
48. Whiteneck GG, Cuthbert JP, Corrigan JD, et al. Prevalence of Self-Reported Lifetime History of Traumatic Brain Injury and Associated Disability: A Statewide Population-Based Survey. J Head Trauma Rehabil 2016;31(1):E55–62.
49. Gordon WA, Brown M, Sliwinksi M. The enigma of "hidden" traumatic brain injury. J Head Trauma Rehabil 1998;13:39–56.
50. Tanielian TL, Jaycox LH, editors. Invisible wounds of war: psychological and cognitive injuries, their consequences, and services to assist recovery. Santa Monica (CA): RAND Corporation; 2008.
51. Fischer HUS. Military casualty statistics: Operation New Dawn, Operation Iraqi Freedom, and Operation Enduring Freedom. Report ID # – RS22452. Congressional Research Service. 02/05/2013. Available at: http://www.fas.org/sgp/crs/natsec/RS22452.pdf. Accessed August 11, 2013.
52. Hoge CW, McGurk D, Thomas JL, et al. Mild traumatic brain injury in U.S. Soldiers returning from Iraq. N Engl J Med 2008;358(5):453–63.
53. Centers for Disease Control and Prevention (CDC). 1991-2021 High School Youth Risk Behavior Survey Data. Available at: http://yrbs-explorer.services.cdc.gov/. Accessed November 20, 2023.
54. Kerr ZY, Chandran A, Nedimyer AK, et al. Concussion Incidence and Trends in 20 High School Sports. Pediatrics 2019;144:e20192180.
55. Gessell LM, Fields SK, Collins CL, et al. Concussions among United States high school and collegiate athletes. J Athl Train 2007;42:495–503.
56. Lindberg MA, Moy Martin EM, Marion DW. Military Traumatic Brain Injury: The History, Impact, and Future. J Neurotrauma 2022;39(17–18):1133–45.
57. Langlois JA, Rutland-Brown W, Wald MM. The epidemiology and impact of traumatic brain injury: a brief overview. J Head Trauma Rehabil 2006;21:375–8.
58. DePadilla L, Miller GF, Jones SE, et al. Self-reported concussions from playing a sport or being physically active among high school students - United States, 2017. MMWR Morb Mortal Wkly Rep 2018;67:82–685.
59. Zuckerman SL, Kerr ZY, Yengo-Kahn A, et al. Epidemiology of sports-related concussion in NCAA athletes from 2009-2010 to 2013-2014: incidence, recurrence, and mechanisms. Am J Sports Med 2015;43:2654–62.
60. Baldwin GT, Breiding MJ, Dawn Comstock R. Epidemiology of sports concussion in the United States. Handb Clin Neurol 2018;158:63–74.
61. Pierpoint LA, Collins C. Epidemiology of Sport-Related Concussion. Clin Sports Med 2021;40(1):1–18.
62. McDaniel M. NFL Admits to Stark Rise in Concussions During 2022 Season. Sports Illustrated. 2023. Available at: https://www.si.com/nfl/2023/02/03/nfl-concussions-up-during-2022-season-injury-totals. Accessed November 20, 2023.
63. Patricios JS, Schneider KJ, Dvorak J, et al. Consensus statement on concussion in sport: the 6th International Conference on Concussion in Sport-Amsterdam, October 2022. Br J Sports Med 2023;57(11):695–711.
64. Eliason PH, Galarneau JM, Kolstad AT, et al. Prevention strategies and modifiable risk factors for sport-related concussions and head impacts: a systematic review and meta-analysis. Br J Sports Med 2023;57(12):749–61.
65. Bello C, Andereggen L, Luedi MM. Beilstein CM. Postcraniotomy Headache: Etiologies and Treatments. Curr Pain Headache Rep 2022;26(5):357–64.

66. Rimaaja T, Haanpää M, Blomstedt G, et al. Headaches after acoustic neuroma surgery. Cephalalgia 2007;27(10):1128–35.
67. Magalhães JE, Azevedo-Filho HR, Rocha-Filho PA. The Risk of Headache Attributed to Surgical Treatment of Intracranial Aneurysms: A Cohort Study. Headache 2013;53(10):1613–23.
68. Rocha-Filho PA, Gherpelli JL, de Siqueira JT, et al. Post-craniotomy headache: characteristics, behaviour and effect on quality of life in patients operated for treatment of supratentorial intracranial aneurysms. Cephalalgia 2008; 28(1):41–8.
69. Kaur A, Selwa L, Fromes G, et al. Persistent headache after supratentorial craniotomy. Neurosurgery 2000;47(3):633–6.
70. Gee JR, Ishaq Y, Vijayan N. Postcraniotomy headache. Headache 2003;43(3): 276–8.
71. Schaller B, Baumann A. Headache after removal of vestibular schwannoma via the retrosigmoid approach: a long-term follow-up study. Otolaryngol Head Neck Surg 2003;387–95.
72. Ducic I, Felder JM 3rd, Endara M. Postoperative headache following acoustic neuroma resection: occipital nerve injuries are associated with a treatable occipital neuralgia. Headache 2012;52(7):1136–45.
73. Shibata Y, Hatayama T, Matsuda M, et al. Epidemiology of post-suboccipital craniotomy headache: A multicentre retrospective study. J Perioper Pract 2023;33(7–8):233–8.
74. Minderhoud JM, Boelens MEM, Huizenga J, et al. Treatment of minor head injuries. Clin Neurol Neurosurg 1980;82:127–40.
75. Couch JR, Lipton RB, Stewart WF, et al. Head or neck injury increases the risk of chronic daily headache: a population-based study. Neurology 2007;69(11): 1169–77.
76. Yamaguchi M. Incidence of headache and severity of head injury. Headache 1992;32:427–31.
77. Couch JR, Bearss C. Chronic daily headache in the posttrauma syndrome: Relation to extent of head injury. Headache 2001;41:559–64.
78. Langer LK, Bayley MT, Lawrence DW, et al. Revisiting the ICHD-3 criteria for headache attributed to mild traumatic injury to the head: Insights from the Toronto Concussion Study Analysis of Acute Headaches Following Concussion. Cephalalgia 2022;42(11–12):1172–83.
79. Headache Classification Committee of the International Headache Society (IHS) The International Classification of Headache Disorders, 3rd edition. Cephalalgia 2018; 38:1–211.
80. Russell MB, Olesen J. Migraine associated with head trauma. Eur J Neurol 1996; 3:424–8.
81. Ashina H, Dodick DW, Barber J, et al. TRACK-TBI Investigators. Prevalence of and Risk Factors for Post-traumatic Headache in Civilian Patients After Mild Traumatic Brain Injury: A TRACK-TBI Study. Mayo Clin Proc 2023;98(10):1515–26.
82. Ashina H, Christensen RH, Al-Khazali HM, et al. White matter hyperintensities and cerebral microbleeds in persistent post-traumatic headache attributed to mild traumatic brain injury: a magnetic resonance imaging study. J Headache Pain 2023;24(1):15.
83. Solomon S. Posttraumatic migraine. Headache 1998;38:772–8.
84. Lucas S, Hoffman JM, Bell KR, et al. A prospective study of prevalence and characterization of headache following mild traumatic brain injury. Cephalagia 2014;34:93–102.

85. Limmroth V, Cutrer FM, Moskowitz MA, et al. Age- and sex-specific incidence rates of migraine with and without visual aura. Am J Epidemiol 1991;134:1111–20.

86. Lew HL, Lin P-H, Fuh J-L, et al. Characteristics and treatment of headache after traumatic brain injury: a focused review. Am J Phys Med Rehabil 2006;85:619–27.

87. Hoffman JM, Lucas S, Dikmen S, et al. Natural history of headache after traumatic brain injury. J Neurotrauma 2011;28(9):1719–25.

88. Theeler BJ, Erickson JC. Mild head trauma and chronic headaches in returning US soldiers. Headache 2009;49(4):529–34.

89. Lieba-Samal D, Platzer P, Seidel S, et al. Characteristics of acute posttraumatic headache following mild head injury. Cephalalgia 2011;31:1618–26.

90. Haas DC. Chronic post-traumatic headaches classified and compared with natural headaches. Cephalalgia 1996;16:486–93.

91. Bettucci D, Aguggia M, Bolamperti L, et al. Chronic post-traumatic headache associated with minor cranial trauma: a description of cephalalgic patterns. Ital J Neurol Sci 1998;19:20–4.

92. Radanov BP, Di Stefano G, Augustiny KF. Symptomatic approach to posttraumatic headache and its possible implications for treatment. Eur Spine J 2001; 10:403–7.

93. Bekkelund SI, Salvesen R. Prevalence of head trauma in patients with difficult headache: the North Norway Headache Study. Headache 2003;43:59–62.

94. Lucas S, Hoffman JM, Bell KR, et al. Characterization of headache after traumatic brain injury. Cephalalgia 2012;32(8):600–6.

95. Xu H, Pi H, Ma L, et al. Incidence of headache after traumatic brain injury in China: a large prospective study. World Neurosurg 2016;88:289–96.

96. Ashina H, Iljazi A, Al-Khazali HM, et al. Persistent post-traumatic headache attributed to mild traumatic brain injury: Deep phenotyping and treatment patterns. Cephalalgia 2020;40(6):554–64.

97. DOD TBI Worldwide Numbers. Health.mil. 2023. Available at: https://health.mil/Military-Health-Topics/Centers-of-Excellence/Traumatic-Brain-Injury-Center-of-Excellence/DOD-TBI-Worldwide-Numbers?type=Articles. Accessed November 24, 2023.

98. Theeler B, Lucas S, Riechers RG 2nd, et al. Post-traumatic headaches in civilians and military personnel: a comparative, clinical review. Headache 2013; 53(6):881–900.

99. Erickson JC. Treatment outcomes of chronic post-traumatic headaches after mild head trauma in US soldiers: an observational study. Headache 2011; 51(6):932–44.

100. Theeler BJ, Flynn FG, Erickson JC. Headaches after concussion in US soldiers returning from Iraq or Afghanistan. Headache 2010;50(8):1262–72.

101. Finkel AG, Ivins BJ, Yerry JA, et al. Which Matters More? A Retrospective Cohort Study of Headache Characteristics and Diagnosis Type in Soldiers with mTBI/Concussion. Headache 2017;57(5):719–28.

102. Theeler BJ, Mercer R, Erickson JC. Prevalence and impact of migraine among US Army soldiers deployed in support of Operation Iraqi Freedom. Headache 2008;48(6):876–82.

103. Mihalik JP, Register-Mihalik J, Kerr ZY, et al. Recovery of posttraumatic migraine characteristics in patients after mild traumatic brain injury. Am J Sports Med 2013;41(7):1490–6.

104. Mihalik JP, Stump JE, Collins MW, et al. Posttraumatic migraine characteristics in athletes following sports-related concussion. J Neurosurg 2005;102(5):850–5.

105. Evans RW. The prevalence of migraine and other neurological conditions among retired National Football League players: A pilot study. Pract Neurol. November/December 2017:21-24. Available at: https://practicalneurology.com/articles/2017-nov-dec/the-prevalence-of-migraine-and-other-neurological-conditions-among-retired-national-football-league-players-a-pilot-study. Accessed November 22, 2023.
106. Evans RW. Sports and Headaches. Headache 2018;58(3):426–37.
107. Rocha-Filho PA. Post-craniotomy headache: a clinical view with a focus on the persistent form. Headache 2015;55(5):733–8.
108. Evans RW. Whiplash injuries. In: Roos RP, editor. Medlink neurology. San Diego (CA): MedLink Corp.; 2023. Available at: www.medlink.com.
109. Pareek AV, Edmondson E, Kung D. Cervicogenic headaches: a literature review and proposed multifaceted approach to diagnosis and management. Neurol Clinic, 2024, in press.
110. Plaschke Bi. In the end, he gave Packers a headache. Los Angeles Times, 1/26/1998. Available at: https://www.latimes.com/archives/la-xpm-1998-jan-26-ss-12339-story.html. Accessed November 22, 2023.
111. Pennington B. SUPER BOWL XXXII; Even a Migraine Doesn't Slow Down Davis on His Way to the M.V.P. New York Times. January 26, 1998.
112. Beitchman JA, Burg BA, Sabb DM, et al. The pentagram of concussion: an observational analysis that describes five overt indicators of head trauma. BMC Sports Sci Med Rehabil 2022;14(1):39.
113. Around the NFL Staff. NFL, NFLPA agree to modify concussion protocols following completion of Tua Tagovailoa investigation. 10/8/22. Available at: https://www.nfl.com/news/nfl-nflpa-agree-to-modify-concussion-protocols-following-completion-of-tuatagov#:~:text=The%20new%20concussion%20protocol%20will,player%20re%2Denters%20a%20game. Accessed November 24, 2023.
114. Oyefus D. How jiu-jitsu can keep Dolphins QB Tua Tagovailoa safe after concussions sidelined him. Miami Herald 9/5/23. Available at: https://www.miamiherald.com/sports/article277475988.html. Accessed November 24, 2023.
115. Staff. Everything you need to know about Zero2 Matrix QB Helmet. American Football Magazine. 7/24/23. available at: https://www.americanfootballmagazine.com/post/zero2-matrix-qb-helmet-with-faqs. Accessed November 24, 2023.
116. Echemendia RJ, Burma JS, Bruce JM, et al. Acute evaluation of sport-related concussion and implications for the sport concussion assessment tool (SCAT6) for adults, adolescents and children: a systematic review. Br J Sports Med 2023;57(11):722–35.
117. Ramsay D, Miller A, Baykeens B, et al. Football (Soccer) as a Probable Cause of Long-Term Neurological Impairment and Neurodegeneration: A Narrative Review of the Debate. Cureus 2023;15(1):e34279.
118. Jensen C. 50 Years Ago, 'Unsafe at Any Speed' Shook the Auto World. New York Times, 11/26/15. Available at: https://www.nytimes.com/2015/11/27/automobiles/50-years-ago-unsafe-at-any-speed-shook-the-auto-world.html.
119. Makdissi M, Critchley ML, Cantu RC, et al. When should an athlete retire or discontinue participating in contact or collision sports following sport-related concussion? A systematic review. Br J Sports Med 2023;57(12):822–30.
120. Romero-Reyes M, Bassiur JP. Temporomandibular joint disorders, bruxism, and headaches. Neurol Clin, 2024, in press.
121. Hecht JS. Occipital nerve blocks in postconcussive headaches: a retrospective review and report of ten patients. J Head Trauma Rehabil 2004;19(1):58–71.

122. Thomas DC, Patil AG, Sood R, et al. Occipital Neuralgia and Its Management: An Overview. Neurol India 2021;69(Supplement):S213–8.

123. Evans RW. Greater occipital neuralgia can cause facial paresthesias. Cephalalgia 2009;29:801.

124. Matthews WB. Footballer's migraine. Br Med J 1972;2(5809):326–7.

125. Soriani S, Cavaliere B, Faggioli R, et al. Confusional migraine precipitated by mild head trauma. Arch Pediatr Adolesc Med 2000;154:90–1.

126. Farooqi AM, Padilla JM, Monteith TS. Acute Confusional Migraine: Distinct Clinical Entity or Spectrum of Migraine Biology? Brain Sci 2018;8(2):29.

127. Weinstock A, Rothner AD. Trauma-triggered migraine: a cause of transient neurologic deficit following minor head injury in children. Neurology 1995; 45(Suppl 4):A347–8.

128. Grangeon L, O'Connor E, Chan CK, et al. New insights in post-traumatic headache with cluster headache phenotype: a cohort study. J Neurol Neurosurg Psychiatry 2020;91(6):572–9.

129. Matharu MS, Goadsby PJ. Posttraumatic chronic paroxysmal hemicranias (CPH) with aura. Neurology 2001;56:273–5.

130. Jacob S, Watson D, Riggs JE. When Treatment Establishes Diagnosis: A Case Report of Posttraumatic Chronic Paroxysmal Hemicrania. Headache 2018;58(6): 894–5.

131. Putzki N, Nirkko A, Diener HC. Trigeminal autonomic cephalalgias: a case of post-traumatic SUNCT syndrome? Cephalalgia 2005;25(5):395–7.

132. Jacob S, Saha A, Rajabally Y. Post-traumatic short-lasting unilateral headache with cranial autonomic symptoms (SUNA). Cephalalgia 2008;28(9):991–3.

133. Evans RW, Lay CL. Posttraumatic hemicrania continua? Headache 2000;40: 761–2.

134. Mathew PG, Cooper W. The Diagnosis and Management of Posttraumatic Headache with Associated Painful Cranial Neuralgias: a Review and Case Series. Curr Pain Headache Rep 2021;25(8):54.

135. Stewart M, Boyce S, McGlone R. Post-traumatic headache: don't forget to test the supraorbital nerve. BMJ Case Rep 2012;2012.

136. Devoti JF, Nicot R, Roland-Billecart T, et al. Characterization of Infraorbital Nerve Sequelae After Orbital Floor or Zygomaticomaxillary Complex Fractures. J Craniofac Surg 2022;33(1):52–6.

137. Fukutake T, Mine S, Yamakami I, et al. Roller coaster headache and subdural hematoma. Neurology 2000;54:264.

138. Scranton RA, Evans RW, Baskin DS. A Motion Simulator Ride Associated With Headache and Subdural Hematoma: First Case Report. Headache 2016; 56(2):372–8.

139. Matsuda W, Sugimoto K, Sato N, et al. Delayed onset of posttraumatic acute subdural hematoma after mild head injury with normal computed tomography: a case report and brief review. J Trauma 2008;65(2):461–3.

140. Kim SW, Kang HG. Delayed-onset subdural hematoma after mild head injury with negative initial brain imaging. J Integr Neurosci 2022;21(2):69.

141. Yamada SM, Tomita Y, Murakami H, et al. Headache in patients with chronic subdural hematoma: analysis in 1080 patients. Neurosurg Rev 2018;41(2): 549–56.

142. Jensen TS, Gorelick PB. Headache associated with ischemic stroke and intracranial hematoma. In: Olesen J, Tfelt-Hansen P, Welch KMA, editors. The headaches. 2nd edition. Philadelphia: Lippincott Williams & Wilkins; 2000. p. 781–7.

143. Radulovic D, Janosevic V, Djurovic B, et al. Traumatic delayed epidural hematoma. Zentralbl Neurochir 2006;67(2):76–80.

144. Milo R, Razon N, Schiffer J. Delayed epidural hematoma. A review. Acta Neurochir 1987;84:13–23.

145. Benoit BG, Russell NA, Richard MT, et al. Epidural hematoma: report of seven cases with delayed evolution of symptoms. Can J Neurol Sci 1982;9:321–4.

146. Pettyjohn EW, Donlan RM, Breck J, et al. Intracranial Hypotension in the Setting of Post-Concussion Headache: A Case Series. Cureus 2020;12(9):e10526.

147. Park JK. Rudofsky Salama. Cranial cerebrospinal fluid leaks. In: UpToDate, Connor RF, editors. UpToDate. Wolters Kluwer; 2023.

148. Griswold DP, Fernandez L, Rubiano AM. Traumatic Subarachnoid Hemorrhage: A Scoping Review. J Neurotrauma 2022;39(1–2):35–48.

149. Keser Z, Meschia JF, Lanzino G. Craniocervical Artery Dissections: A Concise Review for Clinicians. Mayo Clin Proc 2022;97(4):777–83.

150. D'Alise MD, Fichtel F, Horowitz M. Sagittal sinus thrombosis following minor head injury treated with continuous urokinase infusion. Surg Neurol 1998; 49(4):430–5.

151. Kaplan JB, Bodhit AN, Falgiani ML. Communicating carotid-cavernous sinus fistula following minor head trauma. Int J Emerg Med 2012;5(1):10.

152. Ashina H, Porreca F, Anderson T, et al. Post-traumatic headache: epidemiology and pathophysiological insights. Nat Rev Neurol 2019;15(10):607–17.

153. Chen Q, Bharadwaj V, Irvine KA, et al. Mechanisms and treatments of chronic pain after traumatic brain injury. Neurochem Int 2023;171:105630.

154. Graham DI, Saatman KE, Marklund N, et al. Neuropathology of brain injury. In: Evans RW, editor. Neurology and trauma. 2nd edition. New York: Oxford; 2006. p. 45–94.

155. Mavroudis I, Ciobica A, Luca AC, et al. Post-Traumatic Headache: A Review of Prevalence, Clinical Features, Risk Factors, and Treatment Strategies. J Clin Med 2023;12(13):4233.

156. Weyer A. Posttraumatic Headaches and Postcraniotomy Syndromes. Neurol Clin 2022;40(3):609–29.

157. Hu L, Yang S, Jin B, et al. Advanced Neuroimaging Role in Traumatic Brain Injury: A Narrative Review. Front Neurosci 2022;16:872609.

158. Schwedt TJ. Post-traumatic headache due to mild traumatic brain injury: Current knowledge and future directions. Cephalalgia 2021;41(4):464–71.

159. Polich G, Iaccarino MA, Kaptchuk TJ, et al. Nocebo Effects in Concussion: Is All That Is Told Beneficial? Am J Phys Med Rehabil 2020;99(1):71–80.

160. Carriere JS, Pimentel SD, Yakobov E, et al. A systematic review of the association between perceived injustice and painrelated outcomes in individuals with musculoskeletal pain. Pain Med 2020;21:1449–63.

161. Evans RW. Persistent post-traumatic headache, postconcussion syndrome, and whiplash injuries: the evidence for a non-traumatic basis with an historical review. Headache 2010;50:716–24.

162. Obermann M, Keidel M, Diener HC. Post-traumatic headache: is it for real? Crossfire debates on headache: pro. Headache 2010;50(4):710–5.

163. Leininger BE, Gramling SE, Farrell AD, et al. Neuropsychological deficits in symptomatic minor head injury patients after concussion and mild concussion. J Neurol Neurosurg Psychiatry 1990;53:293–6.

164. Weiss HD, Stern BJ, Goldberg J. Posttraumatic migraine: chronic migraine precipitated by minor head or neck trauma. Headache 1991;31:451–6.

165. Packard RC. Posttraumatic headache: permanence and relationship to legal settlement. Headache 1992;32:496–500.
166. Jacobs MS. Psychological factors influencing chronic pain and the impact of litigation. Curr Phys Med Rehabil Rep 2013;1:135–41.
167. Mickeviciene D, Schrader H, Obelieniene D, et al. A controlled prospective inception cohort study on the post-concussion syndrome outside the medico-legal context. Eur J Neurol 2004;11:411–9.
168. Stovner LJ, Schrader H, Mickeviciene D, et al. Headache after concussion. Eur J Neurol 2009;16:112–20.
169. Hadler NM. If you have to prove you are ill, you can't get well. The object lesson of fibromyalgia. Spine 1996;21:2397–400.
170. Carroll LJ, Cassidy JD, Peloso PM, et al. Prognosis for mild traumatic brain injury: results of the WHO Collaborating Centre Task Force on Mild Traumatic Brain Injury. J Rehabil Med 2004;(suppl.43):84–105.
171. Hanks RA, Rapport LJ, Seagly K, et al. Outcomes after Concussion Recovery Education: Effects of litigation and disability status on maintenance of symptoms. J Neurotrauma 2018;36:554–8.
172. Binder LM, Rohling ML. Money matters: a meta-analytic review of the effects of financial incentives on recovery after closed-head injury. Am J Psychiatry 1996;153:7–10.
173. Tsanadis J, Montoya E, Hanks RA, et al. Brain injury severity, litigation status, and self-report of postconcussive symptoms. Clin Neuropsychol 2008;22(6):1080–92.
174. Ruff RM, Wylie T, Tennant W. Malingering and malingering-like aspects of mild closed head injury. J Head Trauma Rehab 1993;8:60–73.
175. Andrikopoulos J. Post-traumatic headache in mild head injured litigants. Headache 2003;43:553.
176. Evans RW, Strutt AM. Medico-Legal Aspects of Concussion. Headache 2020;60(8):1749–60.
177. Hubbard JE, Hodge SD Jr. The Litigation Complexity of Posttraumatic Headaches. Curr Pain Headache Rep 2021;25(6):39.
178. Larsen EL, Ashina H, Iljazi A, et al. Acute and preventive pharmacological treatment of post-traumatic headache: a systematic review. J Headache Pain 2019;20(1):98.
179. Ashina H, Diener HC, Tassorelli C. et al., Guidelines of the International Headache Society for Controlled Trials of Pharmacological Preventive Treatment for Persistent Post-Traumatic Headache (PPTH) attributed to mild traumatic brain injury. Cephalalgia 2024, in press.
180. Tyler GS, McNeely HE, Dick ML. Treatment of posttraumatic headache with amitriptyline. Headache 1980;20:213–6.
181. Packard RC. Treatment of chronic daily posttraumatic headache with divalproex sodium. Headache 2000;40:736–9.
182. Saran A. Antidepressants not effective in headache associated with minor closed head injury. Int J Psychiatry Med 1988;18:75–83.
183. Cushman DM, Borowski L, Hansen C, et al. Gabapentin and Tricyclics in the Treatment of Post-Concussive Headache, a Retrospective Cohort Study. Headache 2019;59(3):371–82.
184. Spierings ELH, Silberstein SD, Najib U, et al. A phase 2 study of fremanezumab as a treatment for posttraumatic headache in adult patients. Headache 2021;61:97–8.

185. Ashina H, Iljazi A, Al-Khazali HM, et al. Efficacy, tolerability, and safety of erenumab for the preventive treatment of persistent post-traumatic headache attributed to mild traumatic brain injury: an open-label study. J Headache Pain 2020;21(1):62.

186. Buture A, Tomkins EM, Shukralla A, et al. Two-year, real-world erenumab persistence and quality of life data in 82 pooled patients with abrupt onset, unremitting, treatment refractory headache and a migraine phenotype: New daily persistent headache or persistent post-traumatic headache in the majority of cases. Cephalalgia 2023;43(6). 3331024231182126.

187. Yerry JA, Finkel AG, Lewis SC, et al. Onabotulinum toxin A for the treatment of chronic post-traumatic headache in service members with a history of mild traumatic brain injury. Cephalalgia 2013;33(11):984–5.

188. Yerry JA, Kuehn D, Finkel AG. Onabotulinum toxin a for the treatment of headache in service members with a history of mild traumatic brain injury: a cohort study. Headache 2015;55(3):395–406.

189. Zirovich MD, Pangarkar SS, Manh C, et al. Botulinum Toxin Type A for the Treatment of Post-traumatic Headache: A Randomized, Placebo-Controlled, Crossover Study. Mil Med 2021;186(5–6):493–9.

190. Gawel MJ, Rothbart P, Lacobs H. Subcutaneous sumatriptan in the acute treatment of acute episodes of PTH headache. Headache 1993;33:96–7.

191. Ashina H, Eigenbrodt AK, Seifert T, et al. Post-traumatic headache attributed to traumatic brain injury: classification, clinical characteristics, and treatment. Lancet Neurol 2021;20(6):460–9.

192. DiTommaso C, Hoffman JM, Lucas S, et al., Medication usage patterns for headache treatment after mild traumatic brain injury. Headache, 2013, in press.

193. Watanabe TK, Bell KR, Walker WC, et al. Systematic review of interventions for post-traumatic headache. Pharm Manag PM R 2012;4(2):129–40.

194. Argyriou AA, Mitsikostas DD, Mantovani E, et al. An updated brief overview on post-traumatic headache and a systematic review of the non-pharmacological interventions for its management. Expert Rev Neurother 2021;21(4):475–90.

195. Lee MJ, Zhou Y, Greenwald BD. Update on Non-Pharmacological Interventions for Treatment of Post-Traumatic Headache. Brain Sci 2022;12(10):1357.

196. Blumenfeld A, Ashkenazi A, Napchan U, et al. Expert consensus recommendations for the performance of peripheral nerve blocks for headaches–a narrative review. Headache 2013;53(3):437–46.

197. Blake P, Burstein R. Emerging evidence of occipital nerve compression in unremitting head and neck pain. J Headache Pain 2019;20(1):76.

198. Wahab S, Kataria S, Woolley P, et al. Literature Review: Pericranial Nerve Blocks for Chronic Migraines. Health Psychol Res 2023;11:74259.

199. Miller S, Lagrata S, Matharu M. Multiple cranial nerve blocks for the transitional treatment of chronic headaches. Cephalalgia 2019;39:1488–99.

200. Stern JI, Chiang CC, Kissoon NR, et al. Narrative review of peripheral nerve blocks for the management of headache. Headache 2022;62(9):1077–92.

201. Natsis K, Baraliakos X, Appell HJ, et al. The course of the greater occipital nerve in the suboccipital region: a proposal for setting landmarks for local anesthesia in patients with occipital neuralgia. Clin Anat 2006;19(4):332–6.

202. Lambru G, Lagrata S, Matharu MS. Cutaneous atrophy and alopecia after greater occipital nerve injection using triamcinolone. Headache 2012;52(10):1596–9.

203. Gabrhelík T, Michálek P, Adamus M. Pulsed radiofrequency therapy versus greater occipital nerve block in the management of refractory cervicogenic headache - a pilot study. Prague Med Rep 2011;112(4):279–87.

204. Huang JH, Galvagno SM Jr, Hameed M, et al. Occipital nerve pulsed radiofrequency treatment: a multi-center study evaluating predictors of outcome. Pain Med 2012;13(4):489–97.

205. Palmisani S, Al-Kaisy A, Arcioni R, et al. A six year retrospective review of occipital nerve stimulation practice - controversies and challenges of an emerging technique for treating refractory headache syndromes. J Headache Pain 2013;14(1):67.

206. Barmherzig R, Kingston W. Occipital Neuralgia and Cervicogenic Headache: Diagnosis and Management. Curr Neurol Neurosci Rep 2019;19(5):20.

207. Li F, Ma Y, Zou J, et al. Micro-surgical decompression for greater occipital neuralgia. Turk Neurosurg 2012;22(4):427–9.

208. Ducic I, Sinkin JC, Crutchfield KE. Interdisciplinary treatment of post-concussion and post-traumatic headaches. Microsurgery 2015;35:603–7.

209. Conidi FX. Post Traumatic Headache: Clinical care of athletes vs non athletes with Persistent Post Traumatic Headache after Concussion: Sports Neurologist and Headache Specialist Perspective. Curr Pain Headache Rep 2020; 24(10):65.

210. World anti-doping code international standard prohibited list 2023. Available at: https://www.wada-ama.org/sites/default/files/2022-09/2023list_en_final_9_september_2022.pdf. Accessed November 24, 2023.

211. National Football League. Policy on performance-enhancing substances. 2023. Available at: https://nflpaweb.blob.core.windows.net/website/Departments/Legal/07-17-2023-FOR-DISTRIBUTION-2023-Policy-on-Performance-Enhancing-Substances-final.pdf. Accessed November 24, 2023.

212. Evans RW. The post-concussion syndrome. In: Evans RW, Baskin DS, Yatsu FM, editors. Prognosis of neurological disorders. New York: Oxford University Press; 1992. p. 97–107.

213. Okun MS, Mayberg HS, DeLong MR. Muhammad Ali and Young-Onset Idiopathic Parkinson Disease—The Missing Evidence. JAMA Neurol 2023; 80(1):5–6.

214. Denker PG. The postconcussion syndrome: prognosis and evaluation of the organic factors. N Y State J Med 1944;44:379–84.

215. Yilmaz T, Roks G, de Koning M, et al. Risk factors and outcomes associated with post-traumatic headache after mild traumatic brain injury. Emerg Med J 2017; 34:800–5.

216. Rimel RW, Giordani B, Barth JT, et al. Disability caused by minor head injury. Neurosurgery 1981;9:221–8.

217. Rutherford WH, Merrett JD, McDonald JR. Symptoms at 1 year following concussion from minor head injuries. Injury 1978;10:225–30.

218. Andersson EE, Bedics BK, Falkmer T. Mild traumatic brain injuries: a 10-year follow-up. J Rehabil Med 2011;43(4):323–9.

219. Ahman S, Saveman BI, Styrke J, et al. Long-term follow-up of patients with mild traumatic brain injury: a mixed-method study. J Rehabil Med 2013;45(8): 758–64.

220. Edna T-H. Disability 3–5 years after minor head injury. J Oslo City Hosp 1987; 37:41–8.

221. Ingebrigtsen T, Waterloo K, Marup-Jensen S, et al. Quantification of post-concussion symptoms 3 months after minor head injury in 100 consecutive patients. J Neurol 1998;245:609–12.
222. Voormolen DC, Haagsma JA, Polinder S, et al. Post-concussion symptoms in complicated vs. uncomplicated mild traumatic brain injury patients at three and six months post-injury: results from theCENTER-TBI study. J Clin Med 2019;8:E1921.
223. Ashina H, Dodick DW, Barber J, et al. Prevalence of and Risk Factors for Post-traumatic Headache in Civilian Patients After Mild Traumatic Brain Injury: A TRACK-TBI Study. Mayo Clin Proc 2023;98(10):1515–26.
224. Aaseth K, Grande RB, Kvaerner KJ, et al. Prevalence of secondary chronic headaches in a population-based sample of 30-44-year-old persons. The Akershus study of chronic headache. Cephalalgia 2008;28:705–13.
225. Aaseth K, Grande RB, Benth JŠ, et al. 3-Year follow-up of secondary chronic headaches: the Akershus study of chronic headache. Eur J Pain 2011;15(2):186–92.

Headache due to Vascular Disorders

John F. Rothrock, MD*

KEYWORDS

• Headache • Stroke • TIA • Intracranial hemorrhage

KEY POINTS

- Headache commonly accomanies acute stroke and may chronically complicate stroke.
- In some instances of presumed acute headache is a key component of diagnosis and management.
- "Thunderclap" headache demands rapid and accurate diagosis.

INTRODUCTION

The association between stroke and headache is complex, ranging from the nonspecific, wherein headache is largely irrelevant, to the highly specific, wherein headache is a key component of diagnosis and management. Headache may accompany the acute stroke process, chronically complicate stroke or, as with migraine, in rare instances even serve a potentially causal role in generating stroke. In this article, I will address the headaches that accompany or follow stroke, those clinical situations when stroke or the risk of stroke may influence headache management and those relatively rare instances when stroke seems to be a direct result of an acute migraine episode.

In terms of mechanism, there are 2 major types of stroke: hemorrhagic and ischemic. Hemorrhagic stroke may be subdivided into 2 types according to the location of the vessel, which ruptures: intracerebral or subarachnoid. Ischemic stroke typically is due to embolism, thrombosis, or vasospasm and may be subdivided further based on the size of the vessel involved and whether that vessel is an artery or vein/sinus. Whether hemorrhagic or ischemic, each mechanistic subtype of stroke can be produced by a myriad of causes. Headache may acutely accompany or chronically complicate all of the stroke subtypes, and especially in the case of ischemic stroke, the likelihood of acute headache often is highly dependent on the specific stroke etiology (eg, headache, facial pain, or both occur much more frequently with

Inova Health/University of Virginia School of Medicine, Migraineur
* Corresponding author: 8081 Innovation Park Drive, Neurology/Suite 900, Fairfax, VA 22301.
E-mail address: rothrockjf@gmail.com

Neurol Clin 42 (2024) 375–388
https://doi.org/10.1016/j.ncl.2023.12.002
0733-8619/24/© 2023 Elsevier Inc. All rights reserved.
neurologic.theclinics.com

internal carotid artery thrombosis from arterial wall dissection than from atherothrombosis).

Because they are commonly accompanied by acute headache, potentially lethal and yet treatable, there are 5 stroke syndromes that medical providers must recognize and manage capably: aneurysmal subarachnoid hemorrhage, basilar artery thrombosis, cerebellar stroke or hemorrhage, cerebral sinus thrombosis (CST), and hypertensive encephalopathy. The last will not be discussed here.

I will address the other 4 syndromes in some detail. In each, headache may be the predominant or even sole symptom reported by the patient in the early stages of the clinical presentation. Early recognition that the headache is *secondary* and reflecting clinically significant vascular disease may assist in early diagnosis, treatment intervention, and a far more favorable outcome. As will be described in the following sections, aneurysmal subarachnoid hemorrhage (SAH) is best treated when a premonitory low volume bleed occurs and not after a clinically devastating early rebleed. Similarly, patients with CST will enjoy a better outcome when they are diagnosed and treated before clot propagation, venous infarction, seizures, and progressive neurologic deficit. Early diagnosis and potential intervention are no less crucial for patients with basilar artery thrombosis or cerebellar stroke/hemorrhage.

HEADACHE AS A SYMPTOM ACCOMPANYING ACUTE STROKE
Headache and Hemorrhagic Stroke

Subarachnoid hemorrhage
The most common cause of spontaneous (ie, nontraumatic) SAH is rupture of a "berry" aneurysm located in or near the circle of Willis, and the hallmark of aneurysmal SAH is sudden, severe headache that often occurs during physical exertion.[1] Because of the aneurysm's location within the subarachnoid space, focal neurologic deficits are generally present acutely only if there is extension of the SAH into the brain parenchyma.

A significant proportion of high volume and clinically devastating aneurysmal SAH is preceded by a so-called sentinel headache that is analogous to the transient ischemic attack (TIA) of ischemic stroke. These sentinel headaches reflect relatively low volume SAH that usually is manifested clinically by sudden, severe headache only, without any alteration of consciousness or other neurologic signs.[2] The importance of identifying aneurysmal SAH at the time of this "sentinel" presentation cannot be overemphasized. Sentinel SAH headache may herald high-volume rebleed. The risk of rebleed is highest during the 72 hours following sentinel headache, and rebleeds characteristically convey a very poor clinical prognosis.

The classic exertional thunderclap headache of aneurysmal SAH may be associated with primary headache disorders that possess a far more benign prognosis (eg, primary headache associated with sexual activity or cough headache) but in those disorders headache duration is typically far shorter (<2 hours for primary cough headache vs weeks or more for SAH).[3] Also contrasting with spontaneous SAH, in these typically benign headache disorders multiple and relatively stereotyped episodes occur during a more extended period.

The sensitivity of noncontrasted brain computed tomography (CT) performed within the first 6 hours following aneurysmal SAH approaches 100%, representing one of the few neurologic situations where CT is superior to MRI. That high sensitivity progressively declines during the ensuing 18 hours. In cases of "thunderclap" headache wherein the suspicion of SAH remains high despite negative brain imaging, lumbar puncture always should be performed. As is the case for many of the cerebrovascular disorders listed in the International Headache Society's International Classification of Headache Disorders (ICHD-3), the notes accompanying the diagnostic criteria for nontraumatic SAH (6.2.2) seem to be of more clinical utility than the criteria themselves. Those notes emphasize the high diagnostic sensitivity of noncontrasted brain CT but go on to advise that "lumbar puncture is essential" when CT results are nondiagnostic.[4]

Unruptured cerebral aneurysms

Sudden and severe headache may develop in a patient with an unruptured cerebral aneurysm, in the absence of SAH. Some authors have theorized that the relevant headache is indicative of acute expansion of the aneurysm and an imminent risk of rupture, whereas others have suggested that the headache reflects thrombosis occurring within a "giant" aneurysm.[5]

More commonly, clinicians will encounter patients whose diagnostic evaluation for another disorder (eg, migraine) has demonstrated an unruptured, incidental, and asymptomatic aneurysm. How to best manage such aneurysms remains an area of some controversy but, generally, the size and location of the aneurysm(s) seem to influence the risk of eventual rupture. Small (<6 mm) aneurysms are less likely to rupture than larger aneurysms, and aneurysms involving the posterior circulation or anterior communicating artery seem to be more likely to rupture than those within the remainder of the anterior circulation.[6–8]

Hemorrhagic stroke/intracerebral hemorrhage

Spontaneous/nontraumatic intracerebral hemorrhage (ICH) is often accompanied by acute headache, but the association is hardly invariable. No more than one-third of patients with ICH who are capable of providing a coherent history report acute headache. Although this is far lower than the incidence of headache in aneurysmal SAH, the combination of headache and vomiting is at least 3 times greater in ICH than in ischemic stroke. While the absence of these symptoms does not exclude ICH, their presence, especially when combined with acute hypertension, focal neurologic deficits, a depressed level of consciousness and an early clinical course characterized by smoothly progressive neurologic deterioration, should encourage strong consideration of the diagnosis.

Headache is more common with lobar hemorrhage than with deep ICH, and in the latter headache occurs more often with putaminal hemorrhage than with hemorrhage involving the caudate nucleus or thalamus.[9–12] Headache is of little value in localizing ICH but, in general, lobar occipital bleeds tend to produce ipsilateral orbital/periorbital pain, with more anteriorly situated hemorrhages causing headache that may be periauricular, temporal, or frontal.[11]

Despite years of clinical investigation, we still lack any therapy of clearly established value for specific intervention in cases of ICH, and the best treatment remains prevention.

Comments accompanying the listed ICHD-3 criteria for spontaneous ICH (6.2.1) include the observations that (infrequently) headache may be the "presenting and prominent feature" of primary ICH, that ICH headache "occasionally" is thunderclap in character, and, interestingly, that in ICH as opposed to ischemic stroke, headache at onset is associated with a higher risk of early mortality.[4]

Finally, the ICHD-3 comments specifically indicate that ICH should be taken to include intracerebellar hemorrhage, emphasize the important point that headache initially may be the prominent feature in cases of intracerebellar hemorrhage and warn that patients with such hemorrhages may require emergent surgical decompression.

Headache Associated with Ischemic Stroke

Ischemic stroke/general considerations

As has been shown by a recent meta-analysis of 20 studies with 33,231 participants, between 6% and 44% of patients report headache accompanying ischemic stroke; this wide range yielded a pooled prevalence rate of 14%.[13] The onset of headache is sudden and acute in the majority of patients but may be delayed in 10% to 15%. Most patients describe nonspecific headaches with features of tension-type headache but associated symptoms may include nausea, vomiting, photophobia, or phonophobia.[13,14] Predictors of headache associated with ischemic stroke are female gender, younger age, major infarctions, and ischemia occurring within the posterior circulation; the frequency of headache complicating posterior circulation stroke has been reported to range between 30% and 75% versus 15% and 60% for anterior circulation stroke.[13–16] As a predictor of clinical outcome, one investigative group found headache at onset of first-ever ischemic stroke to correlate with a more favorable prognosis.[17]

Headache is more common with cortical infarction than with subcortical infarction, and it follows that headache is more frequently reported with cardio-embolic and large vessel stroke than with small vessel/lacunar stroke.[16,18] In lacunar infarction, headache is reported by less than 10% of patients.

Ischemia in the territory of the middle cerebral artery typically causes pain in the eye region, whereas with ischemia from an anterior cerebral artery source the headache is usually bifrontal. Ischemia from posterior circulation compromise produces headaches that are usually diffuse but may be localized to the occiput.

Ischemic stroke may be chronically complicated by chronic headache even in patients with no preexisting primary headache disorder.[19,20] In one recent study involving 550 patients with first-ever ischemic stroke, 10.4% developed persistent (>3 months) headache attributed to the stroke.[20] Variables associated with persistent headache included lack of sleep, absence of a specific cause for the stroke and stroke involving the cerebellum (the site of the majority of the strokes). The clinical phenotypes of the headache were equally divided between migraine and tension-type headache.[20]

Transient ischemic attack

TIAs are often the harbingers of stroke, and as with all subtypes of acute ischemic stroke, TIAs may be accompanied by headache. In an analysis of more than 2000 patients with acute ischemic stroke or TIA, 27% experienced headache at event onset, and headache was equally common in patients with no persistent neurologic deficit.[21] The presence of acute headache correlated with younger age and with an earlier history of migraine, underscoring the potential hazard of attributing acute TIA or minor stroke to "complicated" or "complex" migraine, each a diagnosis absent from the existing ICHD criteria and correspondingly lacking in specificity or clinical utility.

Another factor potentially complicating diagnosis is cortical spreading depression (CSD), the neurophysiologic event considered to be the source of typical migraine aura and, perhaps, the biologic "headwaters" of headache and other migrainous phenomena as well.[22] Although spreading waves of neuronal depolarization/hyperpolarization explain nicely the positive, negative, and dynamic features of the most common aura types, CSD is not unique to migraine. Along with trauma, ischemia may trigger CSD (or its equivalent in the retina), and sources of cortical ischemia as diverse as carotid dissection or cardioembolism from mechanical prosthetic valves may produce paroxysmal visual or sensory symptoms identical to those of migraine aura.

Key points
- Be wary of diagnosing migraine with aura in patients presenting with aura symptoms but lacking an established history of migraine.
- Especially with older patients or any patient with risk factors for vascular disease, be wary of diagnosing new onset aura even when the patient reports an established history of migraine without aura.

A recent study examining the diagnostic specificity of the current ICHD-3 criteria relative to the preexisting beta version of those criteria found that the current criteria are significantly more specific for diagnosing aura and distinguishing aura from TIA in patients presenting with the first episode of *probable* migraine with aura.[23]

Basilar artery thrombosis

Headache is a frequent symptom of clinically evident basilar artery occlusive disease and occurs in 20% to 53% of patients with basilar syndromes.[24] With acute basilar artery occlusion, the headache can resemble headache due to subarachnoid hemorrhage.[25] The headache is most commonly occipital and can be either lateralized or nonlateralized; at times, the headache is localized to the occipitofrontal or frontal areas of the head. The headache may be associated with occipital tenderness, neck stiffness, and neck pain and may be described as throbbing and aggravated by postural changes. Although typically accompanied by neurologic deficits, the headache may persist longer than neurologic signs or other symptoms and even may occur independently.

Cervical arterial dissection

Cervical artery dissection (CAD) involving either the internal carotid or vertebral artery is a common cause of stroke in persons aged younger than 50 years. Headache occurs in up to 90% of patients and may precede the development of cerebrovascular symptoms in half of CAD patients.[26,27]

In the Cervical Artery Dissection Ischemic Stroke Patients Group study of 982 consecutive patients, headache was more frequent in internal carotid artery dissection than in vertebral artery dissection (OR = 1.36 95% CI: 1.01–1.84).[28] Headache can be the only symptom in arterial dissection.[29] In carotid dissection, the pain is localized to the anterior neck and face and radiates to temporal and frontal regions.[30,31] Vertebral artery dissection can lead to isolated neck pain.[32] Pain in CAD is ipsilateral to the dissection and tends to be severe and throbbing in character. The headache associated with vertebral artery dissection is more variable and can even mimic cluster headache.[33] Migraine increases the risk of carotid artery dissection.[34]

The clinical presentation of CAD ranges from incidental discovery in a patient who is entirely asymptomatic to disabling or even fatal stroke. CAD may be "spontaneous" or occur as a consequence of trivial (eg, with sneezing) or major trauma. When TIA or stroke complicates CAD, the interval between the anatomic onset of dissection and the development of cerebrovascular symptoms may extend up to days.

The ICHD-3 diagnostic criteria for CAD are of limited utility and perhaps to some degree diagnostically insensitive. Suffice it to say that the development of uncharacteristic headache accompanied by TIA or stroke in a younger patient with no other compelling cause for TIA/stroke or lateral medullary (Wallenberg) stroke occurring in a younger patient should raise concern for extracranial internal carotid or vertebral artery dissection.

Cerebellar stroke

The typical symptoms of a patient presenting to an emergency department with acute ischemic stroke involving the cerebellum may be nonspecific: headache, "dizziness," nausea, and vomiting. The character and location of any associated headache conveys no diagnostic value; despite the posterior location of the stroke, head pain may be referred to the frontal area.[35]

Even when a large portion of the cerebellar hemisphere undergoes acute ischemic infarction, consequent neurologic deficit may not be apparent until the patient is examined while sitting or standing. Appendicular ataxia may not be present, especially if the examination is conducted with the patient supine and thus with gravitational assistance for heel-to-shin testing, and truncal ataxia cannot be adequately assessed in such circumstances. With sitting or standing, however, the truncal ataxia becomes obvious because the patient will sway or fall consistently toward the side of the affected cerebellar hemisphere.

In contrast to brain CT, brain MRI is extremely effective in demonstrating acute ischemic stroke involving the cerebellum. The diffusion-weighted and FLAIR sequences are of particular value in this regard.

As a delay in diagnosis may lead to severe clinical consequences from edematous swelling of the infarcted tissue, with obstructive hydrocephalus and tonsillar herniation, clinicians must maintain a high index of suspicion for the diagnosis of cerebellar stroke. When the concern for that diagnosis seems justified, an adequate diagnostic evaluation must be performed.

Key points

- If the patient's history suggests acute ischemic stroke of the cerebellum, examine the patient while sitting/standing.
- In confirming suspected acute cerebellar ischemic stroke, brain MRI is far more sensitive than CT.

Arteritis

Giant cell arteritis (GCA), more commonly known as "temporal arteritis," produces anterior ischemic optic neuropathy and acute blindness much more often than it does cerebral infarction, but carotid and vertebrobasilar distribution strokes can occur. When they do, it is usually within the first few weeks of active disease and at times may occur even in patients with a normal erythrocyte sedimentation rate (ESR), a normal temporal artery biopsy and despite concomitant treatment with a corticosteroid.[36] Although stroke generated by GCA typically involves the extracranial portions of the carotid and vertebrobasilar systems, intracranial arteritis may occur.

Patients with GCA are usually aged older than 65 years but may be as young as 50 years. There is roughly a 3:1 female-to-male preponderance. There almost always is associated headache, and the headache either is an unprecedented symptom for the patient or is described as "different" from the patient's usual headaches. The pain typically is constant and most often temporal with radiation to the scalp, face, jaw, or occiput.[37] It may be pulsatile. More than half of patients with GCA have accompanying polymyalgia rheumatica (PMR), and slightly less than half of patients with PMR develop GCA.

The ESR and C-reactive protein level typically are elevated in patients with GCA. Unfortunately, abnormalities of each are notoriously nonspecific, and in at least 5% of biopsy-proven cases the ESR may be normal or only modestly elevated.

In something of a *res ipsa loquitur*, the ICHD-3 criteria for diagnosis of headache attributed to GCA (6.4.1) require an established diagnosis of GCA. More helpful in the accompanying comments is the statement that given the variability in the clinical features of GCA, the diagnosis should be considered in any adult aged older than 60 years with new-onset recent and persisting headache.

A less common inflammatory vascular disorder wherein headache is a near-invariable and prominent symptom is primary angiitis of the central nervous system (PACNS).[38,39] Unusual for being restricted to the central nervous system, PACNS may afflict adult patients of any age. The typical symptom complex involves chronic, nonspecific headache with progressive cognitive decline and recurrent episodes of TIA or stroke. Blood markers of inflammation, routine analyses of cerebrospinal fluid, cerebral arteriography, and even brain/meningeal biopsy are not always sufficient to establish the diagnosis even in cases where PACNS seems highly likely. Given that PACNS may be treated effectively with chronic steroid therapy in combination with cyclophosphamide but with the risks inherent in such treatment, accurate diagnosis is critical.

Cerebral sinus thrombosis

Thrombosis of a cerebral vein or sinus may occur at any age and can be caused by a wide variety of disorders. The clinical presentation is similarly variable but headache is often prominent.

Headache is the most common symptom of CST, occurring in about 90% of cases and more often in women and younger patients.[40] It is the presenting symptom in three-quarters of cases, and it may occur in isolation or herald the development of other neurologic signs and symptoms.[41] The headache's location varies widely from case to case and is of little or no diagnostic value. The head pain typically is persistent, and although in the majority of cases its intensity builds gradually, in about 10% the onset is sudden and severe (thunderclap).[42]

Propagation of thrombus may result in progressive neurologic deterioration, permanent neurologic disability, and even death.[43] Systemic anticoagulation with intravenous unfractionated heparin or subcutaneously administered low-molecular weight heparin is considered first-line therapy for acute CST even when venous infarction and associated hemorrhage are demonstrated by brain imaging.[44] Dabigatran could be an alternative to low-molecular weight heparin.[45] Although endovascular intervention involving intrasinus thrombolysis, mechanical thrombectomy, or both may be considered for patients who do not respond to anticoagulant therapy, in the TO-ACT trial patients with clinically severe CST randomized to endovascular therapy experienced no better outcome than those randomized to intravenous heparin.[46]

In some cases, the increased venous pressure resulting from CST produces intracranial hypertension that results in a chronic headache disorder indistinguishable from idiopathic hypertension (IIH). As with IIH, afflicted patients are at risk for progressive visual loss and blindness.

The headache of CST may mimic that of a variety of other primary and secondary headache disorders, including migraine, hemicrania continua, cluster, primary thunderclap headache, nontraumatic subarachnoid hemorrhage, and intracranial hypotension.[4]

Migraine and Stroke

Although results from many epidemiologic studies have differed in regards to what specific subpopulations of migraineurs may or may not be at risk for stroke, the evidence available clearly demonstrates an association between migraine and stroke.

This association is most prominent in younger women aged 45 years or younger who have migraine with aura.[47–49] When ischemic stroke occurs in an individual with a history of migraine, the stroke may result either from another condition coexisting with migraine and independent of a migraine episode or as a complication of an episode of acute migraine.

When it is the coexisting disorder and not migraine itself that is responsible for producing ischemic stroke, a preponderance of that coexisting disorder in the migraine population relative to the age and gender-matched population free of migraine could account for at least a portion of the migraine:stroke association. For example, some investigators have found evidence of a bidirectional relationship between patent foramen ovale (PFO) and migraine, and in a study of patients with cryptogenic stroke and a history of migraine, just under 80% had evidence of a PFO with right-to-left shunting.[50] In the study by West and colleagues, the prevalence of PFO in patients with cryptogenic stroke and migraine with frequent aura was 93%.[51]

Migraine as a cause of stroke/migrainous infarction

Although the majority of strokes occurring in migraineurs do not occur during an acute migraine episode, at times acute migraine is complicated by brain infarction. The ICHD-3 criteria for a diagnosis of migrainous infarction (1.4.3) require an established history of migraine *with aura*, acute aura symptoms typical of previous migraine episodes, persistence of those symptoms beyond 1 hour, and neuroimaging evidence of infarction involving an area relevant to the symptoms.[4] If migrainous infarction can occur in individuals without a history of aura or involve deficits that do not mimic previous aura symptoms, these criteria may be diagnostically insensitive.[52]

How migraine directly causes stroke remains unclear. Cerebral angiography performed at the time of migrainous infarction or shortly thereafter has demonstrated findings consistent with arterial vasospasm, but such abnormalities have been reported in only a relative handful of cases.[53] Migraine-induced arterial dissection, thrombosis resulting from a migraine-associated chronic arteriopathy, and cerebral oligemia related to the migraine process itself all have been proposed as potential sources of migrainous infarction, but as yet unknown is whether migrainous infarction is the result of a single biologic process or can occur consequent to a variety of independent mechanisms.

TREATMENT OF MIGRAINE ATTACKS IN PATIENTS WITH TRANSIENT ISCHEMIC ATTACK OR STROKE

According to their labels, treatment of acute migraine attacks with triptans is contraindicated in patients with TIA or stroke and in patients with multiple uncontrolled vascular risk factors. Triptans have mild vasoconstrictive properties, and theoretically triptans could lead to further decrease of already reduced blood flow during the oligemic phase of aura; the degree of vasoconstriction observed in humans, however, is not to the level that typically would lead to decreased cerebral blood flow or ischemia.[54] With little scientific evidence to support the concern, ergots are similarly contraindicated due to their putative potential for promoting vasoconstriction and vascular complications.[55] Small molecule calcitonin-gene-related peptide (CGRP) antagonists (gepants) and lasmiditan (ditans), a 5-HT_{1F}-agonist, have no direct vasoconstrictive properties and may be used to treat migraine attacks in patients with vascular comorbidities.[56,57]

Stroke Prevention in Patients with Migraine

Most patients with TIA or ischemic stroke receive antiplatelet treatment. Aspirin lowers stroke risk and has a weak preventive action in migraine.[58,59] In some patients, clopidogrel also may reduce migraine burden.[60] The combination of aspirin plus slow-release dipyridamole is at times used for secondary stroke prevention, and the dipyridamole component may predispose to headache.[61] Anticoagulation with warfarin or the newer oral medications that exert their anticoagulant effect independent of vitamin K oral in individuals chronically at risk for cardioembolism is typically well tolerated by the subset with migraine.

Although stroke induced by propranolol has been reported, patients with hypertension and migraine generally can be treated with β-blockers with proven efficacy in migraine prevention (chiefly propranolol and metoprolol).[62,63] Lisinopril, an angiotensin-converting enzyme inhibitor, and candesartan are at least equivocally effective for migraine prophylaxis.[64,65] OnabotulinumtoxinA is effective in the prevention of chronic migraine and can safely be used in patients with migraine and a history of stroke or TIA.[66] Valproic acid is another option for migraine prophylaxis if the individual is at no risk of pregnancy. Given that CGRP is a potent vasodilator, monoclonal antibodies directed against CGRP or its receptor pose a *theoretical* risk of provoking unopposed vasoconstriction.[67] Although a history of ischemic stroke or subarachnoid hemorrhage does not represent an absolute contraindication to the use of anti-CGRP therapies in patients with migraine, the potential benefit of such treatment should be weighed against this theoretical risk.

In women who have migraine with aura, use of an estrogen-containing oral contraceptive conveys approximately an 8-fold increase in stroke risk. Although even with this substantial increase in relative risk, the *absolute* risk of stroke remains small (consequent to the low stroke incidence in younger individuals generally), in the absence of any compelling need to continue such use, a switch to an alternative means of contraception is recommended (eg, a progesterone-based preparation or a hormone-secreting or non–hormone-secreting intrauterine device).

THUNDERCLAP HEADACHE

The phrase "the worst headache of my life" traditionally has been considered a diagnostic red flag, but coming from a patient with an established history of recurrent headache this frequently means that he or she simply is experiencing a particularly

---

Box 1
Causes of "thunderclap" headache

Secondary
- Aneurysmal subarachnoid hemorrhage
- Reversible cerebral vasoconstriction syndrome
- Cerebral arterial dissection
- Acute intracranial hypotension
- CST
- Posterior reversible leukoencephalopathy syndrome
- Acute hypertensive crisis
- Pituitary "apoplexy"
- Colloid cyst of third ventricle
- Chiari malformation

Primary
- Primary headache associated with sexual activity
- Primary exercise headache
- Primary cough headache
- Primary thunderclap headache
- "Crash" migraine

severe episode of migraine. More concerning is a "thunderclap" headache, implying the sudden onset of severe head pain that rapidly reaches its maximum intensity.[68]

What is perhaps the most clinically worrisome cause of thunderclap headache has been described previously. So-called sentinel headache is the TIA of aneurysmal subarachnoid hemorrhage, auguring a high risk of imminent rebleed. Other causes of thunderclap headache, both primary and secondary, are listed in **Box 1.**

Although migraine headache typically builds over hours to its maximum intensity, in instances of "crash" migraine the pain may reach maximum intensity quite rapidly. Patients with reversible cerebral vasoconstriction syndrome present with thunderclap headache and angiographic evidence of transient cerebral arterial narrowing. Vasospasm also has been observed in patients with headache more typical of migraine but if this transient vasospasm occurs frequently in migraine, it is rarely associated with migrainous infarction. Suffice it to say that although migraine seems to be a primary brain disorder with an increased permeability of meningeal arteries playing a more significant role in generating headache than any spasm or dilation occurring in cranial arteries, this does not obviate the concomitant occurrence of transient changes in the caliber of those cranial vessels.

Clinicians infrequently may encounter patients who experience "idiopathic" recurrent thunderclap headache in the absence of any history of established migraine and without documented acute, transient cerebral vasospasm. Especially with its initial occurrence, and as is the case for any first episode of thunderclap headache, "idiopathic" primary thunderclap headache is a diagnosis of exclusion.

To underscore the absolute necessity of excluding aneurysmal subarachnoid hemorrhage in this clinical setting, the ICHD-3 notes for primary thunderclap headache (4.4) caution that primary thunderclap headache should be considered a "diagnosis of last resort" and that "the search for an underlying cause should be both expedited and exhaustive."[4]

CLINICS CARE POINTS

- As with headache generally, optimal management of stroke requires identification of mechanism and specific etiology.
- "Thunderclap" headache represents a clinical situation wherein such management is especially critical and should be accomplished rapidly.

DISCLOSURE

Nothing to disclose.

REFERENCES

1. Edlow JA, Caplan LR. Avoiding pitfalls in the diagnosis of subarachnoid hemorrhage. N Engl J Med 2000;342(1):29–36.
2. Leblanc R. The minor leak preceding subarachnoid hemorrhage. J Neurosurg 1987;66(1):35–9.
3. Auer L. Unfavorable outcome following early surgical repair of ruptured cerebral aneurysms–a critical review of 238 patients. Surg Neurol 1991;35:152–8.
4. The International Classification of Headache Disorders ICHD-3, 3rd edition. Cephalalgia. 2018;38(1):1-211.

5. Witham TF, Kaufmann AM. Unruptured cerebral aneurysm producing a thunder-clap headache. Am J Emerg Med 2000;18(1):88–90.
6. Lysack JT, Coakley A. Asymptomatic unruptured intracranial aneurysms: approach to screening and treatment. Can Fam Physician 2008;54(11): 1535–8. 7.
7. International Study of Unruptured Intracranial Aneurysms Investigators. Unrup-tured intracranial aneurysms–risk of rupture and risks of surgical intervention. N Engl J Med 1998;339(24):1726–8.
8. UCAS Japan Investigators, Morita A, Kirino T, Hashi K, et al. The natural course of unruptured cerebral aneurysms in a Japanese cohort. N Engl J Med 2012;366: 2474–82.
9. Walshe TM, Davis KR, Fisher CM. Thalamic hemorrhage: a computed tomographic-clinical correlation. Neurology 1977;27(3):217–22.
10. Stein RW, Kase CS, Hier DB, et al. Caudate hemorrhage. Neurology 1984;34(12): 1549–54.
11. Ropper AH, Davis KR. Lobar cerebral hemorrhages: acute clinical syndromes in 26 cases. Ann Neurol 1980;8(2):141–7.
12. Harriott AM, Karakaya F, Ayata C. Headache after ischemic stroke: A systematic review and meta-analysis. Neurology 2020;94(1):e75–86.
13. Seifert CL, Schonbach EM, Magon S, et al. Headache in acute ischaemic stroke: a lesion mapping study. Brain 2016;139(Pt 1):217–26.
14. Kropp P, Holzhausen M, Kolodny E, et al. Headache as a symptom at stroke onset in 4,431 young ischaemic stroke patients. Results from the "Stroke in Young Fabry Patients (SIFAP1) study". J Neural Transm 2013;120(10):1433–40.
15. Koudstaal PJ, van Gijn J, Kappelle LJ. Headache in transient or permanent cere-bral ischemia. Dutch TIA Study Group. Stroke 1991;22(6):754–9.
16. Vestergaard K, Andersen G, Nielsen MI, et al. Headache in stroke. Stroke 1993;1621–4.
17. Chen PK, Chiu PY, Tsai IJ, et al. Onset headache predicts good outcome in pa-tients with first-ever ischemic stroke. Stroke 2013;44(7):1852–8.
18. Arboix A, Garcia-Trallero O, Garcia-Eroles L, et al. Stroke-related headache: a clinical study in lacunar infarction. Headache 2005;45(10):1345–52.
19. Hansen AP, Marcussen NS, Klit H, et al. Pain following stroke: a prospective study. Eur J Pain 2012;16(8):1128–36.
20. Lebedeva ER, Ushenin AV, Gurary NM, et al. Persistent headache after first-ever ischemic stroke: clinical characteristics and factors associated with its develop-ment. J Headache Pain 2022;23:103–13.
21. Tentschert S, Wimmer R, Greisenegger S, et al. Headache at stroke onset in 2196 patients with ischemic stroke or transient ischemic attack. Stroke 2005; 36(2):e1–3.
22. Charles A, Brennan K. Cortical spreading depression-new insights and persistent questions. Cephalalgia 2009;29(10):1115–24.
23. Gobel CH, Karstedt SC, Munte TF, et al. ICHD-3 is significantly more specific than ICHD-3 beta for diagnosis of migraine with aura and with typical aura. J Headache Pain 2020;21(1):2.
24. Williams D, Wilson TG. The diagnosis of the major and minor syndromes of basilar insufficiency. Brain 1962;85:741–74.
25. Mattle HP, Arnold M, Lindsberg PJ, et al. Basilar artery occlusion. Lancet Neurol 2011;10(11):1002–14.
26. Sturzenegger M. Spontaneous internal carotid artery dissection: early diagnosis and management in 44 patients. J Neurol 1995;242(4):231–8.

27. Saeed AB, Shuaib A, Al-Sulaiti G, et al. Vertebral artery dissection: warning symptoms, clinical features and prognosis in 26 patients. Can J Neurol Sci 2000;27(4):292–6.

28. Debette S, Grond-Ginsbach C, Bodenant M, et al. Differential features of carotid and vertebral artery dissections: the CADISP study. Neurology 2011;77(12): 1174–81.

29. Arnold M, Cumurciuc R, Stapf C, et al. Pain as the only symptom of cervical artery dissection. J Neurol Neurosurg Psychiatry 2006;77(9):1021–4.

30. Perez DJ. Spontaneous carotid artery dissection. JAAPA 2017;30(10):27–9.

31. Zetterling M, Carlstrom C, Konrad P. Internal carotid artery dissection. Acta Neurol Scand 2000;101(1):1–7.

32. Kim JG, Choi JY, Kim SU, et al. Headache characteristics of uncomplicated intracranial vertebral artery dissection and validation of ICHD-3 beta diagnostic criteria for headache attributed to intracranial artery dissection. Cephalalgia 2015;35(6):516–26.

33. Lai SL, Chang YY, Liu JS, et al. Cluster-like headache from vertebral artery dissection: angiographic evidence of neurovascular activation. Cephalalgia 2005;25(8):629–32.

34. Rist PM, Diener HC, Kurth T, et al. Migraine, migraine aura, and cervical artery dissection: a systematic review and meta-analysis. Cephalalgia 2011;31(8): 886–96.

35. Searls DE, Pazdera L, Korbel E, et al. Symptoms and signs of posterior circulation ischemia in the new England medical center posterior circulation registry. Arch Neurol 2012;69(3):346–51.

36. Hayreh SS, Podhajsky PA, Raman R, et al. Giant cell arteritis: validity and reliability of various diagnostic criteria. Am J Ophthalmol 1997;123(3):285–96.

37. Ward TN, Levin M. Headache in giant cell arteritis and other arteritides. Neurol Sci 2005;26(Suppl 2):s134–7.

38. Salvarani C, Brown RD Jr, Calamia KT, et al. Primary central nervous system vasculitis: analysis of 101 patients. Ann Neurol 2007;62(5):442–51.

39. de Boysson H, Zuber M, Naggara O, et al. Primary angiitis of the central nervous system: description of the first fifty-two adults enrolled in the French cohort of patients with primary vasculitis of the central nervous system. Arthritis Rheumatol 2014;66(5):1315–26.

40. Ferro JM, Canhao P, Stam J, et al. Prognosis of cerebral vein and dural sinus thrombosis: results of the International Study on Cerebral Vein and Dural Sinus Thrombosis (ISCVT). Stroke 2004;35(3):664–70.

41. Agostoni E. Headache in cerebral venous thrombosis. Neurol Sci 2004;25(Suppl 3):S206–10.

42. de Bruijn SF, Stam J, Kappelle LJ. Thunderclap headache as first symptom of cerebral venous sinus thrombosis. CVST Study Group. Lancet 1996;348(9042): 1623–5.

43. Luo Y, Tian X, Wang X. Diagnosis and Treatment of Cerebral Venous Thrombosis: A Review. Front Aging Neurosci 2018;10:2.

44. Ferro JM, Bousser MG, Canhao P, et al. European Stroke Organization guideline for the diagnosis and treatment of cerebral venous thrombosis - Endorsed by the European Academy of Neurology. Eur Stroke J 2017;2(3):195–221.

45. Ferro JM, Coutinho JM, Dentali F, et al. Safety and Efficacy of Dabigatran Etexilate vs Dose-Adjusted Warfarin in Patients With Cerebral Venous Thrombosis: A Randomized Clinical Trial. JAMA Neurol 2019;76(12):1457–65.

46. Coutinho JM, Zuurbier SM, Bousser MG, et al. Effect of Endovascular Treatment With Medical Management vs Standard Care on Severe Cerebral Venous Thrombosis: The TO-ACT Randomized Clinical Trial. JAMA Neurol 2020;77(8):966–73.

47. Kurth T, Rist PM, Ridker PM, et al. Association of migraine with aura and other risk factors with incident cardiovascular disease in women. JAMA 2020;323(22):2281–9.

48. Schurks M, Rist PM, Bigal ME, et al. Migraine and cardiovascular disease: systematic review and meta-analysis. BMJ 2009;339:b3914.

49. Kurth T. Migraine and ischaemic vascular events. Cephalalgia 2007;27(8):965–75.

50. Schwedt TJ, Demaerschalk BM, Dodick DW. Patent foramen ovale and migraine: a quantitative systematic review. Cephalalgia 2008;28(5):531–40.

51. West BH, Noureddin N, Mamzhi Y, et al. Frequency of Patent Foramen Ovale and Migraine in Patients With Cryptogenic Stroke. Stroke 2018;49(5):1123–8.

52. Rothrock J, North J, Madden K, et al. Migraine and migrainous stroke: risk factors and prognosis. Neurology 1993;43:2473–6.

53. Rothrock JF, Walicke P, Swenson MR, et al. Migrainous stroke. Arch Neurol 1988;45(1):63–7.

54. Amin FM, Asghar MS, Hougaard A, et al. Magnetic resonance angiography of intracranial and extracranial arteries in patients with spontaneous migraine without aura: a cross-sectional study. Lancet Neurol 2013;12(5):454–61.

55. Saxena VK, De Deyn PP. Ergotamine: its use in the treatment of migraine and its complications. Acta Neurologica Napoli 1992;14:140–6.

56. Krege JH, Rizzoli PB, Liffick E, et al. Safety findings from Phase 3 lasmiditan studies for acute treatment of migraine: Results from SAMURAI and SPARTAN. Cephalalgia 2019;39(8):957–66.

57. de Vries T, Villalon CM, MaassenVanDenBrink A. Pharmacological treatment of migraine: CGRP and 5-HT beyond the triptans. Pharmacol Ther 2020;107528. https://doi.org/10.1016/j.pharmthera.2020.107528.

58. Diener HC, Hartung E, Chrubasik J, et al. A comparative study of oral acetylsalicylic acid and metoprolol for the prophylactic treatment of migraine. A randomized, controlled, double-blind, parallel group phase III study. Cephalalgia 2001;21(2):120–8.

59. Bensenor IM, Cook NR, Lee IM, et al. Low-dose aspirin for migraine prophylaxis in women. Cephalalgia 2001;21(3):175–83.

60. Wilmshurst PT, Nightingale S, Walsh KP, et al. Clopidogrel reduces migraine with aura after transcatheter closure of persistent foramen ovale and atrial septal defects. Heart 2005;91(9):1173–5.

61. Davidai G, Cotton D, Gorelick P, et al. Dipyridamole-induced headache and lower recurrence risk in secondary prevention of ischaemic stroke: a post hoc analysis. Eur J Neurol 2014;21(10):1311–7.

62. Mendizabal J, Rothrock J, Greiner. Migrainous stroke causing thalamic infarction and amnesia during treatment with propranolol. Headache 1997;37:594–6.

63. Silberstein SD, for the US Headache Consortium. Practice parameter: evidence-based guidelines for migraine headache (an evidence-based review). Report of the Quality Standards Subcommitee of the American Academy of Neurology. Neurology 2000;55:754–63.

64. Schrader H, Stovner LJ, Helde G, et al. Prophylactic treatment of migraine with angiotensin converting enzyme inhibitor (lisinopril): randomized, placebo controlled, crossover study. BMJ 2001;322:19–22.

65. Stovner LJ, Linde M, Gravdahl GB, et al. A comparative study of candesartan versus propranolol for migraine prophylaxis: A randomised, triple-blind, placebo-controlled, double cross-over study. Cephalalgia 2014;34(7):523–32.
66. Dodick DW, Turkel CC, DeGryse RE, et al. OnabotulinumtoxinA for treatment of chronic migraine: pooled results from the double-blind, randomized, placebo-controlled phases of the PREEMPT clinical program. Headache 2010;50(6): 921–36.
67. Deen M, Correnti E, Kamm K, et al. Blocking CGRP in migraine patients - a review of pros and cons. J Headache Pain 2017;18(1):96.
68. Schwedt TJ, Matharu MS, Dodick DW. Thunderclap headache. Lancet Neurol 2006;5(7):621–31.

Headaches and Vasculitis

David S. Younger, MD, DrPH, MPH, MS[a,b,*]

KEYWORDS

- Vasculitis • Adult • Childhood • Headaches • Blood–brain barrier
- Clinicopathology • Examination • Diagnosis

KEY POINTS

- The systemic vasculitides are heterogeneous clinicopathological disorders that share the common feature of vascular inflammation.
- The classification of diverse forms of vasculitides is based upon the caliber of the vessels involved.
- The underlying pathophysiology reflects diminished blood flow, vascular alterations, and the risk of vessel occlusions with variable ischemia, necrosis, tissue damage.
- Neuroimaging plays a vital role in the diagnosis of primary and secondary vasculitides with a multiplicity of options available to accurately describe the underlying clinical deficits of involved cases.
- Granulomatous angiitis of the nervous system and primary CNS angiitis are equivalent terms for a spectrum of potentially fatal, rare and distinctive adult and childhood disorders of the brain.
- While headache may be a clue to underlying CNS vasculitis and the risk of imminent ischemic tissue injury, proof thereof lies in biopsy of involved brain tissues.
- The decidedly rare childhood primary CNS angiitites and its subtypes, that have historically relied upon the experience of adults remain problematic due to the paucity of epidemiologic, correlative histopathological and neuroradiological, and randomized clinical trial data.
- This article is an overview of the clinical presentation, differential diagnosis, laboratory evaluation and treatment of adult and childhood vasculitides and its relation to headaches.

INTRODUCTION

It may be said that efforts to define a disease are attempts to understand the very concept of the disease. This has been especially evident in systemic and neurologic disorders associated with vasculitis. For the past 100 years, since the first description of

[a] Department of Medicine, Section of Neuroscience, City University of New York School of Medicine, New York, NY, USA; [b] Department of Neurology, White Plains Hospital, White Plains, NY, USA
* 333 East 34th Street, Suite 1J, New York, NY 10016.
E-mail address: youngd01@nyu.edu

Neurol Clin 42 (2024) 389–432
https://doi.org/10.1016/j.ncl.2023.12.003
0733-8619/24/© 2023 Elsevier Inc. All rights reserved.

neurologic.theclinics.com

granulomatous angiitis of the nervous system (GANS) and granulomatous angiitis of the brain (GAB)[1] and polyarteritis nodosa (PAN),[2] central nervous system (CNS) vasculitides have captured the attention of generations of clinical investigators around the globe to reach a better understanding of vasculitides involving the central and peripheral nervous system. Since that time, it has become increasingly evident that this will necessitate an international collaborative effort. Since my earlier review a decade ago,[3] notable progress has been made in vasculitis of the nervous system. This review has been adapted, and in some portions reproduced from a contemporaneously updated textbook chapter on adult and childhood vasculitis of the nervous system.[4]

CLASSIFICATION AND NOSOLOGY

The 2012 Revised International Chapel Hill Consensus Conference (CHCC) Nomenclature of Vasculitides[5] is the most widely used classification for the vasculitides. It categorized the clinicopathologic entities based on the involved vessels and updated the nosology of the vasculitic syndromes, using specific descriptive terminology that conveyed pathophysiologic specificity. The Pediatric Rheumatology European Society and the European League against Rheumatism (EULAR)[6] in collaboration with the Pediatric Rheumatology International Trials Organization reported methodology and overall clinical, laboratory, and radiographic characteristics for several childhood systemic vasculitides followed by a final validated classification[7] also based on vessel size, similar to the CHCC nomenclature.[8]

The classification of vasculitides involving the nervous system with a predilection for headaches is shown in **Box 1**. Small vessel vasculitis (SVV) includes granulomatosis with polyangiitis [GPA; Wegener type]), microscopic polyangiitis (MPA), and eosinophilic granulomatosis with polyangiitis (EGPA; Churg-Strauss syndrome [CSS]), known collectively as antineutrophil cytoplasmic antibody (ANCA)-associated vasculitides (AAV). Vasculitic disorders associated with immune complexes (ICs) include immunoglobulin A (IgA) vasculitis (IgAV; Henoch-Schönlein purpura [HSP]), cryoglobulinemic vasculitis (CV or CryoVas), and hypocomplementemic urticarial vasculitis (HUV) associated with C1q antibodies. Vasculitis without a predominant vessel size and caliber, respectively from small to large, involving arteries, veins, and capillaries, comprises the category of variable vessel vasculitis (VVV) characteristic of Behçet disease (BD) and Cogan syndrome. Medium vessel vasculitides (MVV) includes PAN Kawasaki disease (KD). Large vessel vasculitides (LVV) are represented by giant cell arteritis (GCA), and Takayasu arteritis (TAK). Vascular inflammation confirmed to a single organ system such as vasculitis restricted to the CNS and peripheral nervous system (PNS), and IgG4 related aortitis (IgG4-related disease [RD]), are collectively referred to as single organ vasculitides (SOV).

At the turn of the twentieth century, GANS[9] was the prototypical form of a vasculitis restricted to the CNS, recognized not only for its clinical heterogeneity in association with a variety of comorbid illnesses such as cancer, sarcoidosis, amyloid, human immunodeficiency virus (HIV), and zoster varicella virus infection; but the predilection for cerebral vessels of varying caliber from small meningeal to named cerebral vessels. Salvarani and coworkers[10] provided insights into the caliber of cerebral vessels involved through cerebral angiography and histopathologic examination of brain and meningeal tissue that translated into effective treatment and prognosis of primary CNS vasculitides (PCNSV). Adult[11] and childhood isolated CNS angiitis (IACNS),[12] primary angiitis of the CNS (PACNS),[13] GAB[14] and GANS[9] adult CNS vasculitis (PCNSV)[15] and childhood PACNS (cPACNS)[16] are equivalent terms for a prototypical primary vasculitic disorder restricted to the CNS. The category of cPACNS has recently

---

Box 1
Vasculitides with nervous system involvement predisposing to headaches

Large Vessel Vasculitis
  Giant cell arteritis
  Takayasu arteritis

Medium Vessel Vasculitis
  Polyarteritis nodosa
  Kawasaki disease

Small Vessel Vasculitis
  ANCA-Associated Vasculitis
    Microscopic polyangiitis
    Granulomatosis with polyangiitis (Wegener)
    Eosinophilic granulomatosis with polyangiitis (Churg-Strauss)
  Immune-Complex Vasculitis
    Cryoglobulinemia
    IgA vasculitis (Henoch-Schönlein)
    Hypocomplementemic urticarial vasculitis (anti-C1q)

Variable Vessel Vasculitis
  Behçet disease
  Cogan syndrome

Single Organ Vasculitis
  Primary Angiitis of the CNS
  Idiopathic aortitis (IgG4)

Vasculitis associated with systemic collagen vascular disease
  Systemic lupus erythematosus
  Rheumatoid arthritis

Vasculitis associated with illicit substance abuse
  Amphetamines
  Cocaine
  Heroin

Vasculitis associated with infection
  Acute bacterial meningitis
  Mycobacterial tuberculous infection
  Spirochete disease
  Varicella zoster virus–related vasculopathy
  Fungal infection
  Human immunodeficiency virus/AIDS

---

been subtyped based upon clinical progression and the caliber of vessels involved as predicted by neuroimaging on magnetic resonance angiography (MRA), computed tomography angiography (CTA), and conventional catheter angiography (CA) as angiography-positive nonprogressive (APNP) and angiography-positive progressive (APP)-cPACNS[16] and angiography-negative (AN) small-vessel cPACNS.[17]

BLOOD–BRAIN BARRIER

The past decade has also witnessed extraordinary progress in the understanding of the blood–brain barrier (BBB), which has in turn shed new insights into current understanding of the etiopathogenesis of headache in the vasculitides. The neurovascular unit comprises local neuronal circuits, glia, pericytes, and vascular endothelium that play a vital role in the dynamic modulation of blood flow, metabolism, and electrophysiologic regulation,[18] which together ensure a well-controlled internal environment, provided by cellular exchange mechanisms in the interface between blood, cerebrospinal fluid (CSF), and the brain.[19] Many of the influx and efflux mechanisms of the BBB are present early in the developing brain, encoded by genes at higher levels than in the adult.[20]

In comparison to CNS vasculitides in which loss of BBB integrity that results from disruption of tight junctions, increase in transcytosis, change in transport properties, and increased leukocyte infiltration and trafficking accompanies systemic and CNS inflammation[21] contributes to the secondary headaches, migraine headaches and its reversible premonitory symptoms are unassociated with breakdown or leakage of the BBB during attacks[22] and instead are most closely associated with the release of calcitonin gene–related peptide expressed in peripheral sensory trigeminal neurons that innervates the pain-sensitive dura and meningeal blood vessels.[23]

The molecules implicated in the pathologic breakdown of the BBB include the vasoactive protein vascular endothelial growth factor, the inflammatory cytokines interleukin 1 (IL-1), IL-6, tumor necrosis factor α (TNF-α), metalloproteinase type 2 and 9, and the leukocyte adhesion molecules P-selectin and E-selectin, and immunoglobulin (Ig) superfamily molecules vascular cell adhesion molecule type 1, and intercellular adhesion molecule type 1. The disruption of tight and adherens junctions, enzymatic degradation of the capillary basement membrane or both, leads to altered expression and function of membrane transporters or enzymes, and increased passage of inflammatory cells across the BBB from the blood to the CNS, with dysfunction of astrocytes and other components.[19]

Although transient breakdown is associated with varying neuronal dysfunction and damage, extended BBB disruption leads to aberrant angiogenesis, neuroinflammation, concomitant vasogenic edema, accumulation of toxic substances in the brain interstitial fluid, and oxidative stress. Further investigation is necessary to a more complete understanding of the unique BBB alterations and sequelae that cause or contribute to vascular inflammation, brain tissue injury in primary and secondary CNS vasculitis, and the origin of headaches.

CLINICOPATHOLOGIC CORRELATIONS
Large-Size Vessel Vasculitis

Two disorders, GCA and TAK, which fall under the category of LVV, and a third disorder, isolated aortitis, which affects large vessels but is generally considered in the category of a single-organ vasculitis (SOV), can all be associated with headache.

Giant cell arteritis

Two-thirds of patients with temporal GCA present with headache, often in association with musculoskeletal complaints, in individuals of both genders and age older than 50 years.[24,25] The headache emanates along tender granulomatous lesions of inflamed extracranial vessels, including branches of the external carotid artery, including the superficial temporal, occipital, facial, and internal maxillary arteries, as well as ophthalmic, posterior ciliary, and central retinal vessels, and in the vertebral and carotid arteries to the point of dural investment. There may be tender red cords along the temple, with scalp tenderness or occipital and nuchal pain. Untreated or inadequately recognized unilateral or bilateral blindness, the result of arteritis of the intraorbital posterior ciliary and central retinal arteries, is the commonest dreaded complication, seen in up to one-half of patients. There may be oculomotor disturbances resulting from vasculitis of the extraocular muscles; vertigo and hearing impairment resulting from acute auditory artery involvement; cervical myelopathy resulting from anterior spinal artery involvement; and brainstem strokes and transient ischemic attacks resulting from vasculitic involvement of the proximal intracranial carotid artery and extracranial vertebral artery.

The erythrocyte sedimentation rate (ESR) is typically increased to 100 mm/h or more. Temporal artery biopsy is the only sure way of establishing the diagnosis; however, false-negative findings on the contemplated affected side may be caused by inadvertent sampling of a vasculitic-free length of vessel. Noninvasive imaging using ultrasonography, high-resolution contrast-enhanced MRI, and [18 F]fluorodeoxyglucose (FDG) PET can facilitate recognition of GCA and assist the surgeon in centering on an involved segment of vessel.[26] Ultrasonography may show hypoechoic circumferential wall thickening, which occurs around the arterial lumen, termed the halo sign. Contrast-enhanced high-resolution MRI shows areas of active inflammation. [18F]FDG-PET, which can examine all of the involved vessels with a single examination, shows areas of abnormal vascular uptake typically synonymous with vessel wall inflammation.

The earliest lesions in GCA consist of vacuolization of vascular smooth muscle of the media, with enlargement of mitochondria, infiltration of lymphocytes, plasma cells, and histiocytes. Over time, inflammation extends into the intima and adventitia, leading to segmental fragmentation and necrosis of the elastic lamina, granuloma formation, and proliferation of connective tissue along the vessel wall. The classic histologic picture of granulomatous vasculitis, which is observed in about one-half of affected patients, eventuates in infiltration of vessel cell by giant cells at the junction between the intima and media, leading to thrombosis, intimal hyperplasia, and fibrosis.[27]

Takayasu arteritis

Individuals aged younger than 50 years, particularly women of Asian descent with granulomatous arteritis affecting the aorta and its branches, are most susceptible to TAK.[5] About two-thirds of patients manifest systemic reactions at onset, including malaise, fever, stiffness of the shoulders, nausea, vomiting, night sweats, anorexia, weight loss, and irregularity of menstrual periods weeks to months before the local signs of vasculitis were recognized.[28] Headache is associated with visual loss, absent pulses in the neck and limbs with symptoms of claudication, and syncope on bending of the head backward, caused by vasculitis-related circulatory insufficiency along the aorta and branches to the brain, face, and limbs.[29] Other investigators ascribe headache to associated neck pain and carotid arterial inflammation[30] and increased propensity to migraine.[31] There may be ischemic presentations of amaurosis fugax, monocular blindness, subclavian steal and carotid sinus syndrome, audible neck and limb bruits, and asymmetry of pulses, all resulting from granulomatous vasculitis of the ascending and descending aorta and its major branches.[32,33]

Although arterial biopsy is impractical given the restriction of lesions to the aorta and its branches, cerebral MRA and conventional angiography show vessel irregularities, stenosis, poststenotic dilatations, aneurysmal formation, occlusions, and increased collateralization. Although the mechanism and distribution of headache differs between patients with GCA and TAK, and pervasiveness of headache is greater in GCA than in TAK, there are strong similarities and subtle differences in the distribution of arterial disease on cerebral arteriography that suggest that the 2 disorders likely exist along a spectrum of the same or similar disease.[34]

Immunoglobulin G4-related aortitis

In 1972, Walker and colleagues[35] noted that 10% of 217 patients presenting with abdominal aneurysms at Manchester Royal Infirmary between 1958 and 1969 for resection showed excessive thickening of aneurysm walls and perianeurysmal adhesions at operation. Subsequent histologic examination of the walls of the aneurysms showed extensive active chronic inflammatory changes including plasma-cell infiltration. In the same year, 2008, 3 important observations were made. First, Sakata and colleagues[36] concluded that inflammatory abdominal aortic aneurysm (IAAA) was related to IgG4 sclerosing disease. Second, Kasashima and colleagues[37] concluded that IAAA was an IgG4-related disorder (RD) together with retroperitoneal fibrosis (RPF). Third, Ito and colleagues[38] described a patient with IAAA, hydronephrosis caused by RPF, and high levels of IgG4 in whom treatment with CS led to clinical improvement and reduction in IgG4 levels. Histologic inspection of the aortic wall specimen showed lymphocytoplasmacytic infiltration. Immunohistochemical analysis of the tissue showed IgG4-positive plasma cells.

Isolated noninfectious aortitis comprises disorders characterized by chronic inflammation restricted to the aortic wall and IgG4 infiltrating plasma cells.[39] Headache was an initial feature among 14% of patients with aortitis who had concomitant GCA or TAK,[40] without which the diagnosis of coexisting aortitis might have been overlooked.[41] The clinical features of patients with inflammatory aneurysms differs from those with atherosclerotic disease due to generally younger age by a decade, lower incidence of rupture, lack of claudication of intermittent the limbs and presence of peripheral pulses, less likelihood of unusual presenting features, elevated ESR, and lack of calcification on preoperative abdominal radiographs. The risk factors for aortitis include advanced age, history of connective tissue disease, IgG4-related systemic disease (IgG4-RD), diabetes mellitus, and heart valve pathology.[42] Ultrasound and CT imaging suggests the diagnosis, respectively, in 13.5% and 50% of patients, the former showing a sonolucent halo with clear definition of the aortic wall posterior to the thickened anterior and lateral aortic walls.

Medium-Size Vessel Vasculitis

Two distinct disorders, PAN and KD belong to the category of medium-vessel vasculitis, each of which can have associated headache symptoms.

Polyarteritis nodosa

There are only a few well-documented postmortem series of patients with PAN to investigate the clinicopathologic correlation of the vasculitis and headache. Kernohan and colleagues[43] estimated that 8% of patients with PAN had CNS involvement. In a description of the postmortem findings of 5 pathologically studied patients with PAN, headache was nonetheless a complaint in 4 of them during the course of their illness, with the involvement of epineurial vessels of the PNS, medium vessels of the systemic vasculature, and small meningeal arteries and large named vessels of the CNS, as follows. Patient 1 with weakness and paresthesia of the legs, and lightning pains in the limbs and head showed PAN involvement of epineurial vessels sparing systemic and CNS vasculature. Patient 2, who developed fatal progressive worsening of PAN with associated pain in the legs and suboccipital region had widespread systemic PAN at postmortem examination; however, the brain was not examined. Patient 4, who complained of right supraorbital, mandibular, and aural pain, which was attributed to infected sinuses and nonerupted wisdom tooth, developed confusion, left-sided weakness and sensory loss, followed by stupor and coma before death. Postmortem examination showed near complete obstruction of the right middle cerebral artery (MCA) caused by chronic PAN involvement. Patient 5, who developed severe headache as though his head was in a vise at the onset of PAN died after progressive stupor and coma. Postmortem examination showed diffuse system PAN with the involvement of small meningeal arteries. In these patients, headache, which was a pervasive feature at any stage of the illness, did not always correlate with the observed histopathology.

The neuropathologic changes of PAN include characteristic hyaline-like necrosis of a portion of the media and the internal elastic lamina, followed by extension of the inflammatory process to the adventitia by periarteritis (**Fig. 1**). The perivascular inflammation was secondary thus to the lesion in media of the artery, and although periarteritis developed, there was usually proliferation of the intima, leading to narrowing of the vessel lumen. When present, aneurysms developed during the subacute stage of the disease, leading to the gross nodosa or nodule features. Vasculitic involvement of arterioles, capillaries, and venules, and glomerulonephritis are typically absent, and there is no association with ANCAs, the latter of which proves to be a useful discriminatory feature.

Kawasaki disease

This disorder was named in the honor of the investigator[44] who described acute febrile mucocutaneous syndrome with lymphoid involvement and desquamation of the fingers and toes in children. It affects medium and small arteries, particularly the coronary arteries, leading to aneurysm and ectasia formation.[5] Endothelial damage occurs in the acute stages of the illness.[45] Headache is an associated symptom, along with cough, abdominal pain, arthralgia, and seizures, which are noted in up to one-quarter of untreated patients.[46] Those with abdominal pain and headache are older by a decade or more than those without these symptoms. Migraine and Raynaud phenomenon, which coexist in some patients with KD, may be reflective of similar vascular lesions that indicate the late consequences of extracoronary endothelial cell dysfunction.[47]

Small-Vessel Size Vasculitis

The category of SVV includes several disorders that fall under the designations of AAV and immune complex vasculitis. The category of AAV, which is associated with necrotizing vasculitis with few or no immune deposits, predominantly affects small vessels, including capillaries, venules, arterioles, and small arteries, and is associated with myeloperoxidase (MPO) ANCA or proteinase 3 (PR3) ANCA immunocytochemistry. It includes 3 disorders: MPA, GPA, formerly termed Wegener disease, and EGPA. The other major category of SVV are the immune complex vasculitides, characterized by moderate to marked vessel wall deposits of Ig and complement components all along

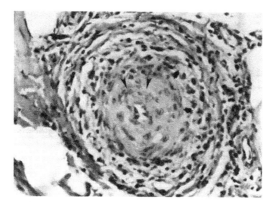

Fig. 1. Polyarteritis nodosa. This small muscular artery from muscle is from a patient with PAN. In the third, or proliferative, phase shown here, chronic inflammatory cells replace the neutrophils of the second phase; there is evidence of necrosis of the media (*arrows*), early intimal proliferation (*arrowheads*), and fibrosis. The lumen is almost completely occluded. In the healing phase, this process is replaced by dense, organized connective tissue (stain, hematoxylin-eosin, original magnification × 250).

small arteries and veins. Immune complex SVV includes the entities of antiglomerular basement membrane disease, CV, HUV mediated by anti-C1q antibodies, and IgAV/HSP.

Microscopic polyangiitis

Fever, arthralgia, purpura, hemoptysis, pulmonary hemorrhage, abdominal pain, and gastrointestinal bleeding precede the explosive phase of systemic necrotizing SVV, which affects the kidney and lungs, with rapidly progressive glomerulonephritis and pulmonary capillaritis. Cerebral signs and symptoms, including headache, was noted at presentation in 18% of patients.[48] Abnormal ANCA serology was noted in up to 80% of patients. Two of five deaths were attributed to CNS involvement by vasculitis during periods of disease at 4 and 8 months, respectively; however, that hypothesis could not be confirmed because postmortem examinations were not performed. MPA is associated with MPO-ANCA in 58% of patients and PR3 in 26%, respectively, attributing disease activity to MPO-AAV and PR3-AAV.[49]

Granulomatosis with polyangiitis

CNS involvement in GPA was recognized by Drachman[49] who described a patient with 1 month of dull bifrontal-vertex headache, which awakened him from sleep for 1 month. This headache was followed by early complaints of rhinitis, nasal obstruction, epistaxis, and sensory and motor mononeuropathy multiplex, and later by disorientation, confusion, and hypertension. Many patients with GPA complain of severe constant headache attributed to destructive sinusitis early in the course of the illness. Other possible causes for concomitant headache and cerebral involvement include vasculitis of large arterial branch vessels, particularly over the surface of the brain; hypertensive encephalopathy as suggested by microscopic infarction in the basal ganglia in close relation to arteries showing fibrinoid impregnation of their walls; and meningeal inflammation due to inflammatory cell infiltration especially plasma cells. Autoantibodies against neutrophil granule serine PR3 are detected in two-thirds of patients, and MPO in 24% of patients, respectively, attributing disease activity to PR3-AAV and MPO-AAV.[49]

Eosinophilic granulomatosis with polyangiitis

In 1951, Churg and Strauss[50] described the clinicopathologic findings of EGPA among 13 patients with so-called allergic granulomatosis, allergic angiitis, and periarteritis nodosa. Clinically, severe asthma, fever, and hypereosinophilia were noted, in association with widespread vascular lesions at postmortem examination, comprising fibrinoid collagen changes and granulomatous proliferation of epithelioid cells and giant cells, the so-called allergic granuloma, both within vessel walls and in connective tissue throughout the body. Other manifestations included cutaneous and subcutaneous nodules and granulomatous lymphadenitis. Contrary to the characterization that CNS involvement was rare in EGPA yet conferred a poorer prognosis,[51] clinical CNS involvement, presumably headache as well, was noted in 8 (62%) of patients, varying from disorientation to convulsions and coma. Three patients with CNS involvement died of cerebral (2 patients) or subarachnoid hemorrhages (1 patient). Involvement of the peripheral nervous system, which is a principal criterion for the diagnosis[52] may provide a clue to the nature of the CNS lesions. Epineurial necrotizing vasculitis noted in 54% of patients of one cohort[53] was typified by CD8-positive suppressive/cytotoxic and CD4-positive helper T-lymphocytes, in addition to eosinophils in inflammatory infiltrates, with only occasional CD20-positive B-lymphocytes, and scare deposits of IgG, C3d complement (C3d), and immunoglobulin E.

Cryoglobulinemia
The presence of one or more serum immunoglobulins that precipitate lower than core body temperatures and redissolve on rewarming is termed cryoglobulinemia.[54] Wintrobue and Buell[55] described the first patient with cryoglobulinemia, a 56-year-old woman who presented with progressive frontal headache; left face and eye pain; and right shoulder, neck, and lumbar discomfort after a bout of shingles. These symptoms were followed by Raynaud symptoms, recurrent nosebleeds, exertional dyspnea and palpitation, and changes in the eye ground attributed to central vein thrombosis. Postmortem examination showed infiltrating myeloma of the humerus and lumbar vertebra, and splenic enlargement. A unique plasma protein was detected, which spontaneously precipitated with cold temperature and solubilized at high temperature and which differed from Bence-Jones proteinuria of other patients with myeloma.

Gorevic and colleagues[56] provided a complete description of the main clinical and biological features of mixed CV in 40 patients, the clinical findings of which included palpable purpura in all patients, polyarthralgia in three-quarters, renal disease in slightly more than half, and deposits of IgG, immunoglobulin M (IgM), and complement, or renal arteritis in one-third. All cryoglobulins have rheumatoid activity consisting of IgM and polyclonal IgG, and one-third had monoclonal IgM κ components. Brouet and colleagues[57] provided modern classifications of cryoglobulinemia among 86 patients, which included type 1, composed of a single monoclonal immunoglobulin; and types II and III as mixed cryoglobulinemia, composed of different immunoglobulins, with a monoclonal component in type II, and polyclonal immunoglobulin in type III. In the absence of well-defined disease, the presence of mixed cryoglobulinemia was termed essential.

Agnello and colleagues[57] reported a strong association with concomitant hepatitis C virus (HCV) infection and a high rate of false-negative serologic tests in type II cryoglobulinemia. The frequency of headache has not been specifically cited in any published cases of cryoglobulinemia. However, headache could be a presenting feature in those with CNS involvement, as noted in 2 patients with lacunar cerebral strokes and associated subcortical white matter changes on brain MRI,[58,59] 2 patients with cortical stroke syndromes and associated cortical gray matter infarction on brain MRI,[60] 1 patient with a temporal arteritis-like syndrome with associated ischemic cerebral infarction,[61] 3 patients with relapsing encephalopathy,[62] 2 patients with cerebral hemorrhage,[59] 2 patients with ischemic subcortical infarcts,[58] and 5 patients with postmortem evidence of CNS involvement clinically alone or pathologically with widespread vasculitis,[56,63] including the brain. With an overall mortality of 8.7% and a 33% fatality rate among those with CNS involvement,[64] the symptom set of CNS involvement including headache seems to be important in prognosis.

Hypocomplementemic urticarial vasculitis
This uncommon disorder presents with recurrent attacks of erythematous, urticarial, and hemorrhagic skin lesions lasting up to 24 hours at a time, associated with recurrent attacks of fever, joint swelling, and variable abdominal distress. Serum complement levels are depressed; however, immunodiffusion against purified preparations of human C1q shows strong reactivity. Skin biopsies show varied patterns of polymorphonuclear infiltration involving the vessel wall characteristic of necrotizing vasculitis, infiltration scattered diffusely through the dermis typical of anaphylactoid purpura, or mild nonspecific perivascular infiltration. Renal biopsy may show mild-to-moderate glomerulonephritis indistinguishable from those seen in other forms of chronic membranoproliferative glomerulonephritis. The differences in HUV from systemic lupus erythematosus (SLE) include more urticarial and purpuric skin lesions, mild or absent

renal involvement, or other visceral involvement. Moreover, serum speckled antinuclear and anti-DNA antibodies, and basement membrane Ig deposits, are characteristically absent in HUV.

Among 14 patients with HUV reported by Wisnieski and colleagues,[65] 1 patient with orbital pseudotumor complained of headache. It is unlikely that the headache in HUV would favor SLE in an individual patient because prospective studies suggest that headache occurs in SLE at a frequency equal to normal controls.[66] Buck and colleagues[67] and Grotz and colleagues[68] cited aseptic meningitis and pseudotumor cerebri, both typified by headache, as a possible neurologic manifestation of HUV.

Immunoglobulin A vasculitis

Osler[69] described cerebral manifestations in association with attacks of purpura in a patient with transient hemiparesis, in 3 others with potentially fatal hemorrhage, including 1 patient with a history of childhood attacks culminating in subdural hemorrhage, and in 2 others who progressed to the comatose state, one of whom had postmortem confirmation of a subdural hemorrhage; however, headache was not mentioned. Green[70] quoted a personal communication from Dr Eli Davis (St Andrew's Hospital, UK) indicating the frequency of blood in CSF in 2 of 1000 patients and reporting a child with headache and xanthochromia that followed onset of fever, malaise, sore throat, arthralgia, rash, and meningeal symptoms after presumed streptococcal illness.

The first mention of headache in this disorder was provided by Lewis and Philpott[71] in the description of 3 patients with neurologic complications of HSP, 2 of whom manifested severe headache concomitant at onset followed shortly afterward by meningeal signs and xanthochromic CSF, which indicates subarachnoid hemorrhage; a third patient without complaints of headache rapidly lapsed into coma after repeated convulsions. Postmortem examination in the only patient who died was limited to the abdominal cavity, which showed subacute nephritis and arteriolitis.

Belman and colleagues[72] estimated the incidence of headache to be 8.9% and noted that it was the presenting symptom in 1 of their 3 reported patients, specifically a child with a prodrome of febrile irritability, colic, nausea, and vomiting, who later developed palpable purpuric rash, hematuria, and skin biopsy, which showed leukocytoclastic vasculitis. The other 2 patients differed in the development of other neurologic signs, which included transient postictal hemiparesis or mononeuropathy multiplex.

Recognized as a distinct entity for more than 200 years, HSP is the commonest vasculitis in children, with an incidence of 10 patients per 100,000 a year and an association with a variety of pathogens, drugs, and other environmental exposures.[73] Positive throat cultures are noted in up to one-third of cases, with group A β-hemolytic *Streptococcus* and titers to anti-streptolysin O increased in up to one-half of cases. Recognized neurologic complications include headache, obtundation, seizures, paresis, cortical blindness, chorea, ataxia, cranial nerve palsies, peripheral neuropathy, and myositis. IgA seems to play a pivotal role in the pathogenesis of anaphylactoid purpura,[74] with IgA-containing immune complexes and rheumatoid factor (RF)[75] and selective deposition of IgA1 so noted in glomerular mesangium in renal biopsies in virtually all patients with HSP nephritis and IgA nephropathy.[76]

Variable-Size Vessel Vasculitis

This category of vasculitis can affect vessels of any size, including those that are small, medium, and large, and of any type, including arteries, veins, and capillaries. BD and Cogan syndrome are 2 examples of a primary VVV with a propensity for vasculitis, CNS involvement, and headache.

Behçet disease

This disorder is characterized by relapsing aphthous ulcers of the mouth, eye, and genitalia.[77] Nervous system involvement has been estimated in 10%[78] to 25%[79] in clinicopathologically confirmed patients, with approximately one-third showing parenchymal involvement and two-thirds vascular involvement. Headache is the commonest neurologic symptom, independent of neurologic involvement in two-thirds of patients and noted to be primary in 38%, with 24% manifesting tension-type, and 15% migraines in one cohort.[80] Frontal and occipital headache and deep-seated pain around the eyes were presenting symptoms in several patients with imminent florid involvement later studied at postmortem examination[81–84] or a clue to silent neurologic involvement in other cohorts.[85]

Siva and Saip[86] classified neurologic involvement into 2 major primary types, one caused by vascular inflammatory mechanisms with focal or multifocal parenchymal involvement, presenting most often as a subacute brainstem syndrome, and another with few symptoms and a more favorable prognosis, caused by isolated cerebral venous sinus thrombosis and intracranial hypertension. A secondary form results instead from cerebral emboli due to cardiac disease, intracranial hypertension from superior vena cava syndrome, and neurotoxicity of specific mediations used in treatment. Mortality among clinicopathologically confirmed cases[79] was 41%, with 59% occurring within 1 year of onset of neurologic involvement. Among nonfatal cases, residual neurologic signs were not uncommon.

The neuropathologic findings in BD in brain biopsies and postmortem examination have been remarkably consistent among patients during the past several decades, showing perivascular cuffing of small meningovascular and parenchymal arteries and veins[79,81,82,84,87] rarely with medium-sized arteries showing fibrinoid degeneration and recanalization, and examples of venous thrombosis.[83] The inflammatory cell infiltrates are generally composed of lymphocytes, both T-cells and B-cells, macrophages, rarely plasma cells and eosinophils, and reactive astrocytosis and microscopic gliosis in neighboring cerebral, cerebellar, and brainstem white matter. Neuroimaging in those with neural parenchymal involvement showed a mesodiencephalic junction lesion, with edema extending along certain long tracts of the brainstem and diencephalon in 46% of patients, with the next most common location of involvement along the pontobulbar region in 40% of cases supporting a small-vessel vasculitis.

Cogan syndrome

Mogan and Baumgartner[88] described a 26-year-old man with recurrent headache-like pain, spasm, and redness of the left eye with photophobia, excessive tearing, and marked conjunctival injection, followed by severe attack of dizziness, tinnitus, vertigo, nausea, vomiting, ringing in the ears, profuse perspiration, and deafness. A diagnosis of recurrent interstitial keratitis (IK) and explosive Menière disease was made. In retrospect, this was probably the first reported patient with Cogan syndrome of nonsyphilitic IK with vestibuloauditory symptoms.[89] Symptoms of IK develop abruptly and gradually resolve, associated with photophobia, lacrimation, and eye pain (which may be unilateral or bilateral), with a tendency to recur periodically for years, before becoming quiescent. Vestibuloauditory dysfunction is manifested by sudden onset of Menière-like attacks of nausea, vomiting, tinnitus, vertigo, and frequently, progressive hearing loss, which characteristically occurs before or after the onset of IK.

With probably fewer than 100 reported patients with this rare childhood disorder, most reported patients with typical Cogan syndrome have appeared as single case reports or patient series, often without pathologic confirmation or evidence of systemic vasculitis in a biopsy or at postmortem examination. Headache was described by

Norton and Cogan[90] during the acute illness or at onset in a patient with atypical Cogan syndrome, who manifested a superior central retinal artery branch occlusion and orbital edema, as well as by Cody[91] and Cody and Williams[92] among 3 of 5 patients with typical Cogan syndrome, and 1 of 2 patients with atypical Cogan syndrome.

More recently, Gluth and colleagues[93] noted headache in 24 of 60 (40%) patients with Cogan syndrome of mean age 38 years (range 9–70 years), whereas Pagnini and colleagues[94] noted headache at onset in 17% of children of mean age 11 years (range 4–18 years) typically in association with other systemic features, including fever, arthralgia, myalgia, arthritis, and weight loss in up to 48% of children. Haynes and colleagues[95] found headache less common in typical Cogan syndrome in 17% of patients at onset, compared with 27% with atypical Cogan syndrome, a finding that correlated with CNS involvement identified in 4% of patients with typical Cogan syndrome compared with 15% with atypical Cogan syndrome, respectively.

Pathologically proven necrotizing vasculitis in association with Cogan syndrome was confirmed at postmortem examination in 3 patients, 838,485 by examination of subcutaneous nodular tissue and amputated limbs, and postmortem examination in 1 patient[96] or examination of biopsy tissue alone in 10 living patients.[97–104] Crawford[97] observed 3 patients with systemic necrotizing vasculitis, both of whom had headache at onset of Cogan syndrome. Postmortem examination in the first patient (case 1) who had frontal headaches and IK before onset of vestibuloauditory symptoms, showed necrotizing arteritis involving small arteries and arterioles of the brain, gastrointestinal tract, and kidneys, in addition to cerebral edema and petechial hemorrhages.

Single-Organ Vasculitis

SOV affects arteries or veins of any size in a single organ without features to indicate that it is a limited expression of a systemic vasculitis.[5] Involvement of small, medium, and large vessels of a single organ can be multifocal or diffuse as in those leading to an isolated organ-related clinicopathologic syndrome of the CNS, kidneys, peripheral nerves, coronary and pulmonary vessels, and retina, or focally in the breast, genitourinary, gastrointestinal system, or aorta, particularly after incidental biopsy or surgical resection because of a related or unrelated vasculitic process.[105]

Primary central nervous system vasculitis

The identification of angiographic beading in 2 patients and a sausage appearance in another patient at sites of presumed arteritis, the sine qua non of cerebral vasculitis was first noted by Hinck and colleagues in GCA[106] and later by Cupps and Fauci[107] in IACNS. The latter observation, along with preliminary efficacy of a combination immunosuppressive regimen of oral cyclophosphamide (CYC) and alternate-day prednisone in 3 patients with IACNS defined angiographically alone, and in one other patient, with histologically proven GANS of the filum terminate, led to prospective diagnostic and therapeutic recommendations.[11] At that time, investigators at the National Institutes of Health regarded IACNS and GANS as equivalent entities, with the former term emphasizing the restricted nature of the vasculitis and the latter the granulomatous histology. Giant cells and epithelioid cells, usually found at autopsy in GANS, were an inconsistent finding in a meningeal and brain biopsy and were therefore considered unnecessary for antemortem diagnosis.

In 1988, Calabrese and Mallek[108] added 8 new cases of so called PACNS, emphasizing both the restricted nature of the cerebral vascular changes as defined by classic angiographic (5 cases), diagnostic histopathological features in biopsy (2 cases) or postmortem tissue (1 case) of the nervous system; and the success of high-dose immunosuppression to achieve remission (7 cases). Among them, Patient 5, a 74-year-old man with headache, mental change, transient hemiparesis and aphasia, had a CSF protein of 169 mg/dL with 38 WBCs. Cerebral angiography showed only tortuosity and some irregularity of the lumen of intracranial vessels without segmental or alternating stenosis and ectasia prompting leptomeningeal and brain biopsy that in fact showed GANS affecting small meningeal veins with proliferation of epithelioid cells along vascular walls sparing the cortex. That case exemplified the problem in the Calabrese and Mallek criteria,[108] that is, of equating cases of medium-vessel and large-vessel vasculitis ascertained by cerebral angiography with others diagnosed by brain biopsy that continues to impact the validity of PACNS and its clinicopathological subtypes. Notwithstanding, the clinical course can be rapidly progressive over days to weeks or at times insidiously over many months, with seemingly prolonged periods of stabilization.

In the same year, 1988, Younger and colleagues[14] added 4 patients with GANS defined by the presence of granulomatous giant cell and epithelioid cell infiltration in the walls of arteries of various caliber from named cerebral vessels to small arteries and veins at postmortem examination (**Fig. 2**). One each was noted in association with Hodgkin lymphoma, herpes zoster, neurosarcoidosis, and no associated disorder. Headache was noted at onset in all 4 patients, as well as in 57% of patients with GANS, and during the course of the disease in 78%. The combination of headache, mental change, increased protein content with or without pleocytosis followed by hemiparesis, quadriparesis, progressive to lethargy, and stupor were predictive of a poor prognosis and mandated the need for combined meningeal and brain biopsy to establish the diagnosis with certainty.

Although there has not been a prospective study of the outcome of GANS and PACNS, undiagnosed and therefore untreated, the outcome of either is poor. Enthusiasm for treatment with combination chemotherapy using CYC has waned with recognition of the apparent risk of fatal side effects and the apparent efficacy at least of corticosteroids and azathioprine in one retrospective analysis summarized in the data shown in **Table 1**.[9]

Among 30 such cases diagnosed by meningeal and brain biopsy, 28 were treated with corticosteroids alone (11 patients) or with oral CYC (16 patients) or azathioprine (1 patient), and followed for up to a year of whom 18 (64%) improved, 7 (25%) were unchanged, and 3 (11%) died (with roughly equally satisfactory outcomes after

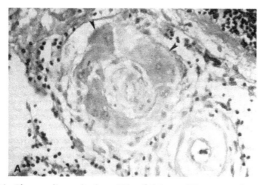

Fig. 2. CNS vasculitis. The media and adventitia of this small leptomeningeal artery have been almost completely replaced by multinucleated giant cells (*arrowheads*). There is intimal proliferation with obliteration of the vascular lumen, and a dense, perivascular, mononuclear inflammatory infiltrate can be seen (stain, hematoxylin-eosin, original magnification × 250).

Table 1					
Outcome of 54 cases of granulomatous angiitis					
Outcome	CS	CS+CYC	CS+AZA	None	Total
Improved	8/0[a]	9/0	1/0	0	18/0
Same	3/0	4/0	0	1/0	8/0
Died[a]	0/6	3/1	0	1/17	4/24

Abbreviations: AZA, azathioprine; CS, corticosteroids; CYC, cyclophosphamide.
[a] Patients diagnosed antemortem in the numerator, and postmortem in the denominator.

treatment with corticosteroids with or without CYC). However, 3 patients diagnosed antemortem died while taking corticosteroids and CYC; and 2 suffered serious sequelae of the therapy including fatal lymphoma, immunosuppression and opportunistic infection, or pneumonia and leukopenia. Comparatively, among 24 patients diagnosed postmortem, 7 (29%) who received treatment with corticosteroids alone (6 patients) or with CYC (1 patient) died, as did 17 (71%) who were untreated. Thus, 17 of 18 (94%) who received no treatment died, indicating that without therapy, the disease was usually fatal. Treatment with corticosteroids alone or in combination with CYC was associated with a considerable reduction in mortality; 24 of 34 (70%) patients so treated survived, and were improved (50%) or clinically unchanged. In this analysis, there was no appreciable benefit in the addition of CYC; however, the numbers were small, unmatched for age, disease activity, or other factors, and follow-up was nonuniform. The authors[9] suggested that CYC be reserved for histologically confirmed cases of PCNSV and GANS, especially those who continue to progress or fail to improve on corticosteroids alone, and who can be monitored closely for serious medication side effects.

Salvarani and colleagues[15] diagnosed PCNSV in 31 patients by histopathology and 70 patients angiographically, in whom 18 had a granulomatous inflammatory pattern, 8 lymphocytic pattern, and 5 acute necrotizing pattern. Headache was the commonest symptom in 63% of patients, followed by abnormal cognition, hemiparesis, and persistent neurologic deficit. Hajj-Ali and Calabrese[109] contrasted GANS and PACNS with the reversible cerebral vasoconstriction syndrome (RCVS), the latter of which was typified by sudden onset of a severe thunderclap-like headache with or without associated neurologic deficits and most reversible angiographic findings not caused by true vasculitis.

Childhood IACNS or childhood PACNS (cPACNS) caused by the involvement of distal small vessels have a gradual onset of persistent headache, cognitive decline, mood disorder, and focal seizures, and involvement of proximal medium and large arteries leads to large arterial stroke and propensity to subarachnoid hemorrhage.[12] The incurred deficit is influenced not only by the size and distribution of the involved vessels but also by the degrees and number of stenosis. Overall, the commonest presenting features of cPACNS are acute severe headaches and stroke features.[16] Children with angiographically positive progressive cPACNS can present with both focal and diffuse neurologic deficits with multifocal MRI lesions and evidence of both proximal and distal vessel stenosis on angiography. Untreated, they progress beyond 3 months, acquiring new neurologic deficits and new angiographically confirmed areas of vessel inflammation. Those with angiographically positive nonprogressive cPACNS often present with focal deficits, unilateral MRI lesions, and proximal angiographic vascular stenoses. Such patients instead have monophasic inflammatory large-vessel disease, which usually fails to progress beyond 3 months.[110]

Angiographically negative, SV-cPACNS vasculitis[110,111], which presents with new onset of severe headaches, seizures, or cognitive decline, warrants prompt consideration of lesional brain biopsy to ascertain the diagnosis before the commencement of immuno-suppressant treatment because both corticosteroids and delay in performance of the biopsy can obscure the histopathologic features. In contrast to adult PCNSV, granuloma-tous inflammation is typically absent. Instead, brain biopsy shows a mixture of lympho-cytes and macrophages, with occasional plasma cells, polymorphonuclear cells, and eosinophils in the walls of small arteries, arterioles, capillaries, and venules in the lepto-meninges, cortex, and subcortical white matter. More than a decade ago, BrainWorks in-vestigators began prospectively recording Canadian children with the umbrella diagnosis of inflammatory brain diseases (IBDs or IBrainDs), included among them, N-methyl-D-aspartate receptor-positive encephalitis and other antineuronal antibody-mediated CNS diseases, and intermixing progressive and nonprogressive large-vessel and small-vessel vasculitis, and its association with infection. They cited an increase primary pediatric IBDs and its toll as a leading cause of new-onset devastating neurological def-icits in children.[112]

Vasculitis Associated with Systemic Collagen Vascular Disease

Specific systemic disorders associated with vasculitis, and in turn with headache, include sarcoidosis and the serologically specific collagen vascular disorders such as SLE and rheumatoid arthritis (RA).

Systemic lupus erythematosus

The early concepts of the collagen vascular disorders introduced by Klemperer[113,114] stemmed from the appreciation of fibrinoid necrosis using collagen staining in patients with SLE. As collagen swells and fragments, it dissolves to form a homogeneous hy-aline and granular periodic acid-Schiff-positive material. The latter fibrinoid material contain immunoglobulins, antigen–antibody complexes, complement, and fibrinogen. The organ-specific responses of the CNS of this fibrinoid material lead to recognizable clinical sequelae caused by vascular and parenchymal damage. Several fluorescent antibody tests provide serologic support of SLE. The antinuclear antibody (ANA) screen produces a homogeneous pattern in most patients, with antibodies to native double-stranded (ds) DNA and reactivity to the Smith (Sm) and ribonucleoprotein an-tigens, the combination of which constitutes the extractable nuclear antigen. Circu-lating IgG and IgM antibodies with an affinity for charged phospholipids, antiphospholipid antibodies (APAs), some of which have procoagulant activity such as the lupus anticoagulant (LAC) and the generic anticardiolipin (ACL) antibody assay using cardiolipin as the antigen probe for APA, are all important determinants of pro-thrombotic events, especially in the CNS, wherein there is a propensity for occlusive microangiopathy.

Borowoy and colleagues[115] noted a prevalence of neuropsychiatric SLE (NPSLE) of 6.4% in a cohort of 1253 patients with SLE defined by the American College of Rheu-matology (ACR)[116] compared with the reported estimates of NPSLE of 14% to 39% in children and adults. Headache was regarded as a nonspecific minor NPSLE manifes-tation of chronic disease, along with mild cognitive impairment and depression. Ac-cording to Tomic-Lucic and colleagues,[117] those with so-called late-onset SLE caused by development of disease after age 50 years had a frequency of NPSLE of 6.6% compared with 36.6% in early onset disease along with a higher prevalence of comorbid conditions and higher Systemic Lupus International Collaborating Clinics/ACR damage index, despite less major organ involvement and a more benign course. Once thought to be an important cause of CNS or cerebral lupus, true vascu-litis was present in only 12% of postmortem examinations in the series by Johnson and Richardson.[118] There was neither mention of headache or CNS vasculitis among the 150 patients with SLE described by Estes and Christian[119] nor mention of headache among 50 clinicopathologic cases of SLE, one-half of whom had CNS lesions, compiled by Devinsky and colleagues.[120] Feinglass and colleagues[121] noted neuropsychiatric manifestations at onset of SLE among 3% of 140 patients compared with 37% in the course of the illness; however, headache was not specifically tabulated.

Cerebral dysfunction in SLE can be caused by large vessel or small vessel involvement or both. In the series by Feinglass and colleagues,[121] vasculitis was noted in 28% of patients, as well as in 46% of those with neuropsychiatric involvement compared with 17% of patients lacking neuropsychiatric involvement. Postmortem examination of the CNS in 10 of the 19 fatalities showed 2 cases of multiple large and small infarcts, one of which showed inflammatory cell infiltrates in the walls of medium-sized vessels and perivascular infiltrates around small arterioles. Although active CNS vasculitis was absent in the brain and spinal tissue of all 50 cases reported by Devinsky and colleagues,[120] 2 cases nonetheless showed inactive healed CNS vasculitis suggested by focal disruption of the elastic lamina and mild intimal proliferation of a single medium-sized artery, one of which had active systemic vasculitis of the PAN type, and both of which showed Libman-Sacks endocarditis and embolic brain infarcts. Focal angiitis of the CNS with cyst-like formation around affected blood vessels was noted at postmortem in the patient described by Mintz and Fraga,[122] with typical SLE rash, cutaneous vasculitis, and active neuropsychiatric involvement.

Trevor and colleagues[123] summarized the literature of large named cerebral vessel occlusions from 1958 to 1965 and noted 1 patient with an MCA stenosis progressing to occlusion and 3 others with angiographic internal carotid artery (ICA) occlusions, adding 3 new patients and suggesting a relation to the occurrence of cerebral arteritis. Two women, one aged 21 years and the other aged 42 years, presented with headache followed by focal neurologic symptoms attributed respectively to left MCA, followed by right ICA occlusions, and a right MCA stenosis progressing to occlusion in 4 months. A third patient had a left ICA occlusion without mention of headache. Johnson and Richardson[118] attributed the vasculitic nature of this process histopathologically to cerebral vasculitis mediated by acute inflammation and necrosis. Younger and colleagues[124] reported large named cerebral vessel occlusion attributed to circulating ACL antibodies in a young man in whom a vasculitis mechanism was not evoked.

The pathogenic mechanisms of cerebral SLE are poorly understood.[125] Immune complex–mediated vasculitis affecting small vessels is thought to account for much of the damage in CNS lupus despite the paucity of cerebral vasculitis evident in the form of inflammatory infiltrates in vessel walls at postmortem examination. In those with discrete vascular infarcts, there is a known association with the presence of circulating pathogenic antibodies, which predisposes some individuals to a high risk of stroke caused by both small-vessel and large-vessel occlusion.[124,126]

Lupus cerebritis and meningoencephalitis are 2 neurologic disturbances that can be associated with preceding headache. These disturbances are noted in up to 75% of patients with SLE depending on criteria,[127] and an etiopathogenesis related to antibody-mediated neuronal dysfunction is likely given the lack of correlation of symptoms of NPSLE and CNS lesions at postmortem examination, together with the transient nature of the disturbance. Patients with SLE are also predisposed to infectious episodes, including those not yet treated because of impaired B-cell function and humoral immunity, in addition to others receiving immunosuppressant medication rendered impaired in T-cell function and cell-mediated immunity.[127]

Rheumatoid arthritis

The ACR and European League Against Rheumatism Collaborative Initiative[128] published classification criteria for RA; and rheumatoid vasculitis (RV) qualifies as an extra-articular manifestation of RA.[129] There remains only a slight excess mortality in patients with RV compared with RA controls after allowance for general risk factors such as age and sex.[130] Three forms of vasculitis occur in RA, affecting all calibers of blood vessels, from dermal postcapillary venules to the aorta, usually in association with circulating IgM and IgG RF as measured by the latex fixation test, decreased complement levels, and a positive ANA test. The first form is a proliferative endarteritis of a few organs, notably the heart, skeletal muscle, and nerves characterized by inflammatory infiltration of all layers of small arteries and arterioles, with intimal proliferation, necrosis, and thrombosis. The second form is a fulminant vasculitis indistinguishable from PAN, with less-severe leukocytosis, myalgia, renal and gastrointestinal involvement, and bowel perforation. The third type takes the form of palpable purpura, arthritis, cryoglobulinemia, and low complement levels.

CNS vasculitis is rare in RV; however, the postmortem findings of 9 such patients have been reported,[131–138] and although not mentioned in any of them, headache would not be an unexpected feature. The duration of RA had a range of 1 to 30 years, with most surviving decades. The neurologic presentations included delirium, confusion, seizures, hemiparesis, Gerstmann-like syndrome, blindness, and peripheral neuropathy. Postmortem examination showed widespread systemic vasculitis in 3 patients.[131,133,134]

Vasculitis Associated with Illicit Substance Abuse

Even although headache in an illicit intravenous drug user (IVDU) should always prompt concern for stroke, hemorrhage, and CNS infection, further separable by neuroimaging and CSF analysis, cerebral vasculitis is rare, with very few histologically documented patients described in the literature. Three observations cast doubt on the frequent association of substance abuse with true cerebral vasculitis. First, most cases have been diagnosed by beading alone on a cerebral angiogram, without pathologic verification. Second, the vascular insult associated with drug abuse is likely caused by contributory factors, including human immunodeficiency virus type 1 (HIV-1) and acquired immunodeficiency syndrome (AIDS), which frequently accompanies drug abuse. Third, necrotizing arteritis itself is not a feature of an experimental animal model, in which vessel beading develops within 2 weeks of potential administration of amphetamine, postmortem examination of which shows per vascular cuffing, not arteritis.

Amphetamines

Parenteral illicit drug use as a cause of CNS vasculitis was first reported in association with amphetamines in 1970 among 14 drug addicts who suffered strokes and intracranial hemorrhage in association with multiple amphetamine and narcotic drug use.[139] Necrotizing arteritis of the polyarteritis type was found in cerebral arteries and arterioles. Many of the patients had complicating factors, including severe hypertension and hepatitis B antigenemia. Two patients, one abbreviated D.G. and the other E.V., who injected methamphetamine intravenously, had arterial lesions in cerebral, cerebellar, and brainstem pontine vessels; however, detailed histopathologic descriptions were not provided. Cerebral vasculitis was identified in a dubious report[140] of a 3-week postpartum woman, who took her first over-the-counter Dexedrine diet pill in many months containing phenylpropanolamine followed 90 minutes later by sudden headache, nausea, and vomiting. Brain CT showed subarachnoid blood with a frontal lobe hematoma, and bilateral carotid angiography showed diffuse segmental narrowing and dilatation of small, medium, and large vessels and branches of the anterior and posterior circulation. Evacuation and histopathologic analysis of the hematoma showed necrotizing vasculitis of small arteries and veins, with infiltration of polymorphonuclear leukocytes particularly prominent in the intima, with fragmentation of the elastic lamina and areas of vessel occlusion. It was unclear whether the findings were related to primary or drug-related CNS vasculitis.

Cocaine

Nine histologically verified patients with cocaine-related vasculitis have been described.[141–147] In all but 1 patient who had a long-standing cocaine habit with abuse sometime in the 6 months before admission, onset of neurologic symptoms immediately followed cocaine use, which was intranasally in 6, intravenously in 2, smoked in 1, and acquired via unknown modality in another. Cerebral vasculitis, associated with cerebral hemorrhage in 3 patients and ischemia in 7, typically began with abrupt onset of headache, focal hemiparesis, confusion or agitation, and grand mal seizures, which progressed to stupor, coma, and death. The underlying pathologic condition of cerebral vasculitis established by brain and meningeal biopsy in 7 patients and postmortem examination in 2 was nonnecrotizing, with transmural mononuclear cell inflammation affecting small arteries and veins or veins alone each in 3 patients, necrosis of small cerebral vessels associated with polymorphonuclear cell inflammation of small arteries and veins or large named vessels in 2 others, and perivascular cuffing of small arteries and veins in another.

Heroin

Neither convincing pathologically confirmed cases of heroin-induced cerebral vasculitis have been described in the literature nor has cerebral vasculitis been suggested as a likely occurrence in heroin abuse,[148–150] or acute heroin overdose.[151] In detailed neuropathologic studies carried out on 134 victims of acute heroin intoxication, including 18 who survived for periods of hours or days[152] with cerebral edema in conjunction with vascular congestion, capillary engorgement, and perivascular bleeding attributed to toxic primary respiratory failure, there was only ischemic nerve cell damage resembling systemic hypoxia without histologic evidence of cerebral vasculitis, and a single focus of lymphocytic perivascular inflammation. The brains of 10 intravenous drug abusers who died of heroin overdoses, including one caused by gunshot injury[153] similarly showed no evidence of cerebral vasculitis at postmortem examination, instead revealing only a few perivascular mononuclear cells associated with pigment deposition.

Vasculitis Caused by Central Nervous System Infection

The category of infection-related vasculitides includes acute bacterial and mycobacterial tuberculous (TB) meningitis, spirochete organisms (notably, neurosyphilis and Lyme neuroborreliosis [LNB]), viral infections (notably, varicella zoster virus [VZV]), mycotic and parasitic infections, and HIV/AIDS. Recognition of a coexistent or preceding infection is important because prompt treatment may avert or lessen the severity of both headache and vasculitis.

Acute bacterial meningitis

Diagnosis of the different forms of purulent bacterial meningitis was possible after the development of modern bacteriologic methods and the introduction of lumbar puncture as a diagnostic tool by Quinke in 1891. However, the relationship between vascular and parenchymatous cerebral changes, including vasculitis, and acute and chronic neurologic symptoms and signs, including headache, has still not been thoroughly resolved in clinicopathologically studied cases of meningitis. Nor have investigators resolved the origin of vasculitis, whether caused by extension of inflammation from inflamed meninges or the passage of vessels through inflammatory exudation. Twelve of 59 infants age younger than 2 years who suffered from meningitis caused by *Hemophilus influenzae*, meningococcemia, or pneumococcemia were reported by Dodge and Swartz[154] noting polymorphonuclear infiltration extending to the subintimal region of small arteries and veins was associated with exudative meningitis and anatomic necrosis of the cerebral cortex in all infants studied. However, occlusion of a major venous sinus was found in only 2 cases, and subarachnoid hemorrhage secondary to necrotizing arteritis was noted in only one case, representing a most unusual pathologic finding, according to the authors. Angiography reflected the localized nature of purulent meningitis in a 6-month-old infant with fatal *H influenzae* meningitis described by Lyons and Leeds[155] in whom cerebral angiography showed vasospasm, stenosis, occlusion, and an extremely slow arteriovenous circulation and collateral blood supply with a marked decrease in the diameter of bilateral supraclinoid internal carotid arteries. Only one area considered to be a mycotic aneurysm as suggested by irregular dilatations was later shown to be caused by histologically confirmed vasculitis, showing the limited nature of cerebral vasculitis in purulent meningitis. Roach and Drake[156] described 5 cases of ruptured cerebral aneurysms as suggested by cerebral angiography caused by septic emboli; 2 of these patients complained of headache; however, none of them had demonstrable vasculitis in histologic examination of the aneurysm specimen after surgery or in postmortem examination of the brain. Focal arteriographic changes in the setting of purulent meningitis may be the result of perivascular inflammation caused by the surrounding exudate.[157]

Mycobacterial tuberculous infection
TB meningitis was the first type of meningitis to be described clinically as dropsy of the brain in 1768 and subsequently shown to be inflammatory when meningeal tubercles and visceral tubercles were found to be identical in 1830. The tuberculoma, once the commonest intracranial tumor, is now exceptionally rare. The chief neurologic signs and symptoms of TB meningitis reflecting meningeal irritation manifested as neck stiffness and a positive Kernig sign; increased intracranial pressure, notably headache and vomiting; and mental changes, seizures, and focal neurologic signs. According to Smith and Daniel,[158] arteritis is the rule in the neighborhood of TB lesions, wherein vessel walls are invaded by mononuclear cells, with the adventitia more heavily involved than the media. The subintimal and intimal regions form a layer of homogeneous fibrinoid material that later involves the media, and the vessel lumen is reduced by inflammatory cell exudation beneath the fibrinoid material, the end results of which are reduction or complete obliteration of the lumen, proliferative endarteritis, and cerebral infarction. The vessels most heavily involved were those at the base of the brain and others in the sylvian fissure.

Headache was a presenting sign in case 7 reported by Smith and Daniel[158] of an 18-year-old girl with fever, confusion, right hemiplegia, back and neck pain for several days, followed by incontinence, complete flaccid paraplegia, delirium dementia, generalized spasticity, and death. Postmortem examination showed advanced TB meningitis with dense basal adhesions, hydrocephalus, and obliteration of the spinal subarachnoid space by adhesions, hemorrhagic infarction, and widespread arteritis with acute fibrinoid necrosis, without tuberculomas.

Headache has been an inconstant feature of TB meningitis, so noted in 2 autopsy-studied pediatric and adult cases,[159] notably including a 4-year-old girl (Case 4) with fever, left arm weakness, and increasing disorientation, which rapidly progressed to coma, nuchal rigidity, and spasticity of the legs. Vertebral angiography showed local widening of a branch of the left posterior cerebral artery (PCA) and a posterior fossa mass. The patient died soon afterward, and at postmortem examination, there was TB meningitis with typical TB vasculitis consisting of inflammatory changes in arteries at the base of the brain, notably in small vessels, with intimal swelling, leading to concentric narrowing of vessel lumina.

Headache was also a presenting symptom in another patient from among 3 others described by Leher,[160] none of whom had a previous history of tuberculosis, and all of whom had diagnostic angiographic abnormalities and histopathologic evidence of TB arteritis. That patient (Case 1) was a 33-year-old man with anorexia and insomnia. Carotid angiography showed narrowing of the supraclinoid ICA as well as narrowing of 2 convexity vessels in the sylvian fissure. At postmortem examination, there was marked eccentric left frontoparietal region arterial narrowing caused by fibroblastic proliferation of the intima, with many inflammatory cells below the elastica. Leher[160] described the radiopathologic triad of ventricular dilatation recognized by sweeping of the pericallosal artery; vessel narrowing, typically of the supraclinoid portion of the ICA caused by compression by thickened leptomeninges and exudation, arteritis and spasm; and narrowing or occlusion of smaller and medium-sized arteries with scanty collaterals, local swelling, and early draining veins. Occlusive TB vasculitis is associated with local areas of cerebral infarction of vessels at the base of the brain and arteritis.

Sudden headache accompanied by visual loss may be presenting features of tuberculosis. Kopsachilis and colleagues[161] described a 39-year-old man without known tuberculosis who developed sudden visual loss in one eye. Fluorescein angiography showed an inferotemporal branch retinal vein occlusion consisting of blockage with areas of hemorrhage, exudation, and late leakage. This occlusion was followed by optic disk swelling and headache. Biopsy of an enlarged cervical and submandibular lymph node showed caseating epithelioid cells confirming tuberculosis. Treatment with anti-TB treatment led to improved visual acuity.

Spirochete disease

Two spirochete diseases, neurosyphilis and neuroborreliosis, can be associated with CNS vasculitis in the course of infection.

Neurosyphilis. Meningovascular syphilis comprises 39% to 61% of all symptomatic cases of neurosyphilis and tends to occur more frequently in patients with concurrent HIV/AIDS. It is characterized by obliterative endarteritis, which affects blood vessels of the brain, spinal cord, and leptomeninges, precipitating substantial ischemic injury. Often referred to as Heubner arteritis, it involves medium-sized to large arteries with lymphoplasmacytic intimal inflammation and fibrosis; however, there is a variant form termed Nissl-Alzheimer arteritis, which characteristically affects small vessels and produces both adventitial and intimal thickening. Both types can lead to vascular thrombotic occlusions and cerebral infarction, with preferential involvement of the MCA. The search for the cause of stroke in young adults should include meningovascular syphilis as a potential cause.

Sudden acute severe headache heralded onset of occlusion of bilateral vertebral and proximal basilar artery was documented by MRA in a 35-year-old African man who responded to thrombectomy with restoration of blood flow but succumbed to fatal pontine and subarachnoid hemorrhages.[162] Postmortem examination showed reactive plasma reagin and a positive Venereal Disease Research Laboratory (VDRL) test in CSF with CNS vasculitis characterized by mural thrombi along the vertebrobasilar arteries with well-defined lines of Zahn of alternating layers of fibrin, platelet, and red blood cell aggregates, and inflammatory cell infiltration of the arterial walls, particularly in the adventitia. Headache of 2 to 3 weeks in duration was the presenting feature of 2 other patients with stroke syndromes,[163] 1 of whom had narrowing of bilateral M1 segments of the MCA, reactive CSF VDRL-positive *Treponema pallidum* hemagglutination assay and fluorescent treponemal antibody-absorption staining in the CSF, similar to the second patient, who presented with a stroke in the territory of the PCA without focal changes on cerebral angiography; neither of these patients was studied pathologically for true vasculitis.

Lyme neuroborreliosis. The term LNB was introduced by Veenendaal-Hilbers and colleagues[164] in 1988 to emphasize CNS involvement caused by *Borrelia burgdorferi* infection, the causative agent of Lyme disease. Among 20 patients described in the literature with neurovascular clinical syndromes ascribed to CNS vasculitis, for whom detailed information was available, including documentation of positive CSF Lyme serology, 3 such patients[165] presented with headache and were noted to have histopathologically confirmed vasculitis. Patient 3 reported by Oksi and colleagues[165] was an 11-year-old boy with headache and hyperactivity syndrome who developed gait difficulty concomitantly with a stroke visualized on brain MRI. Subsequent craniotomy and biopsy of the area of enhancement disclosed lymphocytic vasculitis of small vessels without fibrinoid necrosis, and CSF *B burgdorferi* serology was positive. Headache improved with intravenous antimicrobial therapy. A second patient (Case 2) reported by Topakian and colleagues[166] presented with headache, fatigue, malaise, nausea, and vomiting, first considered migrainous and then psychosomatic until subsequent MRI disclosed ischemic brain infarctions; MRA was compatible with diffuse vasculitis, and CSF showed lymphocytic pleocytosis with positive oligoclonal bands, and diagnostic CSF and serum *B burgdorferi* serology. Brain biopsy showed vasculitis involving leptomeningeal arteries comprising lymphoplasmacytic vessel wall infiltration with focal necrosis. Epithelioid cells were beaded in multiple granuloma-like formations in the leptomeninges. There was symptomatic improvement after a course of intravenous antimicrobial therapy. A third patient reported by Miklossy and colleagues[167] of a 50-year-old man with leg spasticity and CSF pleocytosis for 15 months progressed to hemiparesis and ventilatory support, and was later found to have diagnostic *B burgdorferi* serology in serum and CSF. Postmortem examination showed perivascular lymphocytic inflammation of leptomeningeal vessels, some of which showed infiltration of the vessel walls, duplication of the elastic lamina, narrowing of lumina, and complete obstruction of some leptomeningeal vessels by organized thrombi.

However, among 17 other reported patients with presumed CNS vasculitis caused by *B burgdorferi* infection of the CNS, only 9 presented with headache.[164,168–173] Neither was headache mentioned in the case report of 8 others[174–177] none of whom had histologically proven CNS vasculitis.

Varicella zoster virus-related vasculopathy. VZV causes chickenpox in childhood and most children manifest only mild neurologic sequelae. After it resolves, the virus becomes latent in neurons of cranial and spinal ganglia of nearly all individuals and reactivates in adult elderly and immunocompromised individuals, to produce shingles. An uncommon but serious complication of virus reactivation is ischemic and hemorrhagic stroke caused by VZV vasculopathy, which affects both immunocompetent and immunocompromised individuals presenting with headache and mental status changes with or without focal neurologic deficits and a spectrum of vascular damage from vasculopathy to vasculitis, with stroke.[178,179] Both large and small vessels can be involved, and MRI shows multifocal ischemic lesions, commonly at gray–white matter junctions. The diagnosis of VZV can be missed when symptoms and signs occur months after zoster, or in the absence of a typical zoster rash.

Fourteen patients with VZV-related vasculopathy have been described in the literature for whom detailed clinicopathologic data were available. Only one patient presented with headache, fever, mental status change, and focal neurologic deficits, and focal narrowing of the ICA, anterior cerebral artery (ACA) and MCA, with antibody to VZV in CSF, without a rash[180]; VZV deoxyribonucleic acid (DNA) and VZV-specific antigen was found in 3 of 5 cerebral arteries examined with histologically confirmed CNS vasculitis involving the circle of Willis. Among the other literature cases, Patient 1 reported by Eidelberg and colleagues,[181] who presented with headache and herpes zoster ophthalmicus (HZO) rash, was deemed to have CNS vasculitis based on complete occlusion of the MCA; however, postmortem examination showed no evidence of vasculitis. Headache was not mentioned in 5 other patients despite histologically proven widespread small-vessel granulomatous angiitis associated with lymphoma in 2 patients[182] and basilar branch vessel involvement of granulomatous angiitis in another.[183] Another patient with contralateral hemiplegia 1 month after HZO was found at postmortem examination to have endarteritis of unilateral ACA, MCA, and PCA[184] with VZV DNA from the involved vessels. Neither headache nor supporting histopathology was present in 7 other patients with VZV vasculopathy, including 5 patients with HZO and contralateral hemiparesis[185] and 2 patients with HZO and contralateral delayed hemiparesis.[186]

More recently, Nagel and colleagues[187] analyzed virus-infected cerebral and temporal arteries from 3 patients with VZV vasculopathy. Several characteristic histopathological findings were noted in all VZV-infected arteries studied, including disrupted internal elastic lamina, hyperplastic intima composed of cells expressing smooth muscle actin and smooth muscle myosin heavy chain but not endothelial cells expressing CD31, and decreased medial smooth muscle cells. The location of VZV antigen, degree of neointimal thickening, and disruption of the media were related to the duration of disease, wherein the presence of VZV primarily in adventitia occured early in infection, and in the media and intima later. These findings supported the hypothesis of VZV reactivation from ganglia and its spread transaxonally to arterial adventitia and thence transmurally.

Stroke in VZV vasculopathy seems to result from changes in arterial caliber and contractility produced in part by abnormal accumulation of smooth muscle cells and myofibroblasts in thickened neointimal and disruption of the media.[187] Nagel and colleagues[188] studied the immune characteristics of virus-infected temporal arteries 3 days after onset of ischemic optic neuropathy, and in the MCA after 10 months of protracted CNS disease. In both early and later VZV vasculopathy, T-cells, activated macrophages, and rare B-cells were found in adventitia and intima, whereas neutrophils and VZV antigen were abundant along with a thickened intima associated with inflammatory cells in vasa vasorum vessels. In the media of late VZV vasculopathy, viral antigen but not leukocytes was found and VZV was not found in inflammatory cells.

Fungal infection. Four fungal species, *Aspergillus*, *Candida*, *Coccidioides*, and *Mucormycetes*, can lead to opportunistic infection in immunocompromised and severely disabled hosts and have the capacity to invade arteries of the CNS. Cysticercosis, the most common parasitic infection of the nervous system caused by the tapeworm *Taenia solium*, leads to tissue cysts in the CNS within the subarachnoid space and basal cisterns, producing an arachnoiditis and small-vessel angiitis with resulting tissue infarction. Histopathologically confirmed fungal arteritis of cerebral vasculitis has rarely been reported; however, Shigenaga and colleagues[189] described a 62-year-old farmer with palpitation, shortness of breath, dizziness, malaise, and aplastic anemia treated with corticosteroids. Two months later he developed frontal headache, fever, tetraplegia, and fatal coma. Postmortem examination showed thromboendarteritis of the circle of Willis arteries, leptomeningitis, meningoencephalitis, and softening of the brain. The ACA and MCA showed aspergillotic arteritis involving all layers of the vessel wall by polymorphonuclear leukocytes, lymphocytes, and plasma cells, with complete occlusion of the lumen, distention and thinning of the walls, and extension of the inflammatory reaction to the adventitia.

Headache was not mentioned in the case description by Davidson and Robertson[190] of a 75-year-old farmer who lapsed into sudden fatal unconsciousness and was found to have a mycotic basilar artery aneurysm. Microscopic examination of the affected vessel showed focal necrosis of all layers and heavy infiltration by neutrophils and occasional mononuclear cells admixed with thrombus of varying ages and *Aspergillus* hyphae situated parallel to the vessel wall.

Frontal headache was the presenting symptom of a 74-year-old man described by Wollschlaeger and colleagues[191] who was later found to have an intrasellar mass on cerebral angiography, biopsy of which showed *Aspergillus* granuloma of the pituitary gland, which infiltrated the ICA within the cavernous sinus, with branching hyphae of septated fungus extending into the lumen of the artery and forming a massive organizing thrombus.

Human immunodeficiency virus/acquired immunodeficiency syndrome

Early in the HIV/AIDS epidemic, it was clear that many infected persons were IVDUs. Their associated risk behavior exposed them to infection through sharing of contaminated needles, thereby increasing the risk of spread of HIV and other blood-borne infections. The 2 postulated periods in the neurobiology of HIV when autoimmune disease manifestations can occur that seem to be significant for the development of cerebral vasculitis are shortly after seroconversion and before the spread of productive infection, and after initiation of highly active antiretroviral therapy (HAART) in association with the immune reconstitution inflammatory syndrome (IRIS).[192] The timing of early HIV invasion has been difficult to ascertain based on the presence of one or more well-recognized clinicopathologic HIV/AIDS syndromes, including HIV encephalitis, HIV-associated dementia, and AIDS dementia complex,[193–195] all of which indicate symptomatic infection.

Headache associated with irritation and confusion was the presenting feature of a 42-year-old homosexual man without evidence of immunodeficiency who developed cerebral granulomatous angiitis in association with human T-lymphotropic virus type III.[196] At postmortem examination, there was evidence of fibrous intimal scarring and marked luminal narrowing of the ACA, MCA, and PCA and their proximal branches, with mononuclear cell infiltration of the vessel walls and numerous multinucleated giant cells near the internal elastic lamina.

However, headache was neither mentioned in the description of 6 presymptomatic HIV-seropositive IVDUs reported by Gray and colleagues[153] with nonnecrotizing cerebral vasculitis studied at postmortem examination nor mentioned in the clinicopathologic description of 23 IVDUs from the Edinburgh HIV Autopsy Cohort described by Bell and colleagues[197] who died suddenly after seroconversion, but while still in the presymptomatic stage of HIV infection, compared to 10 HIV-negative IVDUs, 12 non-IVDU controls, and 9 patients with full-blown AIDS, who also died suddenly.

Among the presymptomatic HIV-positive patients, 7 showed infiltration of T-cells in the walls of veins in association with low-grade lymphocytic meningitis; 7 others showed isolated lymphocytic meningitis, and 1 patient had focal perivascular lymphocytic cuffing and macrophage collections throughout the central white matter tissue of the brain and in basal ganglia. Headache was not a conspicuous complaint in early HIV-associated hemophilia[198] even among patients who died suddenly of intracranial hemorrhage and liver cirrhosis with comparable neuropathologic changes of gliosis, occasional microglial nodules, perivascular mononuclear infiltrates, and leptomeningeal meningitis, without multinucleated giant cells or evidence of HIV in the brain. The introduction of HAART has changed the incidence, course, and prognosis of the neurologic complications of HIV infection concomitant with almost undetectable viral load in plasma and an increase in circulating T-lymphocytes. Yet, headache was not mentioned in the only pathologically confirmed patient with cerebral vasculitis and IRIS described by van der Ven and colleagues.[199]

DIAGNOSIS

There is general agreement on 4 principles in the diagnosis of vasculitis. First, vasculitis is a potentially serious disorder with a propensity for permanent disability because of tissue ischemia and infarction; recognition of the neurologic manifestations is important in developing a differential causative diagnosis. Second, undiagnosed and untreated, the outcome of vasculitis is potentially fatal. Third, a favorable response to an empirical course of immunosuppressive and immunomodulating therapy should never be considered a substitute for the absolute proof of the diagnosis of vasculitis. Fourth, histopathologic confirmation of vasculitis in the nervous system should be obtained for accurate diagnosis, via brain and meninges tissue biopsy when there is CNS involvement, or analysis of nerve and muscle biopsy specimens when PNS involvement is postulated. The laboratory evaluation of vasculitis of the CNS is summarized in **Box 2**.

Serologically-specific serum studies should be obtained in all patients guided by the clinical presentation and postulated causative diagnosis to avoid excessive cost and spurious results. Electrodiagnostic studies are useful in the initial investigation of systemic vasculitis because they can identify areas of asymptomatic involvement and sites for muscle and nerve biopsy and distinguish the various neuropathic syndromes associated with peripheral nerve and muscle involvement. A thorough sampling of distal and proximal nerves and muscles, using standard recording and needle electrodes for the performance of nerve conduction studies (NCS) and needle electromyography (EMG), at core skin temperatures of 34°C, with comparison to normative data may suggest a pattern of mononeuritis multiplex (MNM). Other presentations including a rapid and stepwise progression of coalescing axonopathic severe deficits along with the involvement of systemic organs warrants consideration of necrotizing arteritis that should be confirmed with biopsy of involved nerve and muscle tissue before commencing immunosuppressive therapy.

Open biopsy of a cutaneous nerve to ascertain proof of necrotizing arteritis was first recommended by Harry Lee Parker in a discussion of PAN by Woltman and Kernohan in 1938.[43] Biopsy of the superficial peroneal musculocutaneous nerve and peroneus brevis muscle was later implemented in the histopathologic diagnosis of PAN in several patients with mononeuritis multiplex.[200,201] A quarter century later, a series of investigations established the importance of cutaneous nerve biopsy in the definition of peripheral nerve vasculitis (PNV).[202–204] The Peripheral Nerve Society has published guidelines for the histopathologic diagnosis of PNV.[205]

Box 2
Laboratory evaluation of systemic and nervous system vasculitides

Studies in Blood, Urine, and Body Fluids

CBC, chemistry panel, ANA, ANCA by IIF; ANCA ELISA serology specific for PR3 and MPO (in those with IIF ANCA seropositivity, other cytoplasmic fluorescence, and ANA that results in homogeneous or peripheral nuclear fluorescence); ESR, CK, T- and B-cell subset panel, circulating IC, acute and convalescent viral, retroviral, bacterial, fungal, TB, syphilis and Lyme serology; quantitative immunoglobulins, IFE, C1q, complement proteins, RF, cryoglobulins, anticardiolipin and aPL, LAC, dsDNA antibodies, and appropriate HLA haplotypes; urinalysis for spot and 24-h collection for chemical and cellular microscopic analysis; bronchoscopy (in those with lung lesions) for lavage; lumbar CSF analysis for protein, glucose, cell count, IgG level, oligoclonal bands, cytology, VDRL, bacterial Gram stain and culture; India ink, cryptococcal antigen and fungal culture; acid-fast and TB culture; viral encephalitis panel for real-time PCR analysis of DNA and RNA viruses; paired analysis of serum and CSF for autoantibody-mediated encephalopathy, and Lyme index with *B burgdorferi* and HIV serology.

Neuroradiological Studies

Screening color Doppler ultrasonography of the temporal arteries and great vessels, 3-T brain and spinal cord MRI and high field MRA or CTA and DSA of the brain and other vascular beds and major vessels; 18FDG body PET-CT, and nuclear medicine cerebral perfusion with SPECT.

Histopathological and Neurophysiological Studies

Bronchoscopy or needle tissue biopsy of lung lesion and endoscopic biopsy of kidney tissue; USG-guided temporal artery biopsy; EMG-NCS of the legs and arms; 3 mm punch skin biopsy for ENF density and histology using PLP 9.5, with IF of vessel walls and microscopic analysis for leukocytoclasia; open sural nerve and soleus muscle or superficial fibular nerve and peroneus muscle tissue biopsies for epineurial and epimysial vasculitic foci; and en bloc open or stereotactic-guided biopsy of cortical brain and leptomeningeal tissues for vasculitic foci in arteries and veins.

Abbreviations: 18FDG body PET-CT, Fluorodeoxyglucose positron emission tomography fused with CT; ANA, antinuclear antibody; ANCA, antineutrophil cytoplasmic antibody; aPL, antiphospholipid; CBC, complete blood count; CK, creatine kinase; CSF, cerebrospinal fluid; CT and CTA, computed tomography and computed tomography angiography; DNA and RNA, deoxyribonucleic and ribonucleic acid; ds, double-stranded; DSA, digital subtraction angiography; ELISA, enzyme-linked immunosorbent assay; EMG-NCS, electromyography and nerve conduction studies; ENF, epidermal nerve fiber; ESR, erythrocyte sedimentation rate; IC, HIV-1, human immunodeficiency virus type 1; HLA, human leukocyte antigen; IFE, immunofixation electrophoresis; Ig, immunoglobulin; immune complexes; IIF, indirect immunofluorescence; dsDNA, LAC, lupus anticoagulant; MRA, magnetic resonance angiography; MPO, myeloperoxidase; PCR, polymerase chain reaction; PLP9; 5, protein gene product 9.5; PR3, proteinase 3; RBC and WBC, red and white blood cells; RF, rheumatoid factor; SPECT, single photon emission CT; T and B, thymus and bone marrow derived cells; TB, tuberculosis; USG, ultrasonography; VDRL, Venereal Disease Research Laboratory.

Electroencephalography (EEG), brain neuroimaging, and CSF studies are also integral to the diagnostic evaluation of most CNS disorders, including vasculitis. Although there are no typical electrographic findings in CNS vasculitis, EEG should be performed to screen for epileptogenic foci. MRI is more sensitive than CT but both methods lack specificity in histologically confirmed cases. The most common MRI findings are multiple bilateral cortical and deep white matter signal abnormalities and enhancement of the meninges after gadolinium. MRA and functional imaging of the brain provide complementary findings to conventional MRI (**Fig. 3**). The former is useful in the evaluation of medium-vessel and large-vessel disease but miss fine-vessel contours better seen on cut-film or digital subtraction angiography. The abnormal diffuse and focal perfusion patterns seen on single-photon emission CT (SPECT) do not always correlate with

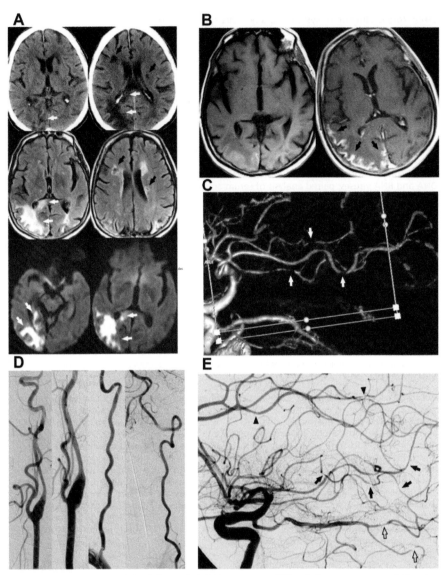

Fig. 3. (*A–E*) Primary angiitis of the CNS. (*A*) Noncontrast CT (*top*) demonstrates multifocal regions of low attenuation. Those in the right frontal subcortical white matter and left basal ganglia (*black arrows*) are sharply defined, without mass effect and likely reflect old infarctions. Both the cortex and underlying white matter of the right occipital lobe are involved as is the right splenium of the corpus callosum (*white arrows*). In these locations, the margins are more ill-defined, and there is subtle mass effect characterized by sulcal and ventricular effacement, suggesting acute ischemia in the right PCA territory. MRI FLAIR imaging (*middle*) demonstrates central low and peripheral high signal intensity within the frontal and periventricular white matter lesions (*black arrows*) consistent with chronic encephalomalacia from old infarctions. The FLAIR hyperintense signal within the right occipital lobe is more confluent and extends to the posterior temporal lobe and splenium, involving both cortex and white matter (*white arrows*) and better delineates the extent of the acute infarct. DWI (*bottom*) demonstrates restricted diffusion consistent with acute ischemia. (*B*) T1-weighted imaging

neurologic symptoms or distinguish vasculitic from nonvasculitic vasculopathy. Beading of vessels, the sine qua non of cerebral vasculitis, is probably found in no more than a third of patients with histologically proven CNS vasculitis, and may also be seen in CNS infection, atherosclerosis, cerebral embolism, and vasospasm of diverse cause. Multiple microaneurysms, often seen on visceral angiography in systemic vasculitis, are rare in CNS vessels. Whole body FDG PET-CT is a useful adjunct to standard neuro-imaging to reveal areas of abnormal vascular uptake correlative with vessel wall inflammation particularly in LVVs. In the author's experience, three dimensional (3D) surface projections of FDG PET imaging normalized to the whole brain, and fused with non-contrast MRI (PET MRI) for volumetric analysis, have the potential to reveal insights into premorbid brain neuropathology particularly in patients with hypometabolism in widespread cerebral areas and concordant volume loss. Such findings appear to be related to a combination of the dysregulated immune response and brain microglial that transition from surveilling mode to a reactive state change.

Properly performed, lumbar puncture for CSF analysis carries minimal risk and provides potentially useful information regarding possible underlying vasculitis, as suggested by CSF pleocytosis in excess of 5 cells/mm^3, increase in protein level greater than 100 mg/dL, and evidence of intrathecal synthesis of immunoglobulin or oligoclonal bands. Molecular genetic, immunoassay, and direct staining techniques to exclude spirochetal, fungal, mycobacterial, and viral infections, as well as cytospin examination of CSF for possible malignant cells, should be performed.

Combined cortical and meningeal biopsies are the gold standard for the diagnosis of CNS vasculitis but false-negative results occur because of focal lesions and sampling errors. Radiographic studies may guide the biopsy site toward areas of abnormality probably improve the sensitivity but this has not been formally studied. The risk of serious morbidity related to biopsy is probably less than 2.0% at most centers, which is probably less than the cumulative risk of an empirical course of long-term immunosuppressive therapy. There are no certain guidelines as to when to proceed to brain and meningeal biopsy. However, it would certainly be warranted if there were no other explanation for the progressive syndrome of fever, headache, encephalopathy, and focal cerebral signs, in association with CSF pleocytosis, and protein content increase greater than 100 mg/dL, which is suggestive of GANS.

TREATMENT

When headache is a result of cerebral vasculitis, it remits along with other features of CNS involvement, such that it is a useful feature to follow with presumptively effective vasculitis therapy. The systematic approach to the treatment of CNS vasculitis in the setting of headache is shown in **Box 3**.

◄───

pregadolinium and postgadolinium demonstrates extensive leptomeningeal enhancement along the cortical surface of the posterior temporal and occipital lobes. (C) CTA demonstrates multifocal vascular narrowing within several branches of the MCA (*white arrows*) with intervening regions of normal appearing vasculature. At the bottom of the image vascular narrowing within the PCA (not marked) is present. (*D* and *E*) CA reveals completely normal extracranial vasculature. The anterior cerebral (*black arrowheads*), middle cerebral (*black arrows*) and PCA (*black outlined arrows*) demonstrate mild-to-severe short segment stenoses. CA, catheter angiography; CT, computed tomography; CTA, computed tomographic angiography; DWI, diffusion-weighted imaging; FLAIR, fluid attenuation inversion recovery; MCA, middle cerebral artery.

Box 3
Recommendations for the treatment of vasculitis in the literature

Large Vessel Vasculitis
  GCA: EULAR[212]; CS[213,214]; AZA[215]; MTX[216–218]; infliximab[219]; or MMF.[220]
  TAK: EULAR[212]; CS[221]; AZA[222]; RTX[223]; infliximab[224]; anti-TNF-a, anti-IL-6[225]; and TCZ.[226,227]

Medium Vessel Vasculitis
  PAN: FVSG[228]; CS and CYC[229]; MMF[230,231]; infliximab[232]; PE.[233]
  KD: SHARE[234]; ASA + IVIg[235]; CS.[236,237]

Small Vessel Vasculitis
  AAV
    GPA and MPA: EULAR[238]; CS[239]; Induction with CS + CYC[240]; CS + RTX[241–244];
    CS + MMF[245,246]; RTX[247–250]; or MTX,[251] maintenance with AZA or MTX[252,253], and AZA or
    MMF,[254] PE[233,255,256]; IVIg.[257]
    EGPA: EGPA Consensus Task Force[258]; CS[259]; mepolizumab.[260,261]
  Childhood AAV:[262,263]; Remission induction: CS, CYC, MTX or RTX, and remission
  maintenance AZA MMF MTX CYC.[264]

Immune-Complex Vasculitis
  CryoVas[265]; RTX[266–268]; RTX + belimumab[269]
  MC:[269–271], French[272]
  IgAV: SHARE[273]; CS[274]; RTX[275]; MMF[276,277]
  Hypocomplementic-C1q: FVSG[278]; omalizumab[279]

Variable Vessel Vasculitis
  Cogan: CS[93]
  Behçet: CS[280]; MM[281]; colchicine or anti-TNF-a[282,283]

Single Organ Vasculitis
  Adult PACNS: CS alone or with CYC for induction of remission[284–286]; CS-sparing with CYC,
  RTX, MTX, AZA[287]
  cPACNS
    SV/AN: CS with CYC induction followed by CS taper and AZA or MMF maintenance[288]
    LV: CS induction with ASA/clopidogrel followed by CS taper and MMF maintenance[209,289]
    APNP/APP: CS with CYC induction and acute AC followed by CS taper, APT, MMF[209]

Vasculitis associated with systemic disease
  SLE: CS,[117] AC[124]
  RV: CS[134]; RTX[290,291]; infliximab[292,293]; and AZA or MTX[294]

Vasculitis associated with illicit substance abuse: avoidance of illicit substance

Vasculitis associated with infection: appropriate antimicrobial agents chosen specifically to
treat a given causative organism

Abbreviations: AAV, antineutrophil cytoplasmic antibody-associated vasculitis; AC, anticoagulation; AN, angiography-negative; APNP, angiography-positive nonprogressive; APP, angiography-positive progressive; APT, antiplatelet therapy; ASA, aspirin; AZA, azathioprine; BD, Behçet disease; CryoVas, cryoglobulinemia vasculitis; CS, corticosteroids; CYC, cyclophosphamide; EGPA, eosinophilic granulomatosis with polyangiitis; EULAR, European Alliance of Associations for Rheumatology; French, Vasculitis Study Group; GCA, giant cell arteritis; GPA, granulomatosis with polyangiitis; HCV, hepatitis C virus; IgAV, IgA vasculitis; IL, interleukin; INF, interferon; IVIg, intravenous immune globulin; KD, Kawasaki disease; LV, large-vessel; MC, mixed cryoglobulinemia; MMF, mycophenolate mofetil; MPA, microscopic polyangiitis; MTX, methotrexate; PACNS, primary angiitis of the central nervous system; PAN, polyarteritis nodosa; PE, plasma exchange; RTX, rituximab; RV, rheumatoid vasculitis; SHARE, Single Hub and Access point for pediatric Rheumatology in Europe; SLE, systemic lupus erythematosus; SV, small-vessel; TAK, takayasu arteritis; TNF, tumor necrosis factor.

In general, physicians treating adults with clinically-presumptive or histologically-definite primary or secondary adult vasculitides may choose the sequence, route of administration, and constituents of induction and maintenance immunosuppression agents guided by collaborative evidence-based randomized clinical trials (RCTs) or observational cohorts undertaken by the French Vasculitis Study Group (FVSG) database, United States-Canadian Vasculitis Clinical Research Consortium, European Vasculitis Study Society, the EULAR, The French Vasculitis Cohort of Patients with Primary Vasculitis of the Central Nervous System, and the Diagnostic and Classification Criteria in Vasculitis Study (DCVAS). The available therapeutic agents used alone and in combination include corticosteroid preparations, CYC, azathioprine (AZA), methotrexate (MTX), mycophenolate mofetil (MMF), the pyrimidine synthesis inhibitor leflunomide (LEF), plasma exchange (PE), high-dose intravenous immune globulin (IVIg), and diverse biological therapies including humanized monoclonal antibodies (mAbs) including the anti-CD20 mAb rituximab (RTX); the anti-TNF-α agents infliximab, etanercept, and adalimumab; and the anti-IL-6 receptor agent tocilizumab (TCZ).

By comparison, the treatments of pediatric AAV and related primary and secondary CNS vasculitides, that are decidedly uncommon, have historically relied on the experience in adults.[206] Attesting to the rarity of PCNSV, the DCVAS identified 42 (0.6%) cases of PCNSV among registrant pool of 6991 subjects with diverse forms of systemic and single organ vasculitis among 136 sites from 2011 to 2017 based on standard criteria endorsed by ACR and EULAR.[207] Yet, it is unclear why there is no incidence or prevalence data for cPACNS especially if it is one of the commonest inflammatory brain disease (IBrainD).[208] In the absence of clear epidemiologic data and RCTs in comparison to PCNSV,[208] the treatment of cPACNS and its subtypes remain problematic.[209] PedVas, the Pediatric Vasculitis Initiative[210] and ARCHiVe Investigators collaborating on the multicenter international pilot Registry for Childhood Vasculitis: e-entry; in association DCVAS; and members of the Childhood Arthritis and Rheumatology Research Alliance; and the web-based network, BrainWorks, in an International Childhood CNS Vasculitis Outcome Study, have been collecting clinical and biobank data of registered pediatric cases of AAV, TAK, PAN, cPACNS, and unclassified vasculitis since January 2013 to elucidate their presentation, classfication, and initial treatment.[211]

CLINICS CARE POINTS

- Headaches alone are insufficient to accurately diagnose any give form of vasculitis.
- Misdiagnosis and delayed diagnosis of headache and a relationship to purported CNS vasculitis is relatively common.
- Notwithstanding, a delay in diagnosis of either impacts prognosis by delaying effective treatment.
- Comprehensive educational efforts surrounding the clinical presentation of systemic and CNS vasculitides and its relationship to headache will prevent misdiagnoses, and incorrect or insufficient treatment.

DISCLOSURE

The author has nothing to disclose.

REFERENCES

1. Harbitz F. Unknown forms of arteritis with special reference to their relation to syphilitic arteritis and periarteritis nodosa. Am J Med Sci 1922;163:250–72.

2. Kussmaul A, Maier R. Ueber eine bisher nicht beschriebene eigenthümliche arterienerkrankung (periarteritis nodosa), die mit morbus brightii und rapid fortschreitender allgemeiner muskellähmung einhergeht. Deutsche Arch klin Med 1866;1:484–551.

3. Younger DS. Headaches and vasculitis. Neurol Clin 2014 May;32(2):321–62.

4. Younger DS. Adult and childhood vasculitis of the nervous system. Chapter 14. In: Younger DS, editor. Motor disorders. Maryland: Roman and Littlefield; 2022.

5. Jennette JC, Falk RJ, Bacon PA, et al. 2012 revised International Chapel Hill Consensus Conference Nomenclature of Vasculitides. Arthritis Rheum 2013; 65:1–11.

6. Ozen S, Ruperto N, Dillon MJ, et al. EULAR/PRES endorsed consensus criteria for the classification of childhood vasculitides. Ann Rheum Dis 2006;65:936–41.

7. Ruperto N, Ozen S, Pistorio A, et al. EULAR/PRINTO/PRES criteria for Henoch-Schonlein purpura, childhood polyarteritis nodosa, childhood Wegener granulomatosis and childhood Takayasu arteritis: Ankara 2008. Part I: Overall methodology and clinical characterisation. Ann Rheum Dis 2010;69:790–7.

8. Jennette JC, Falk RJ, Bacon PA, et al. 2012 revised International Chapel Hill Consensus Conference Nomenclature of Vasculitides. Arthritis Rheum 2013; 65:1–11.

9. Younger DS, Calabrese LH, Hays AP. Granulomatous angiitis of the nervous system. Neurol Clin 1997;15:821–34.

10. Salvarani C, Brown RD Jr, Christianson TJ, et al. Adult primary central nervous system vasculitis treatment and course: analysis of one hundred sixty-three patients. Arthritis Rheumatol 2015b;67:1637–45.

11. Cupps TR, Moore PM, Fauci AS. Isolated angiitis of the central nervous system. Prospective diagnostic and therapeutic experience. Am J Med 1983;74:97–105.

12. Lanthier S, Lortie A, Michaud J, et al. Isolated angiitis of the CNS in children. Neurology 2001;56:837–42.

13. Calabrese LH, Mallek JA. Primary angiitis of the central nervous system. Report of 8 new cases, review of the literature, and proposal for diagnostic criteria. Medicine (Baltim) 1988;67:20–39.

14. Younger DS, Hays AP, Brust JC, et al. Granulomatous angiitis of the brain. An inflammatory reaction of diverse etiology. Arch Neurol 1988;45:514–8.

15. Salvarani C, Brown RD Jr, Calamia KT, et al. Primary central nervous system vasculitis: analysis of 101 patients. Ann Neurol 2007;62:442–51.

16. Benseler SM. Central nervous system vasculitis in children. Curr Rheumatol Rep 2006;8:442–9.

17. Benseler SM, deVeber G, Hawkins C, et al. Angiography-negative primary central nervous system vasculitis in children: a newly recognized inflammatory central nervous system disease. Arthritis Rheum 2005;52:2159–67.

18. Neuwelt EA, Bauer B, Fahlke C, et al. Engaging neuroscience to advance translational research in brain barrier biology. Nat Rev Neurosci 2011;12:169–82.

19. Benarroch EE. Blood-brain barrier. Recent developments and clinical correlations. Neurology 2012;78:1268–74.

20. Ek CJ, Dziegielewska KM, Habgood MD, et al. Barriers in the developing brain and neurotoxicology. Neurotoxicology 2012;33:586–604.

21. Daneman R. The blood brain barrier in health and disease. Ann Neurol 2012;72: 648–72.

22. Edvinsson L, Tfelt-Hansen P. The blood-brain barrier in migraine treatment. Cephalalgia 2008;28:1245–58.

23. Charles A. The evolution of a migraine attack–a review of recent evidence. Headache 2013;53:413–9.
24. Blair RJ, Ross JJ, Morris A, et al. A sleeping giant. N Engl J Med 2011;365:72–7.
25. Hunder GG, Bloch DA, Michel BA, et al. The American College of Rheumatology 1990 criteria for the classification of giant cell arteritis. Arthritis Rheum 1990;33: 1122–8.
26. Blockmans D, Bley T, Schmidt W. Imaging for large-vessel vasculitis. Curr Opin Rheumatol 2009;21:19–28.
27. Salvarani C, Cantini F, Boiardi L, et al. Polymyalgia rheumatica and giant-cell arteritis. N Engl J Med 2002;347:261–71.
28. Nakao K, Ikeda M, Kimata SI, et al. Takayasu's arteritis: clinical report of eighty-four cases and immunologic studies of seven cases. Circulation 1967;35:1141–55.
29. Riehl JL, Brown J. Takayasu's disease. Arch Neurol 1965;12:92–7.
30. Kerr GS, Hallahan CW, Giordano J, et al. Takayasu arteritis. Ann Intern Med 1994;120:919–29.
31. Graham JR. Migraine (clinical aspects). Handb Clin Neurol 1968;5:45–58.
32. Manno RL, Levine SM, Gelber AC. More than meets the eye. Semin Arthritis Rheum 2011;40:324–9.
33. Arend WP, Michel BA, Bloch DA, et al. The American College of Rheumatology 1990 criteria for the classification of Takayasu arteritis. Arthritis Rheum 1990;33: 1129–34.
34. Grayson PC, Maksimowicz-McKinnon K, Clark TM, et al. Distribution of arterial lesions in Takayasu's arteritis and giant cell arteritis. Ann Rheum Dis 2012;71: 1329–34.
35. Walker DI, Bloor K, Williams G, et al. Inflammatory aneurysms of the abdominal aorta. Br J Surg 1972;59:609–14.
36. Sakata N, Tashiro T, Uesugi N, et al. IgG4-positive plasma cells in inflammatory abdominal aortic aneurysm: the possibility of an aortic manifestation of IgG4-related sclerosing disease. Am J Surg Pathol 2008;32:553–9.
37. Kasashima S, Zen Y, Kawashima A, et al. Inflammatory abdominal aortic aneurysm: close relationship to IgG4-related periaortitis. Am J Surg Pathol 2008;32: 197–204.
38. Ito H, Kaizaki Y, Noda Y, et al. IgG4-related inflammatory abdominal aortic aneurysm associated with autoimmune pancreatitis. Pathol Int 2008;58:421–6.
39. Stone JR. Aortitis, periaortitis, and retroperitoneal fibrosis, as manifestations of IgG4-related systemic disease. Curr Opin Rheumatol 2011;23:88–94.
40. Pipitone N, Salvarani C. Idiopathic aortitis: an underrecognized vasculitis. Arthritis Res Ther 2011;13:119.
41. Gornik HL, Creager MA. Aortitis. Circulation 2008;117:3039–51.
42. Stone JH, Khosroshahi A, Deshpande V, et al. IgG4-related systemic disease accounts for a significant proportion of thoracic lymphoplasmacytic aortitis cases. Arthritis Care Res 2010;62:316–22.
43. Kernohan JW, Woltman HW. Periarteritis nodosa: a clinicopathologic study with special reference to the nervous system. Arch Neurol 1938;39:655–86.
44. Kawasaki T. Acute febrile mucocutaneous syndrome with lymphoid involvement with specific desquamation of the fingers and toes in children. Arerugi 1967;16: 178–222 [in Japanese].
45. Hirose S, Hamashima Y. Morphological observations on the vasculitis in the mucocutaneous lymph node syndrome. A skin biopsy study of 27 patients. Eur J Pediatr 1978;129:17–27.

46. Yun SH, Yang NR, Park SA. Associated symptoms of Kawasaki disease. Korean Circ J 2011;41:394–8.

47. Constantinescu CS. Migraine and Raynaud phenomenon: possible late complications of Kawasaki disease. Headache 2002;42:227–9.

48. Savage CO, Winearls CG, Evans DJ, et al. Microscopic polyarteritis: presentation, pathology and prognosis. QJM 1985;220:467–83.

49. Hagen EC, Daha MR, Hermans J, et al. Diagnostic value of standardized assays for anti-neutrophil cytoplasmic antibodies in idiopathic systemic vasculitis: EC/BCR Project for ANCA Assay Standardization. Kidney Int 1998;53:743–53.

50. Churg J, Strauss L. Allergic granulomatosis, allergic angiitis, and periarteritis nodosa. Am J Pathol 1951;27:277–301.

51. North I, Strek ME, Leff AR. Churg-Strauss syndrome. Lancet 2003;361:587–94.

52. Masi AT, Hunder GG, Lie JT, et al. The American College of Rheumatology 1990 criteria for the classification of Churg-Strauss syndrome (allergic granulomatosis and angiitis). Arthritis Rheum 1990;33:1094–100.

53. Hattori N, Ichimura M, Nagamatsu M, et al. Clinicopathological features of Churg-Strauss syndrome-associated neuropathy. Brain 1999;122:427–39.

54. Ferri C, Sebastiani M, Giuggioli D, et al. Mixed cryoglobulinemia: demographic, clinical, and serologic features and survival in 231 patients. Semin Arthritis Rheum 2004;33:355–74.

55. Wintrobe MM, Buell MV. Hyperproteinemia associated with multiple myeloma. With report of a case in which an extraordinary hyperproteinemia was associated with thrombosis of the retinal veins and symptoms suggesting Raynauds disease. Bull Johns Hopkins Hosp 1933;52:156–65.

56. Gorevic PD, Kassab HJ, Levo Y, et al. Mixed cryoglobulinemia: clinical aspects and long-term follow-up of 40 patients. Am J Med 1980;69:287–308.

57. Brouet JC, Clauvel JP, Danon F, et al. Biologic and clinical significance of cryoglobulins: a report of 86 cases. Am J Med 1974;57:775–88.

58. Origgi L, Vanoli M, Carbone A, et al. Central nervous system involvement in patients with HCV-related cryoglobulin. Am J Med Sci 1998;315:208–10.

59. Cacoub P, Sbai A, Hausfater P, et al. Atteinte neurologique central et infection par le virus de l'hèpatite. Gastroenterol Clin Biol 1998;22:631–3 [in French].

60. Petty GW, Duffy J, Huston J. Cerebral ischemic in patients with hepatitis C virus infection and mixed cryoglobulinemia. Mayo Clin Proc 1996;71:671–8.

61. Díaz de Entre-Sotos FZ, Pérez-Aloe MT, Pérez-Tovar JF. Stroke and limb ischaemia in hepatitis C virus-related cryoglobulinaemia. Ir J Med Sci 2004;173:57.

62. Ince PG, Duffey P, Cochrane HR, et al. Relapsing ischemic encephalopathy and cryoglobulinemia. Neurology 2000;55:1579–81.

63. Abramsky O, Slavin S. Neurological manifestations in patients with mixed cryoglobulinemia. Neurology 1974;24:245–9.

64. Ramos-Cassals M, Robles A, Brito-Zeron P, et al. Life-threatening cryoglobulinemia: clinical and immunological characterization of 29 cases. Semin Arthritis Rheum 2006;36:189–96.

65. Wisnieski JJ, Baer AN, Christensen J, et al. Hypocomplementemic urticarial vasculitis syndrome. Clinical and serological findings in 18 patients. Medicine 1995;74:24–41.

66. Katsiari CG, Vikelis M, Paraskevopoulou ES, et al. Headache in systemic lupus erythematosus vs multiple sclerosis: a prospective comparative study. Headache 2011;51:1398–407.

67. Buck A, Christensen J, McCarty M. Hypocomplementemic urticarial vasculitis syndrome. A case report and literature review. J Clin Aesthet Dermatol 2012; 5:36–46.
68. Grotz W, Baba HA, Becker JU, et al. Hypocomplementemic urticarial vasculitis syndrome. Dtsch Arztebl Int 2009;106:756–63.
69. Osler W. The visceral lesions of purpura and allied conditions. BMJ 1914;1: 517–25.
70. Green B. Schöenlein-Henoch purpura with blood in the cerebrospinal fluid. Br Med J 1946;1:836.
71. Lewis IC, Philpott MG. Neurologic complications in the Schöenlein-Henoch purpura syndrome. Arch Dis Child 1956;31:369–71.
72. Belman AL, Leicher CR, Moshe SL, et al. Neurologic manifestations of Schoenlein-Henoch purpura: report of three cases and review of the literature. Pediatrics 1985;75:687–92.
73. Saulsbury FT. Clinical update: Henoch-Schönlein purpura. Lancet 2007;369: 976–8.
74. Trygstad CW, Stiehm ER. Elevated serum IgA globulin in anaphylactoid purpura. Pediatrics 1971;47:1023–8.
75. Levinsky RJ, Barratt TM. IgA immune complexes in Henoch-Schönlein purpura. Lancet 1979;2:1100–3.
76. Conley ME, Cooper MD, Michael AF. Selective deposition of immunoglobulin A 1 in immunoglobulin A nephropathy, anaphylactoid purpura nephritis, and systemic lupus erythematosus. J Clin Invest 1980;66:1432–6.
77. Behcet H, Matteson EL. On relapsing, aphthous ulcers of the mouth, eye and genitalia caused by a virus. 1937. Clin Exp Rheumatol 2010;28:S2–5.
78. Gökçay F, Celebisoy N, Gökçay A, et al. Neurological symptoms and signs in Behcet disease: a Western Turkey experience. Neurol 2011;17:147–50.
79. Wolf SM, Schotland DL, Phillips LL. Involvement of nervous system in Behçet's syndrome. Arch Neurol 1965;12:315–25.
80. Saip S, Siva A, Altintas A, et al. Headache in Behçet's syndrome. Headache 2005;45:911–9.
81. McMenemey WH, Lawrence TJ. Encephalomyelopathy in Behçet's disease. Report of necropsy findings in two cases. Lancet 1957;273:353–8.
82. Rubinstein LJ, Urich H. Meningo-encephalitis of Behçet's disease. Case report with pathological findings. Brain 1963;86:151–60.
83. Kawakita H, Nishimura M, Satoh Y, et al. Neurological aspects of Behçet's disease. A case report and clinico-pathological review of the literature in Japan. J Neurol Sci 1967;5:417–39.
84. Arai Y, Kohno S, Takahashi Y, et al. Autopsy case of neuro-Behçet's disease with multifocal neutrophilic perivascular inflammation. Neuropathology 2006;26:579–85.
85. Koseoglu E, Yildirim A, Borlu M. Is headache in Behçet's disease related to silent neurologic involvement? Clin Exp Rheumatol 2011;29:S32–7.
86. Siva A, Saip S. The spectrum of nervous system involvement in Behçet's syndrome and its differential diagnosis. J Neurol 2009;256:513–29.
87. Hadfield MG, Aydin F, Lippman HR, et al. Neuro-Behçet's disease. Clin Neuropathol 1997;16:55–60.
88. Mogan RF, Baumgarten CJ. Meniere's disease complicated by recurrent interstitial keratitis: excellent results following cervical ganglionectomy. West J Surg 1934;42:628.
89. Cogan DG. Syndrome of nonsyphilitic interstitial keratitis and vestibuloauditory symptoms. Arch Ophthalmol 1945;33:144–9.

90. Norton EW, Cogan DG. Syndrome of nonsyphylitic interstitial keratitis and vestibu-loauditory symptoms. A long-term follow-up. Arch Ophthalmol 1959;61:695–7.

91. Cody DT, Williams HL. Cogan's syndrome. Laryngoscope 1960;70:447–78.

92. Cody DT, Williams HL. Cogan's syndrome. Proc Staff Meet Mayo Clin 1962;37: 372–5.

93. Gluth MB, Baratz KH, Matteson EL, et al. Cogan syndrome: a retrospective re-view of 60 patients throughout a half century. Mayo Clin Proc 2006;81:483–8.

94. Pagnini I, Zannin ME, Vittadello F, et al. Clinical features and outcome of Cogan syndrome. J Pediatr 2012;160:303–7.

95. Haynes BF, Kaiser-Kupfer MI, Mason P, et al. Cogan's syndrome: studies in thir-teen patients, long-term follow-up, and a review of the literature. Medicine 1980; 59:426–41.

96. Fisher ER, Hellstrom HR. Cogan's syndrome and systemic vascular disease. Analysis of pathological features with reference to its relationship to thromboan-giitis obliterans (Buerger). Arch Pathol 1961;72:572–92.

97. Crawford WJ. Cogan's syndrome associated with polyarteritis nodosa. A report of three cases. Pa Med J 1957;60:835–8.

98. Eisenstein B, Taubenhaus M. Nonsyphilitic interstitial keratitis and bilateral deaf-ness (Cogan's syndrome) associated with cardiovascular disease. N Engl J Med 1958;258:1074–9.

99. Oliner L, Taubenhaus M, Shapira TM, et al. Nonsyphilitic interstitial keratitis and bilateral deafness (Cogan's syndrome) associated with essential polyangiitis (periarteritis nodosa). A review of the syndrome with consideration of a possible pathogenic mechanism. N Engl J Med 1953;248:1001–8.

100. Leff TL. Cogan's syndrome: ocular pathology. N Y State J Med 1967;67: 2249–57.

101. Gelfand ML, Kantor T, Gorstein F. Cogan's syndrome with cardiovascular involvement: aortic insufficiency. Bull N Y Acad Med 1972;48:647–60.

102. Cheson BD, Bluming AZ, Alroy J. Cogan's syndrome: a systemic vasculitis. Am J Med 1976;60:549–55.

103. Del Caprio J, Espinozea LR, Osterland SK. Cogan's syndrome in HLA Bw 17. [letter]. N Engl J Med 1976;295:1262–3.

104. Pinals RS. Cogan's syndrome with arthritis and aortic insufficiency. J Rheumatol 1978;5:294–8.

105. Hernandez-Rodriguez J, Hoffman GS. Updating single-organ vasculitis. Curr Opin Rheumatol 2012;24:38–45.

106. Hinck V, Carter C, Rippey C. Giant cell (cranial) arteritis. A case with angiographic abnormalities. Am J Roentgenol Radium Ther Nucl Med 1964;92:769–75.

107. Cupps T, Fauci A. Central nervous system vasculitis. Major Probl Intern Med 1981;21:123–32.

108. Calabrese HL, Mallek JA. Primary angiitis of the central nervous system: report of 8 new cases, review of the literature, and proposal for diagnostic criteria. Medicine 1988;67:20–39.

109. Hajj-Ali RA, Calabrese LH. Central nervous system vasculitis. Curr Opin Rheu-matol 2009;21:10–8.

110. Benseler SM, deVerber G, Hawkins C, et al. Angiographically-negative primary central nervous system vasculitis in children: a newly recognized inflammatory central nervous system disease. Arthritis Rheum 2005;52:2159–67.

111. Elbers J, Halliday W, Hawkins C, et al. Brain biopsy in children with primary small-vessel central nervous system vasculitis. Ann Neurol 2010;68:602–10.

112. Twilt M, Sheikh S, Cellucci T, et al. Recognizing childhood inflammatory brain diseases in Canada. Presse Med 2013;42:670.
113. Klemperer P. Diseases of the collagen system. Bull N Y Acad Med 1947;23: 581–8.
114. Klemperer P. The pathogenesis of lupus erythematosus and allied conditions. Ann Intern Med 1948;28:1–11.
115. Borowoy AM, Pope JE, Silverman E, et al. Neuropsychiatric lupus: the prevalence and autoantibody associations depend on the definition: results from the 100 Faces of Lupus Cohort. Semin Arthritis Rheum 2012;42:179–85.
116. The American College of Rheumatology nomenclature and case definitions for neuropsychiatric lupus syndrome. Arthritis Rheum 1999;42:599–608.
117. Tomic-Lucic A, Petrovic R, Radak-Perovic M, et al. Late-onset systemic lupus erythematosus: clinical features, course, and prognosis. Clin Rheumatol 2013;32: 1053–8.
118. Johnson RT, Richardson EP. The neurological manifestations of systemic lupus erythematosus. Medicine 1968;47:337–69.
119. Estes D, Christian CL. The natural history of systemic lupus erythematosus by prospective analysis. Medicine 1971;50:85–95.
120. Devinsky O, Petito CK, Alonso DR. Clinical and neuropathological findings in systemic lupus erythematosus: the role of vasculitis, heart emboli, and thrombotic thrombocytopenic purpura. Ann Neurol 1988;23:380–4.
121. Feinglass EJ, Arnett FC, Dorsch CA, et al. Neuropsychiatric manifestations of systemic lupus erythematosus: diagnosis, clinical spectrum, and relationship to other features of the disease. Medicine 1976;55:323–39.
122. Mintz G, Fraga A. Arteritis in systemic lupus erythematosus. Arch Intern Med 1965;116:55–66.
123. Trevor RP, Sondheimer FK, Fessel WJ, et al. Angiographic demonstration of major cerebral vessel occlusion in systemic lupus erythematosus. Neuroradiology 1972;4:202–7.
124. Younger DS, Sacco R, Levine SR, et al. Major cerebral vessel occlusion in SLE due to circulating anticardiolipin antibodies. Stroke 1994;25:912–4.
125. Khamashta MA, Cervera R, Hughes GR. The central nervous system in systemic lupus erythematosus. Rheumatol Int 1991;11:117–9.
126. Levine SR, Welch KM. The spectrum of neurologic disease associated with antiphospholipid antibodies. Arch Neurol 1987;44:876–83.
127. McCaffrey LM, Petelin A, Cunha BA. Systemic lupus erythematosus (SLE) cerebritis versus Listeria monocytogenes meningoencephalitis in a patient with systemic lupus erythematosus on chronic corticosteroid therapy: the diagnostic importance of cerebrospinal fluid (CSF) of lactic acid levels. Heart Lung 2012; 41:394–7.
128. Aletaha D, Neogi T, Silman AJ, et al. 2010 rheumatoid arthritis classification criteria. An American College of Rheumatology/European League Against Rheumatism Collaborative Initiative. Arthritis Rheum 2010;62:2569–81.
129. Turesson C. Extra-articular rheumatoid arthritis. Curr Opin Rheumatol 2013;25: 360–6.
130. Voskuyl AE, Zwinderman AH, Westedt ML, et al. The mortality of rheumatoid vasculitis compared with rheumatoid arthritis. Arthritis Rheum 1996;39:266–71.
131. Pirani CL, Bennett GA. Rheumatoid arthritis; a report of three cases progressing from childhood and emphasizing certain systemic manifestations. Bull Hosp Joint Dis 1951;12:335–67.

132. Kemper JW, Baggenstoss AH, Slocumb CH. The relationship of therapy with cortisone to the incidence of vascular lesions in rheumatoid arthritis. Ann Intern Med 1957;46:831–51.

133. Sokoloff L, Bunim JJ. Vascular lesions in rheumatoid arthritis. J Chronic Dis 1957;5:668–87.

134. Johnson RL, Smyth CJ, Holt GW, et al. Steroid therapy and vascular lesions in rheumatoid arthritis. Arthritis Rheum 1959;2:224–49.

135. Steiner JW, Gelbloom AJ. Intracranial manifestations in two cases of systemic rheumatoid disease. Arthritis Rheum 1959;2:537–45.

136. Ouyang R, Mitchell DM, Rozdilsky B. Central nervous system involvement in rheumatoid disease. Neurology 1967;17:1099–105.

137. Ramos M, Mandybur TI. Cerebral vasculitis in rheumatoid arthritis. Arch Neurol 1975;32:271–5.

138. Watson P, Fekete J, Deck J. Central nervous system vasculitis in rheumatoid arthritis. Can J Neurol Sci 1977;4:269–72.

139. Citron BP, Halpern M, McCarron M, et al. Necrotizing angiitis associated with drug abuse. N Engl J Med 1970;283:1003–11.

140. Glick R, Hoying J, Cerullo L, et al. Phenylpropanolamine: an over-the-counter drug causing central nervous system vasculitis and intracerebral hemorrhage. Case report and review. Neurosurgery 1987;20:969–74.

141. Krendel DA, Ditter SM, Frankel MR, et al. Biopsy-proven cerebral vasculitis associated with cocaine abuse. Neurology 1990;40:1092–4.

142. Fredericks RK, Lefkowitz DS, Challa VE, et al. Cerebral vasculitis associated with cocaine abuse. Stroke 1991;22:1437–9.

143. Murrow PL, McQuillen JB. Cerebral vasculitis associated with cocaine abuse. J Forensic Sci 1993;38:732–8.

144. Tapia JF, Schumacher JM. Case records of the Massachusetts General Hospital. Weekly clinicopathological exercises. Case 27-1993. A 32-year-old man with the sudden onset of a right-sided headache and left hemiplegia and hemianesthesia. N Engl J Med 1993;329:117–24.

145. Merkel PA, Koroschetz WJ, Irizarry MC, et al. Cocaine-associated cerebral vasculitis. Semin Arthritis Rheum 1995;25:172–83.

146. Martinez N, Diez-Tejedor E, Frank A. Vasospasm/thrombus in cerebral ischemia related to cocaine abuse. Stroke 1996;27:147–8 [letter].

147. Diez-Tejedor E, Frank A, Gutierrez M, et al. Encephalopathy and biopsy-proven cerebrovascular inflammatory changes in a cocaine abuser. Eur J Neurol 1998; 5:103–7.

148. Caplan LR, Hier DB, Banks G. Current concepts of cerebrovascular disease-stroke: stroke and drug abuse. Stroke 1982;13:869–72.

149. Richter RW, Pearson J, Bruun B, et al. Neurological complications of addictions to heroin. Bull N Y Acad Med 1973;49:4–21.

150. Louria DB, Hensle T, Rose J. The major medical complications of heroin addiction. Ann Intern Med 1967;67:1–22.

151. Sporer KA. Acute heroin overdose. Ann Intern Med 1999;130:584–90.

152. Oehmichen M, Meibner C, Reiter A, et al. Neuropathology in non-human immunodeficiency virus-infected drug addicts: hypoxic brain damage after chronic intravenous drug abuse. Acta Neuropathol 1996;91:642–6.

153. Gray F, Marie-Claude L, Keohane C, et al. Early brain changes in HIV infection: neuropathological study of 11 HIV seropositive, non-AIDS cases. J Neuropathol Exp Neurol 1992;51:177–85.

154. Dodge PR, Swartz MN. Bacterial meningitis–a review of selected aspects. II. Special neurologic problems, postmeningitic complications and clinicopathological correlations (concluded). N Engl J Med 1965;272:1003–10.

155. Lyons EL, Leeds NE. The angiographic demonstration of arterial vascular disease in purulent meningitis. Radiology 1967;88:935–8.

156. Roach MR, Drake CG. Ruptured cerebral aneurysms caused by micro-organisms. N Engl J Med 1965;273:240–4.

157. Ferris EJ, Rudikoff JC, Shapiro JH. Cerebral angiography of bacterial infection. Radiology 1968;90:727–34.

158. Smith HV, Daniel P. Some clinical and pathological aspects of tuberculosis of the central nervous system. Tuberculosis 1947;28:64–80.

159. Greitz T. Angiography in tuberculous meningitis. Acta Radiol 1964;2:369–77.

160. Lehrer H. The angiographic triad in tuberculous meningitis. A radiographic and clinicopathologic correlation. Radiology 1966;87:829–35.

161. Kopsachilis N, Brar M, Marinescu A, et al. Central nervous system tuberculosis presenting as branch retinal vein occlusion. Clin Exp Optom 2013;96:121–3.

162. Feng W, Caplan M, Matheus M, et al. Meningovascular syphilis with fatal vertebrobasilar occlusion. Am J Med Sci 2009;338:169–71.

163. Adagio N, Muayqil T, Scozzafava J, et al. The re-emergence in Canada of meningovascular syphilis: 2 patients with headache and stroke. CMAJ (Can Med Assoc J) 2007;176:1699–700.

164. Veenendaal-Hilbers JA, Perquin WV, Hoogland PH, et al. Basal meningovasculitis and occlusion of the basilar artery in two cases of Borrelia burgdorferi infection. Neurology 1988;38:1317–9.

165. Oksi J, Kalimo H, Marttila RJ, et al. Inflammatory brain changes in Lyme borreliosis: a report on three patients and review of literature. Brain 1996;119:2143–54.

166. Topakian R, Stieglbauer K, Nussbaumer K, et al. Cerebral vasculitis and stroke in Lyme neuroborreliosis. Two case reports and review of current knowledge. Cerebrovasc Dis 2008;26:455–61.

167. Miklossy J, Kuntzer T, Bogousslavsky J, et al. Meningovascular form of neuroborreliosis: similarities between neuropathological findings in a case of Lyme disease and those occurring in tertiary neurosyphilis. Acta Neuropathol 1990;80:568–72.

168. Schmiedel J, Gahn G, von Kummer R, et al. Cerebral vasculitis with multiple infarcts caused by Lyme disease. Cerebrovasc Dis 2004;17:79–81.

169. May EF, Jabbari B. Stroke in neuroborreliosis. Stroke 1990;21:1232–5.

170. Wilke M, Eiffert H, Christen HJ, et al. Primary chronic and cerebrovascular course of Lyme neuroborreliosis: case reports and literature review. Arch Dis Child 2000;83:67–71.

171. Chehrenama M, Zagardo MT, Koski CL. Subarachnoid hemorrhage in a patient with Lyme disease. Neurology 1997;48:520–3.

172. Uldry PA, Regli F, Bogousslavsky J. Cerebral angiopathy and recurrent strokes following Borrelia burgdorferi infection. J Neurol Neurosurg Psychiatry 1987;50:1703–4.

173. Klingebiel R, Benndorf G, Schmitt M, et al. Large cerebral vessel occlusive disease in Lyme neuroborreliosis. Neuropediatrics 2002;33:37–40.

174. Heinrich A, Khaw A, Ahrens N, et al. Cerebral vasculitis as the only manifestation of Borrelia burgdorferi infection in a 17-year old patient with basal ganglia infarction. Eur Neurol 2003;50:109–12.

175. Cox MG, Wolfs TF, Lo TF, et al. Neuroborreliosis causing focal cerebral arteriopathy in a child. Neuropediatrics 2005;36:104–7.

176. Meurers B, Kohlhepp W, Gold R, et al. Histopathological findings in the central and peripheral nervous system in neuroborreliosis. J Neurol 1990;237:113–6.

177. Lebas A, Toulgoat F, Saliou G, et al. Stroke due to Lyme neuroborreliosis: changes in vessel wall contrast enhancement. J Neuroimaging 2012;22:210–2.

178. Kleinschmidt-DeMasters BK, Gilden DH. Varicella-zoster virus infections of the nervous system: clinical and pathologic correlates. Arch Pathol Lab Med 2001; 125:770–80.

179. Kleinschmidt-DeMasters BK, Amliee-Lefond C, Gilden DH. The patterns of varicella zoster virus encephalitis. Hum Pathol 1996;27:927–38.

180. Gilden DH, Kleinschmidt-DeMasters BK, Wellish M, et al. Varicella zoster virus, a cause of waxing and waning vasculitis: the New England Journal of Medicine case 5-1995 revisited. Neurology 1996;47:1441–6.

181. Eidelberg D, Sotrel A, Horoupian S, et al. Thrombotic cerebral vasculopathy associated with herpes zoster. Ann Neurol 1985;19:7–14.

182. Rosenblum WI, Hadfield MG. Granulomatous angiitis of the nervous system in cases of herpes zoster and lymphosarcoma. Neurology 1972;22:348–54.

183. Linnemann CC, Alvira MM. Pathogenesis of varicella-zoster angiitis in the CNS. Arch Neurol 1980;37:329–40.

184. Melanson M, Chalk C, Georgevich L, et al. Varicella-zoster virus DNA in CSF and arteries in delayed contralateral hemiplegia: evidence for viral invasion of cerebral arteries. Neurology 1996;47:569–70.

185. Amlie-LeFond C, Kleinschmidt-DeMasters BK, Mahalingam R, et al. The vasculopathy of varicella-zoster virus encephalitis. Ann Neurol 1995;37:784–90.

186. Reshef E, Greenberg SB, Jankovic J. Herpes zoster ophthalmicus followed by contralateral hemiparesis: report of two cases and review of literature. J Neurol Neurosurg Psychiatry 1985;48:122–7.

187. Nagel MA, Traktinskiy I, Azarkh Y, et al. Varicella zoster virus vasculopathy. Analysis of virus-infected arteries. Neurology 2011;77:364–70.

188. Nagel MA, Traktinskiy I, Stenmark KR, et al. Varicella-zoster virus vasculopathy: immune characteristics of virus-infected arteries. Neurology 2013;80:62–8.

189. Schigenaga K, Okabe M, Etoh K. An autopsy case of Aspergillus infection of the brain. Kumamoto Med J 1975;28:135–44.

190. Davidson P, Robertson DM. A true mycotic (Aspergillus) aneurysm leading to fatal subarachnoid hemorrhage in a patient with hereditary hemorrhagic telangiectasia. Case report. J Neurosurg 1971;35:71.

191. Wollschlaeger G, Wollschlaeger PB, Lopez VF, et al. A rare cause of occlusion of the internal carotid artery. Neuroradiology 1970;1:32–8.

192. Nachega JB, Morroni C, Chaisson RE, et al. Impact of immune reconstitution inflammatory syndrome on antiretroviral therapy adherence. Patient Prefer Adherence 2012;6:887–91.

193. Sharer LR, Kapila R. Neuropathologic observations in acquired immunodeficiency syndrome (AIDS). Acta Neuropathol 1985;66:188–98.

194. McArthur JC, Haughey N, Gartner S, et al. Human immunodeficiency virus-associated dementia: an evolving disease. J Neurovirol 2003;9:205–21.

195. Price RW, Brew B, Sidtis J, et al. The brain in AIDS: central nervous system HIV-1 infection and AIDS dementia complex. Science 1988;239:586–92.

196. Yankner BA, Skolnik PR, Shoukimas GM, et al. Cerebral granulomatous angiitis associated with isolation of human T-lymphotropic virus type III from the central nervous system. Ann Neurol 1986;20:362–4.

197. Bell JE, Busuttil A, Ironside JW, et al. Human immunodeficiency virus and the brain: investigation of virus load and neuropathologic changes in pre-AIDS subjects. J Infect Dis 1993;168:818–82.
198. Esiri MM, Scaravilli F, Millard PR, et al. Neuropathology of HIV infection in hemophiliacs: comparative necropsy study. BMJ 1989;299:1312–5.
199. van der Ven AJ, Van Oostenbrugge RJ, Kubat B, et al. Cerebral vasculitis after initiation antiretroviral therapy. AIDS 2002;16:2362–4.
200. Bleehan SS, Lovelace RE, Cotton RE. Mononeuritis multiplex in polyarteritis nodosa. Q J Med 1962;32:193–209.
201. Lovelace RE. Mononeuritis multiplex in polyarteritis nodosa. Neurology 1964;14:434–42.
202. Wees SJ, Sunwood LN, Oh SJ. Sural nerve biopsy in systemic necrotizing vasculitis. Am J Med 1981;71:525–32.
203. Kissel JT, Slivka AP, Warmolts JR, et al. The clinical spectrum of necrotizing angiopathy of the peripheral nervous system. Ann Neurol 1985;18:251–7.
204. Said G, Lacroix-Ciaudo C, Fujimura H, et al. The peripheral neuropathy of necrotizing arteritis: a clinicopathologic study. Ann Neurol 1988;23:461–5.
205. Collins MP, Dyck JB, Gronseth GS, et al. Peripheral Nerve Society Guideline on the classification, diagnosis, investigation, and immunosuppressive therapy of non-systemic vasculitic neuropathy: executive summary. J Peripher Nerv Syst 2010;15:176–84.
206. Westwell-Roper C, Lubieniecka JM, Brown KL, et al. Clinical practice variation and need for pediatric-specific treatment guidelines among rheumatologists caring for children with ANCA-associated vasculitis: an international clinician survey. Pediatr Rheumatol Online J 2017;15:61.
207. Craven A, Robson J, Ponte C, et al. ACR/EULAR-endorsed study to develop Diagnostic and Classification Criteria for Vasculitis (DCVAS). Clin Exp Nephrol 2013;17:619–21.
208. Twilt M, Benseler SM. Central nervous system vasculitis in adults and children. Handb Clin Neurol 2016;133:283–300.
209. Beelen J, Benseler SM, Dropol A, et al. Strategies for treatment of childhood primary angiitis of the central nervous system. Neurol Neuroimmunol Neuroinflamm 2019;6:e567.
210. ClinicalTrials.gov Identifier: NCT02006134.
211. Cabral DA, Uribe AG, Benseler S, et al. Classification, presentation, and initial treatment of Wegener's granulomatosis in childhood. Arthritis Rheum 2009;60:3413–24.
212. Hellmich B, Agueda A, Monti S, et al. 2018 Update of the EULAR recommendations for the management of large vessel vasculitis. Ann Rheum Dis 2020;79:19–30.
213. Yates M, Loke YK, Watts RA, et al. Prednisolone combined with adjunctive immunosuppression is not superior to prednisolone alone in terms of efficacy and safety in giant cell arteritis: meta-analysis. Clin Rheumatol 2014;33:227–36.
214. Chandran A, Udayakumar PD, Kermani TA, et al. Glucocorticoid usage in giant cell arteritis over six decades (1950 to 2009). Clin Exp Rheumatol 2015;33:S98–102.
215. Boureau AS, Faucal Pd, Espitia O, et al. Utilisation de l'azathioprine dans le traitement de l'artérite à cellules géantes [Place of azathioprine in the treatment of giant cell arteritis]. Rev Med Interne 2016;37:723–9.
216. Spiera RF, Mitnick HJ, Kupersmith M, et al. A prospective, double-blind, randomized, placebo-controlled trial of methotrexate in the treatment of giant cell arteritis (GCA). Clin Exp Rheumatol 2001;19:495–501.

217. Jover JA, Hernandez-Garcia C, Morado IC, et al. Combined treatment of giant-cell arteritis with methotrexate and prednisone. a randomized, double-blind, placebo-controlled trial. Ann Intern Med 2001;134:106–14.
218. Hoffman GS, Cid MC, Hellmann DB, et al. A multicenter, randomized, double-blind, placebo-controlled trial of adjuvant methotrexate treatment for giant cell arteritis. Arthritis Rheum 2002;46:1309–18.
219. Hoffman GS, Cid MC, Rendt-Zagar KE, et al. Infliximab for maintenance of glucocorticosteroid-induced remission of giant cell arteritis: a randomized trial. Ann Intern Med 2007;146:621–30.
220. Sciascia S, Piras D, Baldovino S, et al. Mycophenolate mofetil as steroid-sparing treatment for elderly patients with giant cell arteritis: report of three cases. Aging Clin Exp Res 2012;24:273–7.
221. Shirai T, Sato H, Fujii H, et al. The feasible maintenance dose of corticosteroid in Takayasu arteritis in the era of biologic therapy. Scand J Rheumatol 2021;50:462–8.
222. Ohigashi H, Haraguchi G, Konishi M, et al. Improved prognosis of Takayasu arteritis over the past decade–comprehensive analysis of 106 patients. Circ J 2012;76:1004–11.
223. Kamisawa T, Okazaki K, Kawa S, et al. Japanese consensus guidelines for management of autoimmune pancreatitis: III. Treatment and prognosis of AIP. J Gastroenterol 2010;45:471–7.
224. Campochiaro C, Tomelleri A, Sartorelli S, et al. A Prospective Observational Study on the Efficacy and Safety of Infliximab-Biosimilar (CT-P13) in Patients With Takayasu Arteritis (TAKASIM). Front Med 2021;8:723506.
225. Regola F, Uzzo M, Toniati P, et al. Novel Therapies in Takayasu Arteritis. Front Med 2021;8:814075.
226. Nakaoka Y, Isobe M, Tanaka Y, et al. Long-term efficacy and safety of tocilizumab in refractory Takayasu arteritis: final results of the randomized controlled phase 3 TAKT study. Rheumatology 2020;59:2427–34.
227. Salvarani C, Hatemi G. Management of large-vessel vasculitis. Curr Opin Rheumatol 2019;31:25–31.
228. Terrier B, Darbon R, Durel CA, et al. French recommendations for the management of systemic necrotizing vasculitides (polyarteritis nodosa and ANCA-associated vasculitides). Orphanet J Rare Dis 2020;15:351.
229. Guillevin L, Cohen P, Mahr A, et al. Treatment of polyarteritis nodosa and microscopic polyangiitis with poor prognosis factors: a prospective trial comparing glucocorticoids and six or twelve cyclophosphamide pulses in sixty-five patients. Arthritis Rheum 2003;49:93–100.
230. Erden A, Batu ED, Sonmez HE, et al. Comparing polyarteritis nodosa in children and adults: a single center study. Int J Rheum Dis 2017;20:1016–22.
231. Brogan PA, Arch B, Hickey H, et al. Mycophenolate Mofetil Versus Cyclophosphamide for Remission Induction in Childhood Polyarteritis Nodosa: An Open-Label, Randomized, Bayesian Noninferiority Trial. Arthritis Rheumatol 2021;73:1673–82.
232. Ginsberg S, Rosner I, Slobodin G, et al. Infliximab for the treatment of refractory polyarteritis nodosa. Clin Rheumatol 2019;38:2825–33.
233. Regent A, Mouthon L, Guillevin L, et al. Role of therapeutic plasma exchanges in systemic vasculitis. Transfus Apher Sci 2020;59:102992.
234. de Graeff N, Groot N, Ozen S, et al. European consensus-based recommendations for the diagnosis and treatment of Kawasaki disease - the SHARE initiative. Rheumatology 2019;58:672–82.

235. Durongpisitkul K, Gururaj VJ, Park JM, et al. The prevention of coronary artery aneurysm in Kawasaki disease: a meta-analysis on the efficacy of aspirin and immunoglobulin treatment. Pediatrics 1995;96:1057–61.
236. Furukawa T, Kishiro M, Akimoto K, et al. Effects of steroid pulse therapy on immunoglobulin-resistant Kawasaki disease. Arch Dis Child 2008;93:142–6.
237. Newburger JW, Sleeper LA, McCrindle BW, et al. Randomized trial of pulsed corti-costeroid therapy for primary treatment of Kawasaki disease. N Engl J Med 2007; 356:663–75.
238. Yates M, Watts RA, Bajema IM, et al. EULAR/ERA-EDTA recommendations for the management of ANCA-associated vasculitis. Ann Rheum Dis 2016;75:1583–94.
239. Pagnoux C, Guillevin L. Treatment of granulomatosis with polyangiitis (Wege-ner's). Expert Rev Clin Immunol 2015;11:339–48.
240. Hoffman GS, Kerr GS, Leavitt RY, et al. Wegener granulomatosis: an analysis of 158 patients. Ann Intern Med 1992;116:488–98.
241. Stone JH, Merkel PA, Spiera R, et al. Rituximab versus cyclophosphamide for ANCA-associated vasculitis. N Engl J Med 2010;363:221–32.
242. Jones RB, Tervaert JW, Hauser T, et al. Rituximab versus cyclophosphamide in ANCA-associated renal vasculitis. N Engl J Med 2010;363:211–20.
243. Jayne D. S2. Rituximab for ANCA-associated vasculitis: the UK experience. Presse Med 2013;42:532–4.
244. Charles P, Guillevin L. S3. Rituximab for ANCA-associated vasculitides: the French experience. Presse Med 2013;42:534–6.
245. Han F, Liu G, Zhang X, et al. Effects of mycophenolate mofetil combined with corticosteroids for induction therapy of microscopic polyangiitis. Am J Nephrol 2011;33:185–92.
246. Silva F, Specks U, Kalra S, et al. Mycophenolate mofetil for induction and main-tenance of remission in microscopic polyangiitis with mild to moderate renal involvement–a prospective, open-label pilot trial. Clin J Am Soc Nephrol 2010; 5:445–53.
247. Specks U, Merkel PA, Seo P, et al. Efficacy of remission-induction regimens for ANCA-associated vasculitis. N Engl J Med 2013;369:417–27.
248. Benard V, Farhat C, Zarandi-Nowroozi M, et al. Comparison of Two Rituximab In-duction Regimens for Antineutrophil Cytoplasm Antibody-Associated Vasculitis: Systematic Review and Meta-Analysis. ACR Open Rheumatol 2021;3:484–94.
249. Cartin-Ceba R, Golbin JM, Keogh KA, et al. Rituximab for remission induction and maintenance in refractory granulomatosis with polyangiitis (Wegener's): ten-year experience at a single center. Arthritis Rheum 2012;64:3770–8.
250. Smith RM, Jones RB, Guerry MJ, et al. Rituximab for remission maintenance in relapsing antineutrophil cytoplasmic antibody-associated vasculitis. Arthritis Rheum 2012;64:3760–9.
251. De Groot K, Rasmussen N, Bacon PA, et al. Randomized trial of cyclophospha-mide versus methotrexate for induction of remission in early systemic antineutro-phil cytoplasmic antibody-associated vasculitis. Arthritis Rheum 2005;52:2461–9.
252. Gopaluni S, Smith RM, Lewin M, et al. Rituximab versus azathioprine as therapy for maintenance of remission for anti-neutrophil cytoplasm antibody-associated vasculitis (RITAZAREM): study protocol for a randomized controlled trial. Trials 2017;18:112.
253. Pagnoux C, Mahr A, Hamidou MA, et al. Azathioprine or methotrexate mainte-nance for ANCA-associated vasculitis. N Engl J Med 2008;359:2790–803.

254. Hiemstra TF, Walsh M, Mahr A, et al. Mycophenolate mofetil vs azathioprine for remission maintenance in antineutrophil cytoplasmic antibody-associated vasculitis: a randomized controlled trial. JAMA 2010;304:2381–8.

255. Jayne DR, Gaskin G, Rasmussen N, et al. Randomized trial of plasma exchange or high-dosage methylprednisolone as adjunctive therapy for severe renal vasculitis. J Am Soc Nephrol 2007;18:2180–8.

256. Walsh M, Merkel PA, Peh CA, et al. Plasma exchange and glucocorticoid dosing in the treatment of anti-neutrophil cytoplasm antibody associated vasculitis (PEXIVAS): protocol for a randomized controlled trial. Trials 2013;14:73.

257. Jayne DR, Chapel H, Adu D, et al. Intravenous immunoglobulin for ANCA-associated systemic vasculitis with persistent disease activity. QJM 2000;93:433–9.

258. Groh M, Pagnoux C, Baldini C, et al. Eosinophilic granulomatosis with polyangiitis (Churg-Strauss) (EGPA) Consensus Task Force recommendations for evaluation and management. Eur J Intern Med 2015;26:545–53.

259. Raffray L, Guillevin L. Updates for the treatment of EGPA. Presse Med 2020;49:104036.

260. Bel EH, Wenzel SE, Thompson PJ, et al. Oral glucocorticoid-sparing effect of mepolizumab in eosinophilic asthma. N Engl J Med 2014;371:1189–97.

261. Ortega HG, Liu MC, Pavord ID, et al. Mepolizumab treatment in patients with severe eosinophilic asthma. N Engl J Med 2014;371:1198–207.

262. Jariwala M, Laxer RM. Childhood GPA, EGPA, and MPA. Clin Immunol 2020;211:108325.

263. Calatroni M, Consonni F, Allinovi M, et al. Prognostic Factors and Long-Term Outcome with ANCA-Associated Kidney Vasculitis in Childhood. Clin J Am Soc Nephrol 2021;16:1043–51.

264. Morishita KA, Moorthy LN, Lubieniecka JM, et al. Early Outcomes in Children With Antineutrophil Cytoplasmic Antibody-Associated Vasculitis. Arthritis Rheumatol 2017;69:1470–9.

265. Perez-Alamino R, Espinoza LR. Non-infectious cryoglobulinemia vasculitis (CryoVas): update on clinical and therapeutic approach. Curr Rheumatol Rep 2014;16:420.

266. De Vita S, Quartuccio L, Isola M, et al. A randomized controlled trial of rituximab for the treatment of severe cryoglobulinemic vasculitis. Arthritis Rheum 2012;64:843–53.

267. Sneller MC, Hu Z, Langford CA. A randomized controlled trial of rituximab following failure of antiviral therapy for hepatitis C virus-associated cryoglobulinemic vasculitis. Arthritis Rheum 2012;64:835–42.

268. Lesniak K, Rymarz A, Lubas A, et al. Noninfectious, Severe Cryoglobulinemic Vasculitis with Renal Involvement - Safety and Efficacy of Long-Term Treatment with Rituximab. Int J Nephrol Renovasc Dis 2021;14:267–77.

269. Saadoun D, Ghembaza A, Riviere S, et al. Rituximab plus belimumab in noninfectious refractory cryoglobulinemia vasculitis: A pilot study. J Autoimmun 2021;116:102577.

270. Giuggioli D, Sebastiani M, Colaci M, et al. Treatment of HCV-Related Mixed Cryoglobulinemia. Curr Drug Targets 2017;18:794–802.

271. Ferri C, Cacoub P, Mazzaro C, et al. Treatment with rituximab in patients with mixed cryoglobulinemia syndrome: results of multicenter cohort study and review of the literature. Autoimmun Rev 2011;11:48–55.

272. Terrier B, Marie I, Lacraz A, et al. Non-HCV-related infectious cryoglobulinemia vasculitis: Results from the French nationwide CryoVas survey and systematic review of the literature. J Autoimmun 2015;65:74–81.

273. Ozen S, Marks SD, Brogan P, et al. European consensus-based recommendations for diagnosis and treatment of immunoglobulin A vasculitis-the SHARE initiative. Rheumatology 2019;58:1607–16.

274. Weiss PF, Feinstein JA, Luan X, et al. Effects of corticosteroid on Henoch-Schonlein purpura: a systematic review. Pediatrics 2007;120:1079–87.

275. Hernandez-Rodriguez J, Carbonell C, Miron-Canelo JA, et al. Rituximab treatment for IgA vasculitis: A systematic review. Autoimmun Rev 2020;19:102490.

276. Ren P, Han F, Chen L, et al. The combination of mycophenolate mofetil with corticosteroids induces remission of Henoch-Schonlein purpura nephritis. Am J Nephrol 2012;36:271–7.

277. Nikibakhsh AA, Mahmoodzadeh H, Karamyyar M, et al. Treatment of severe Henoch-Schonlein purpura nephritis with mycophenolate mofetil. Saudi J Kidney Dis Transpl 2014;25:858–63.

278. Jachiet M, Flageul B, Deroux A, et al. The clinical spectrum and therapeutic management of hypocomplementemic urticarial vasculitis: data from a French nationwide study of fifty-seven patients. Arthritis Rheumatol 2015;67:527–34.

279. Navarro-Navarro I, Jimenez-Gallo D, Villegas-Romero I, et al. Use of omalizumab in the treatment of hypocomplementemic urticarial vasculitis. Dermatol Ther 2020;33:e13237.

280. Noel N, Wechsler B, Boutin DLTH, et al. Outcome of neuro-Behçet: analysis of a large cohort. Presse Med 2013;42:692.

281. Shugaiv E, Tuzun E, Mutlu M, et al. Mycophenolate mofetil as a novel immunosuppressant in the treatment of neuro-Behçet's disease with parenchymal involvement: presentation of four cases. Clin Exp Rheumatol 2011;29:S64–7.

282. Hatemi G, Merkel PA, Hamuryudan V, et al. Outcome measures used in clinical trials for Behcet syndrome: a systematic review. J Rheumatol 2014;41:599–612.

283. Nanthapisal S, Eleftheriou D, Hong Y, et al. Behçet disease in children: the Great Ormond Street Hospital experience. Presse Med 2013;42:651.

284. Salvarani C, Brown RD Jr, Christianson TJH, et al. Long-term remission, relapses and maintenance therapy in adult primary central nervous system vasculitis: A single-center 35-year experience. Autoimmun Rev 2020;19:102497.

285. de Boysson H, Arquizan C, Touze E, et al. Treatment and Long-Term Outcomes of Primary Central Nervous System Vasculitis. Stroke 2018;49:1946–52.

286. de Boysson H, Zuber M, Naggara O, et al. Primary angiitis of the central nervous system: description of the first fifty-two adults enrolled in the French cohort of patients with primary vasculitis of the central nervous system. Arthritis Rheumatol 2014;66:1315–26.

287. Schuster S, Ozga AK, Stellmann JP, et al. Relapse rates and long-term outcome in primary angiitis of the central nervous system. J Neurol 2019;266:1481–9.

288. Hutchinson C, Elbers J, Halliday W, et al. Treatment of small vessel primary CNS vasculitis in children: an open-label cohort study. Lancet Neurol 2010;9:1078–84.

289. Walsh S, Knofler R, Hahn G, et al. Childhood primary large vessel CNS vasculitis: single-centre experience and review of the literature. Clin Exp Rheumatol 2017;35(Suppl 103):213–20.

290. Puéchal X, Gottenberg JE, Berthelot JM, et al. Rituximab therapy for systemic vasculitis associated with rheumatoid arthritis: results from the autoimmunity and rituximab registry. Arthritis Care Res 2012;64:331–9.

291. Buch MH, Smolen JS, Betteridge N, et al. Updated consensus statement on the use of rituximab in patients with rheumatoid arthritis. Ann Rheum Dis 2011;70: 909–20.
292. Bartolucci P, Ramanoelina J, Cohen P, et al. Efficacy of the anti-TNF-α antibody infliximab against refractory systemic vasculitides: an open pilot study on 10 patients. Rheumatology 2002;41:1126–32.
293. Puéchal X, Miceli-Richard C, Mejjad O, et al. Anti-tumor necrosis factor treatment in patients with refractory systemic vasculitis associated with rheumatoid arthritis. Ann Rheum Dis 2008;67:880–4.
294. Puéchal X. Rheumatoid arthritis vasculitis. Presse Med 2013;42:527–30.

The Pseudotumor Cerebri Syndrome

Deborah I. Friedman, MD, MPH*

KEYWORDS

- Pseudotumor cerebri • Idiopathic intracranial hypertension • Obesity
- Optical coherence tomography • Papilledema

KEY POINTS

- The 2013 diagnostic criteria are designed to make an accurate diagnosis while avoiding overdiagnosis.
- All individuals with suspected idiopathic intracranial hypertension (IIH) require an ophthalmic assessment including visual acuity, perimetry, ocular motility, and fundoscopy—these may be supplemented with fundus photography and optical coherence tomography.
- The patient's visual status determines the medical and surgical approaches used to lower cerebrospinal fluid (CSF) pressure.
- Medical and surgical weight loss can potentially normalize intracranial pressure.
- Recent insights into the pathophysiology of IIH are being translated into new therapies.

DIAGNOSIS

The diagnostic criteria for the pseudotumor cerebri syndrome (PTCS; **Box 1**)[1] include minimum cerebrospinal fluid (CSF) pressure parameters that differ for adults and children. The limit of 250 mm of CSF in adults was established in a 1983 study of 116 patients with acute PTCS.[2] Ninety percent of patients had measurements of 250 mm CSF or greater and values between 200 and 249 mm CSF were nondiagnostic.

A study in 2022 evaluated 35 individuals with idiopathic intracranial hypertension (IIH) and papilledema and 116 adults controls.[3] The mean pressure was 18.7 cm CSF in the controls (range 1–30.5 cm CSF, SD 5.2) with 95% below 29 cm CSF. The IIH group had a mean CSF pressure of 37.7 cm CSF (range 29.5–66.0 cm CSF, SD 8.2, $P < .0005$) with 95% of individuals having values above 31 cm CSF. Another study showed similar findings with an upper limit of normal of 30 cm CSF in men and 27.5 cm CSF in women with a body mass index (BMI) greater than 31 kg/m².[4]

Normative values for children are based on larger cohorts.[5,6] The 90th percentile for all children in the reference population was 28 cm CSF, and abnormally low pressure

Yellow Rose Headache and Neuro-Ophthalmology
* 12740 Hillcrest Road, Dallas TX 75230.
E-mail address: DeborahFriedman@tx.rr.com

Neurol Clin 42 (2024) 433–471
https://doi.org/10.1016/j.ncl.2024.02.001
0733-8619/24/© 2024 Elsevier Inc. All rights reserved.

Box 1
Diagnostic criteria for pseudotumor cerebri syndrome

A diagnosis of PTCS is "definite" if the patient fulfills criteria A to E. The diagnosis is considered "probable" if criteria A to D are met, but the measured CSF pressure is less than specified for a "definite" diagnosis.
1. Required for diagnosis of the PTCS
   A. Papilledema
   B. Normal neurologic examination except for cranial nerve abnormalities
   C. Neuroimaging: Normal brain parenchyma without evidence of hydrocephalus, mass, or structural lesion and no abnormal meningeal enhancement on MRI, with and without gadolinium, for typical patients (female and obese), and MRI, with and without gadolinium, and MRV for others. If MRI is unavailable or contraindicated, contrast-enhanced CT may be used.
   D. Normal CSF composition
   E. Elevated LP opening pressure (>250 mm CSF in adults and >280 mm CSF in children [250 mm CSF if the child is not sedated and not obese]) in a properly performed LP.
2. Diagnosis of PTCS without papilledema
   • In the absence of papilledema, a diagnosis of PTCS can be made if B to E are satisfied and, in addition, the patient has a unilateral or bilateral abducens nerve palsy.
   • In the absence of papilledema or sixth nerve palsy, a diagnosis of PTCS can be "suggested" but not made if B to E are satisfied and, in addition, at least 3 of the following neuroimaging criteria are satisfied:
      i. Empty sella
      ii. Flattening of the posterior aspect of the globe
      iii. Distention of the perioptic subarachnoid space with or without a tortuous optic nerve
      iv. Transverse venous sinus stenosis.

Source: The Pseudotumor Cerebri Syndrome, NCL 32.2, P363-396, MAY 2014.

---

below the 10th percentile was 11.5 cm CSF. Children undergoing moderate-to-deep sedation and those with an elevated BMI had higher pressures (5 cm CSF greater when adjusted for age and BMI). Post hoc analysis revealed that the 90th percentile in those receiving minimal or no sedation who were not obese was 25 cm CSF, forming the basis for the 2013 diagnostic criteria.

There is no physiologic rationale for the disparity of opening pressure in children (particularly adolescents) and adults, and many factors influence CSF pressure measurements (see "Therapeutic lumbar punctures" section). Values defining normal and elevated opening pressure overlap to some extent, with some healthy subjects having CSF pressures well above 30 cm CSF. This emphasizes the critical importance of diagnosing the disorder in the appropriate clinical context and not relying solely on opening pressure.

EPIDEMIOLOGY

The incidence of IIH in the United States is generally cited as 1 to 2 per 100,000 in the general population, increasing to 19 per 100,000 in overweight women of childbearing age.[7] These estimates were published over 25 years ago, and the rate of obesity has dramatically increased worldwide since then. Consequently, subsequent studies indicate a global rise in incidence. A meta-analysis and systemic review in 2018 found a marked preponderance of women: 87% with a mean age of 29.8 years.[8] The pooled incidence was 1.20 per 100,000, ranging from 0.03 to 2.36, reflecting country-specific prevalences of obesity. Based on these and other studies, the incidence has at least doubled over recent decades. Onset after age 45 years is rare.

A retrospective case–control study in the northeastern United States found that women with IIH were more likely to be Black (Odds Ratio [OR] 3.96, 95% 1.71–2.95) or Hispanic (OR 2.23, 95% confidence interval [CI] 1.14 to 4.36) and more likely to live in low-income tracts or "food swamps" (neighborhoods with a high density of high-calorie fast food and junk food options) and "food deserts" (neighborhoods with low access to healthy food options).[9]

Among a cohort of candidates for bariatric surgery screened with nonmydriatic fundus imaging, 4 of 532 patients (0.8%) had confirmed findings of IIH on neuro-ophthalmic examination and 3 underwent lumbar punctures (LPs) confirming a diagnosis of IIH.[10] The number of confirmed cases represents a 300 fold increase over the expected value in the general population and a 30 fold increase for the at-risk population. However, it does not justify extensive screening of this population for IIH.

The epidemiology of IIH in children is less well established although the prevalence clearly rises with increasing age and weight. Obesity is not a risk factor in prepubertal children. In one multicenter study of 233 cases, the average patient was more likely to be overweight at diagnosis starting at age 6.7 years in girls and 8.7 years in boys.[11] Overall, boys tended to present earlier than girls (9.95 vs 13.1 years) and were less likely to be overweight (BMI z-score 30.2 vs 24.7 kg/m^2). Boys accounted for 64% of children aged younger than 8 years, decreasing to 32% of those aged 8 to 13 years and 14% of participants aged older than 13 years. Available data regarding pubertal status in 57 participants revealed a female-to-male ratio in prepubertal children of 10:2, rising to 43:2 in pubertal children. The percentage of pediatric obesity increased with age overall, accounting for 77% of girls aged older than 12.5 years and 63% of boys aged over 12.4 years. Severe obesity at diagnosis was present in 37% of female individuals and 28% of male individuals.

The marked female predominance of IIH raises questions of its incidence in trans-gender individuals. Of the 22 reported cases, thus far, 16 of 19 transgender male individuals developed IIH while taking gender-affirming testosterone therapy.[12–14] Three individuals (including 1 individual with recurrent IIH) completed testosterone therapy 10 to 18 months prior to symptom onset; all 3 were obese. Three obese trans-gender female individuals developed IIH including 2 taking oral estradiol and spirono-lactone and another who completed hormonal therapy 4 to 6 years prior. Almost all patients had improvement or resolution using conventional medical and surgical therapy without changing exogenous hormone treatments. The predominance of cases associated with testosterone therapy is consistent with androgen excess in biological female individuals with IIH.[15]

PATHOPHYSIOLOGY

The underlying cause of IIH must explain its predilection to affect obese women of childbearing age and lack of ventriculomegaly. Regarding the latter, the role of the cerebral vasculature in IIH was recognized in Dandy's initial description in 1937.[16] He postulated that spinal fluid accumulating in the brain substance could account for the small ventricles and opined that "the very rapid increase and decrease of the decompression....in two to 3 minutes–from one extreme to the other–could hardly occur except from changes in the vascular bed; certainly the change is much too rapid for an increase or decrease in cerebrospinal fluid."

Farb and colleagues substantiated Dandy's observations with a case series demonstrating cerebral venous sinus stenosis IIH.[17] Dural puncture with CSF removal to reduce intracranial pressure (ICP) reversed the stenotic changes almost immediately, leading to the conclusion that the venous stenosis was secondary to accumulation of

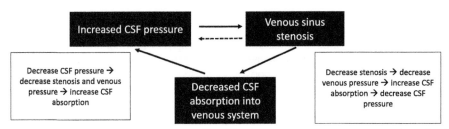

Fig. 1. Feed-forward loop of intracranial hypertension, venous sinus stenosis, and cerebral venous hypertension and areas for intervention.

fluid in the brain, rather than the converse. However, not all patients with venous sinus stenosis showed improvement in venous diameter following the removal of CSF, suggesting that the venous system was the primary cause in some cases. In summary,

- The volumes of the CSF and the vascular spaces in the brain have a reciprocal relationship.
- As cerebral venous sinus pressure rises, CSF absorption into the venous system decreases leading to further increases in CSF pressure (**Fig. 1**).
- Although the initiating factor remains unclear, there is a feed-forward loop involving cerebral venous pressure and ICP.

Regarding the association with obesity, female predilection, and high incidence of polycystic ovary syndrome (PCOS) in women with IIH, recent research focuses on metabolic substrates involved in weight regulation.[18] Similar to PCOS, evidence suggests that IIH is disease of androgen excess with preferential truncal adipose deposition, insulin resistance, and increased cardiovascular risk.[18] Compared to obese controls, the subcutaneous abdominal adipocytes in patients with IIH are dysregulated and geared for lipogenesis.[18] 11β-hydroxysteroid dehydrogenase type 1 (11β-HSD1), an intracellular enzyme that increases local glucocorticoid activity by converting inactive cortisone to active cortisol, is expressed in the choroid plexus epithelial cells, and its activity decreases with weight reduction.[18] Measurements of subcutaneous adipose 11β-HSD1 in patients with IIH undergoing bariatric surgery showed elevated 11β-HSD1 compared to controls.[18]

Glucagon-like peptide-1 (GLP-1) is an incretin secreted in the small intestine. GLP-1 receptor agonists are used to lower body weight in patients with and without type 2 diabetes and improve glycemic control while avoiding hypoglycemia. The choroid plexus epithelium in rats and humans contains GLP-1 receptors and CSF secretion decreases in rats after treatment of GLP-1 receptor.[19] An international randomized clinical trial of exenatide, a GLP-1 receptor agonist, for IIH commenced in 2022 (IIH-Evolve) but was terminated early for financial reasons.[20] However, early results were promising, and incretins are increasingly prescribed for weight loss in patients with IIH in clinical practice.[21]

SECONDARY CAUSES

Over 100 medications and medical conditions are reportedly associated with PTCS.[22] The best-documented conditions are found in **Box 2**. Obesity and weight gain demonstrated in observational studies and generalized fluid retention (orthostatic edema) in women with IIH support a systemic process.[23,24] While some medications, such as tetracyclines and retinoids, likely have a direct effect, medications producing weight

Box 2
Associated conditions

Obstruction to cerebral venous drainage

Cerebral venous sinus thrombosis
  Aseptic (hypercoagulable state)
  Septic (middle ear or mastoid infection)

Bilateral radical neck dissection with jugular vein ligation

Jugular vein tumor

Superior vena cava syndrome

Brachiocephalic vein thrombosis

Increased right heart pressure

Following embolization of arteriovenous malformation

Endocrine disorders

Addison disease

Hypoparathyroidism

Obesity, recent weight gain

Orthostatic edema

Exogenous agents

Amiodarone

Cytarabine

Chlordecone (kepone)

Corticosteroids (particularly withdrawal)

Cyclosporine

Growth hormone

Leuprorelin acetate (LH-RH analog)

Lithium carbonate

Nalidixic acid

Sulfa antibiotics

Tetracycline and related compounds
  Minocycline
  Doxycycline

Vitamin A
  Vitamin supplements, liver
  Cis-retinoic acid (Accutane)
  All-trans-retinoic acid (for acute promyelocytic leukemia)

Infectious or postinfectious

HIV infection

Lyme disease

Other viruses Coronavirus

Following childhood varicella

Other medical conditions

Antiphospholipid antibody syndrome

Behçet disease

Occult craniosynostosis

Polycystic ovary syndrome

Sarcoidosis

Obstructive sleep apnea

Systemic lupus erythematosis

Turner syndrome

Source: The Pseudotumor Cerebri Syndrome, NCL 32.2, P363-396, MAY 2014, Box 3

gain as a side effect are also implicated. Cases of PTCS were also associated with coronavirus infection.[25–28]

SYMPTOMS
Headache

The Idiopathic Intracranial Hypertension Treatment Trial (IIHTT) studied 165 adults (161 female and 4 male) to determine whether acetazolamide was more effective than placebo for improving visual field loss when combined with dietary weight loss management.[29,30] Participants with papilledema with mild visual field loss on automated perimetry enrolled within 2 weeks of diagnosis. Data were captured at baseline and monthly until the 6 month primary outcome timepoint.[31] Headache features were manually reviewed and phenotyped according to the International Classification for Headache Disorders 3–beta version (ICHD-3b).[32]

Headache is the most common manifestation of IIH, affecting over 80% of patients at diagnosis. For many individuals, headache is the most debilitating aspect of the disease[33] and the greatest contributor to reduced quality of life.[33–35] The mean Headache Impact Test-6 score at baseline in the IIHTT was 59.7 ± 9.0, reflecting substantial to severe impact.[31] However, headache characteristics in IIH vary considerably with no "typical" headache location or phenotype.

Eight-four percent (n = 139) of IIHTT enrollees had headache at baseline, of whom 38 had chronic (≥15 days monthly) or daily headaches.[31] The headache phenotype was migraine without aura (52%) or probable migraine (16%), tension type headache (22%), probable tension type headache (4%), and unclassifiable (7%). Half of those with a migraine phenotype, and 29% with a nonmigrainous phenotype, had a history of migraine without or with aura.

The headache was located anteriorly in most participants with frontal pain in 68% and ocular pain in 47%.[31] However, other locations were reported more commonly than previously recognized including posterior (39%), global (36%), unilateral (30%), and nuchal (47%). Headache characterization was pressure-like in 47% and throbbing in 42%. Migraine-associated symptoms were common and 5% experienced photophobia without headache. Most participants also had other symptoms of IIH but 20 patients had headache alone.

Acute medication overuse was present in 37% of enrollees with headache, most commonly with simple analgesics, nonsteroidal anti-inflammatory drugs, or over-the-counter combination analgesics, with 12.9% taking opioids or butalbital.[31] A study in the United Kingdom found that women with IIH were twice as likely to receive prescriptions for opioids (20% in the first year after diagnosis) compared to migraine controls.[36]

Headaches persist even after controlling CSF pressure and resolution of papilledema in at least two-thirds of patients.[33,37,38] Most patients with persistent headache in one study had no prior history of headache.[38] The mechanism is unknown but postulated to be related to central sensitization of the trigeminovascular system in the acute phase of IIH.[39]

Transient visual obscurations

Transient visual obscurations (TVOs) are the second most common symptom of IIH, occurring in 68% of participants in the IIHTT.[40] They may be unilateral or bilateral and typically last between seconds and a few minutes, occurring up to numerous times daily. Patients may experience complete or partial visual loss, described as black-out, gray-out, white-out, cloudy, or hazy vision. Attacks are often provoked by arising after bending over or rolling the eyes upward. They are attributed to optic nerve ischemia due to compression of the vascular supply by CSF in the perioptic subarachnoid space. Although the vision almost always returns to baseline, the attacks are a source of anxiety and disability as they occur unpredictably. After headache and neck pain, TVOs had the greatest impact on quality of life in the IIHTT; many patients avoided driving because of them.[35] Optic disc drusen, producing pseudopapilledema, can also cause TVOs.[41]

Auditory manifestations

Patients with IIH may experience pulsatile (pulse-synchronous) or nonpulsatile tinnitus. Pulsatile tinnitus was present at baseline in 52% and nonpulsatile tinnitus was present in 23% of participants in the IIHTT; one-third of patients had daily tinnitus.[40] The symptom is distressing and often interferes with hearing and sleeping. Pulsatile tinnitus may arise from vascular (eg, arterial abnormalities and fistulas) and nonvascular causes (eg, sigmoid sinus dehiscence and encephalocele).[42–45] Intracranial hypertension per se is likely not the cause of tinnitus in IIH as it is not present in other conditions producing elevated CSF pressure, such as hydrocephalus, trauma, and tumors. Sensorineural hearing at low, medium, or high frequencies may also occur.[46]

Impaired cognition

Patients with IIH often report impaired cognitive function or "brain fog." Subjective cognitive dysfunction was reported in 21% of IIHTT participants and negatively correlated with measures of physical and visual quality of life.[35] Cognitive dysfunction may result from intracranial hypertension, head pain, medications, depression, anxiety, fear of blindness, or a combination of factors. A prospective, case–control study of 31 patients with IIH found significantly impaired reaction time, processing speed, executive function, and visual memory in patients with IIH compared to controls.[47] Most patients were newly diagnosed and some domains improved when retested 3 months later. However, 71% of the patients with IIH had headaches and 26% endorsed depression, both potential confounders. No patients took acetazolamide, topiramate, opioids, or tranquilizers during testing. Another prospective study of 31 patients with IIH (mean disease duration 5.7 ± 4.1 years) found mild cognitive dysfunction overall compared to population norms, most notably in executive function, visual spatial function, and information processing speed.[48] None were being treated for anxiety or depression and 8 patients took acetazolamide. Although cognitive dysfunction in IIH is likely multifactorial, it may considerably impact work, driving, school, and functioning at home.

Visual loss

Thirty-two percent of IIHTT participants reported subjective visual loss, distinct from TVOs, at baseline and subjective visual loss occurs in more than 60% of patients in some series.[40,49,50] Patients may experience tunnel vision (peripheral visual field loss), temporal shadows (physiologic blind spot enlargement), hazy, cloudy, or blurred vision. Central visual loss (with decreased visual acuity) is more worrisome. Metamorphopsia (visual distortion, monocular diplopia, or monocular polyopia) suggests macular edema or exudates from high-grade papilledema. Both of these symptoms portend a poor prognosis and warrant urgent treatment. The tempo of visual loss is usually progressive but abrupt visual decline suggests superimposed optic nerve or retinal ischemia. Functional visual loss may occur at presentation or follow-up, producing visual field constriction resembling pattern of IIH.[51] Failure to recognize functional visual loss may lead to unnecessary procedures and surgery.

Diplopia
Binocular diplopia occurs in one-third to two-thirds of patients at presentation and was reported by 18% of patients in the IIHTT, being the presenting symptom in 2%.[24,40,52] Most commonly, the images are separated horizontally owing to a unilateral or bilateral abducens nerve palsy. A mild esophoria may produce incomplete diplopia with overlapping or elongated images.

Other symptoms and no symptoms
Back pain, including radicular pain, occurred in 53% of IIHTT participants, and 20% reported isolated radicular pain at any spinal level without back pain.[40] Other symptoms affecting over 20% of patients included nausea, vomiting, dizziness, and paresthesia. Atypical presenting symptoms include ataxia, facial paresis, arthralgias, trigeminal neuropathy (paresthesia or hypoesthesia), facial palsy, hemifacial spasm, olfactory dysfunction (hyposmia), torticollis, neck stiffness, tongue weakness, and seizures (from temporal lobe meningoencephalocele).[53]

IIH occasionally manifests as a skull base or spinal CSF leak. Papilledema is often absent in such cases. Brain MRI typically demonstrates an empty sella, and patients are at risk for developing symptomatic IIH when the leak is surgically repaired.[54,55]

IIH is sometimes discovered incidentally in children and adults when a routine eye examination reveals papilledema.[56,57] Those with incidentally discovered disease were less likely to experience headache, TVOs or diplopia, and also significantly less likely to need medical or surgical treatment than symptomatic patients.[58] They had better visual acuity and perimetry findings, less severe papilledema and lower CSF opening pressures than symptomatic patients with a favorable outcome.

SIGNS

Preserving vision is the most important aspect of managing patients with PTCS or IIH. Collaboration with an ophthalmologist or neuro-ophthalmologist is invaluable for assessing and following these patients.

Papilledema
Papilledema is the hallmark sign of intracranial hypertension. Thus, all patients being evaluated for headaches or pulsatile tinnitus require a fundoscopic examination. Papilledema is rarely unilateral, so viewing one normal-appearing optic disc does not ensure that the contralateral disc is normal.[54] High-grade papilledema is readily detected with a direct ophthalmoscope but mild papilledema may be difficult to discern, even for experienced examiners. Multiple techniques are available to complement the fundoscopic examination in such cases, including those described in the next section.

Papilledema is graded as 0 to 5 using the Frisén scale, with zero being normal and higher numbers representing more severe papilledema.[59] The Frisén scale is most useful in acute to subacute disease, as chronic or resolved disc edema often includes a component of optic atrophy. The Frisén scale and examples of various stages are displayed in **Box 3** and **Figs. 2–8**.

Important clinical concepts regarding the evaluation of papilledema include

- Fewer residents and medical students receive adequate training in fundoscopy than in the past. While the technologies below are helpful, they may not be available in the acute situation and some require expertise to correctly interpret them. There is still a role for fundoscopy!
- Competence in direct ophthalmoscopy takes practice. For examiners who are unable to view with each eye, the PanOptic ophthalmoscope offers a larger field

---

Box 3
Papilledema grading system (Frisén scale)

Stage 0: Normal optic disc
A. Blurring of nasal, superior, and inferior poles in inverse proportion to disc diameter
B. Radial nerve fiber layer (NFL) without NFL tortuosity
C. Rare obscuration of a major vessel, usually on the upper pole

Stage 1: Very early papilledema
A. Obscuration of the nasal border of the disc
B. No elevation of disc borders
C. Disruption of the normal radial NFL arrangement with grayish opacity accentuating nerve fiber bundles
D. Normal temporal disc margin
E. Subtle grayish halo with temporal gap (best seen with indirect ophthalmoscope or photography)
F. Concentric or radial retinochoroidal folds

Stage 2: Early papilledema
A. Obscuration of all borders
B. Elevation of the nasal border
C. Complete peripapillary halo

Stage 3: Moderate papilledema
A. Obscuration of all borders
B. Elevation of all borders
C. Increased diameter of the optic nerve head
D. Obscuration of one or more segments of major blood vessels leaving the disc
E. Peripapillary halo: irregular outer fringe with fingerlike extensions

Stage 4: Marked papilledema
A. Elevation of entire nerve head
B. Obscuration of all borders
C. Peripapillary halo
D. Total obscuration on the disc of a segment of a major blood vessel

Stage 5: Severe papilledema
A. Dome-shaped protrusions, representing anterior expansion of the optic nerve head
B. Peripapillary halo is narrow and smoothly demarcated
C. Total obscuration of a segment of a major blood vessel may or may not be present
D. Obliteration of the optic cup

From Frisén L. Swelling of the optic nerve head: a staging scheme. J Neurol Neurosurg Psychiatry 1982;45:13–8; with permission. Adapted from The Pseudotumor Cerebri Syndrome, NCL 32.2, P363-396, MAY 2014,

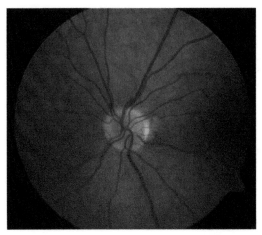

Fig. 2. Normal (stage 0) optic nerve. There is no peripapillary halo, obscuration of a major vessel crossing the disc margin, or disruption of the retinal nerve fiber layer (RNFL). This patient has no physiologic cup, a normal variant. (*Courtesy* of IIHTT Photography Reading Center, Rochester, NY.)

of view through an undilated pupil than direct ophthalmoscopy, gives a sense of depth, and may be used with the examiner's dominant eye alone.

- This reference[60] offers a practical guide to the bedside or office neuro-ophthalmic examination, including step-by-step instructions for performing fundoscopy.[60]
- Papilledema is only one cause of a swollen optic disc. Inflammation, acute ischemia, infiltration, and conditions causing pseudopapilledema (eg, optic disc drusen, tilted optic discs, and myelinated nerve fiber layer) mimic papilledema. Consider the appearance of the disc in the appropriate clinical context and be aware that pseudopapilledema may be difficult to distinguish from true papilledema using fundoscopy alone (**Figs. 9–11**).
- The most dramatic findings of papilledema, such as hemorrhages, exudates, vascular tortuosity, and cotton wool spots, are not included in the Frisén scale because they can occur in different papilledema grades.
- Atrophic optic nerves typically do not observably swell and cannot be used as a barometer of ICP (**Fig. 12**).
- Papilledema and optic disc drusen can coexist.[61]

The presence of spontaneous venous pulsations, which are best viewed over the disc with a direct ophthalmoscope, indicate that the CSF pressure is 190 mm CSF or less.[62] The converse is not true; many people with normal CSF pressure lack spontaneous venous pulsations. Advances in cell phone technology and deep learning may improve the detection of spontaneous venous pulsations in the future.[63,64]

Idiopathic Intracranial Hypertension Without Papilledema

Why might papilledema be absent in patients with IIH?

- The patient had previously undetected papilledema that resolved.
- A pre-existing optic neuropathy precluded the development of papilledema.

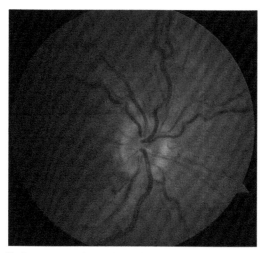

Fig. 3. Stage 1 papilledema. Note the C-shaped halo with a temporal gap. There is disruption of the normal RNFL and a normal temporal disc margin. (*Courtesy* of IIHTT Photography Reading Center, Rochester, NY.)

- CSF pressure was not sufficiently elevated or prolonged to produce papilledema.
- Recurrence of previous IIH associated with papilledema (gliotic changes in the nerve fiber layer from resolved papilledema precluded further disc swelling).

In the absence of papilledema, a definite diagnosis can be made if the other criteria are met plus a unilateral or bilateral abducens nerve palsy. Only a *suggested* diagnosis is possible incorporating 3 of the 4 neuroimaging findings:[1]

- Empty sella (pituitary flattening)
- Flattening of the posterior aspect of the globe

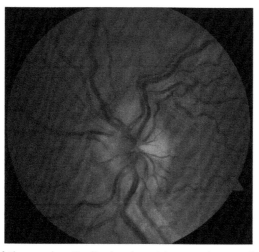

Fig. 4. Elevation of the nasal optic disc border with no major vessel obscuration and a circumferential peripapillary halo are characteristics of stage 2 papilledema. (*Courtesy* of IIHTT Photography Reading Center, Rochester, NY.)

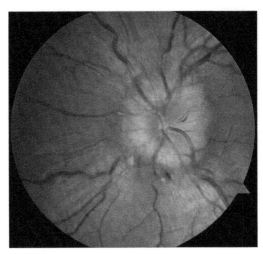

Fig. 5. Obscuration of one or more segments of a major blood vessel leaving the disc margin and elevation of all optic disc borders are seen in stage 3 papilledema. The outer fringe of the peripapillary halo is irregular with fingerlike extensions. (*Courtesy* of IIHTT Photography Reading Center, Rochester, NY.)

- Distention of the perioptic subarachnoid space with or without a tortuous optic nerve
- Transverse venous sinus stenosis

The initial validation study revealed that any 3 of the 4 MRI features was nearly 100% specific with a sensitivity of 64%.[65] Subsequent studies found similar results.[66,67] Transverse venous sinus stenosis had a sensitivity of 53.3% (95% CI 43.9%–62.4%) and specificity of 97.4% (95% CI 86.5%–99.5%) on MR venography (MRV)

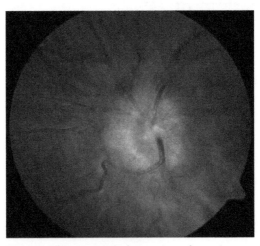

Fig. 6. Stage 4 papilledema. There is total obscuration of a major vessel on the optic disc with elevation of the entire optic nerve head and a complete peripapillary halo. (*Courtesy* of IIHTT Photography Reading Center, Rochester, NY.)

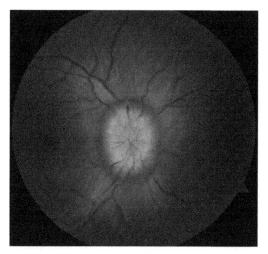

Fig. 7. Partial obscuration of all vessels leaving the disc and at least one vessel on the disc with diffuse optic nerve elevation and a complete peripapillary halo define stage 5 papilledema. (*Courtesy* of IIHTT Photography Reading Center, Rochester, NY.)

and a sensitivity of 45.5% (95% CI 34.8%–56.5%) and specificity of 100% (95% CI 83.2%–100%) on CT venography.[66]

The diagnosis of IIH without papilledema is controversial and likely overdiagnosed. Of 353 patients seen in a neuro-ophthalmology unit from 1990 to 2003 with a confirmed diagnosis of IIH, 20 (5.7%) had IIH without papilledema.[68] Compared with 20 patients with papilledema, matched for age and gender, those with papilledema had mean opening pressure of 373 mm CSF (range 260–550) and patients without papilledema had mean opening pressure of 309 mm CSF (range 260–420). The most common symptom in both groups was headache. Examination revealed spontaneous venous pulsations in 75% of patients without papilledema. Seventy

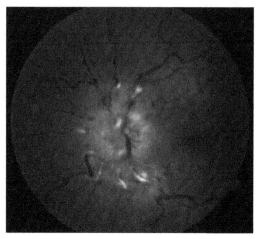

Fig. 8. Stage 4 papilledema with retinal exudates. (*Courtesy* of IIHTT Photography Reading Center, Rochester, NY.)

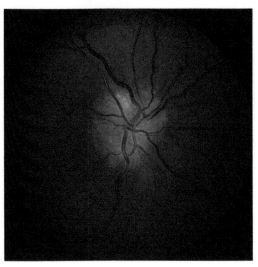

Fig. 9. The "lumpy-bumpy" irregular contour of optic disc drusen may simulate papilledema. (*Courtesy* of Valerie Biousse, MD, Atlanta, GA.)

percent had normal perimetry and 20% had nonphysiologic visual field constriction. Patients without papilledema were more refractory to diuretics and migraine treatment, had more LPs, and 4 underwent shunting to treat intractable headaches.

Another study diagnosed IIH in only 1 of 18 patients referred to a neuro-ophthalmology center with headache and a normal optic nerve appearance.[69] Most of the referred patients were overweight women leading to subconscious cognitive error and intuitive overdiagnosis. A subsequent study of 296 patients undergoing brain

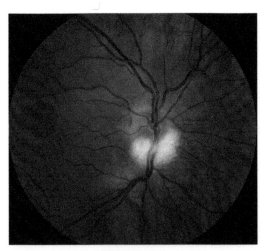

Fig. 10. Myelinated optic nerve fibers. The optic disc is surrounded inferiorly by myelinated, feathery nerve fibers. (*Courtesy* of Anil D. Patel, MD, FRCSC, FACS, Oklahoma City, OK.)

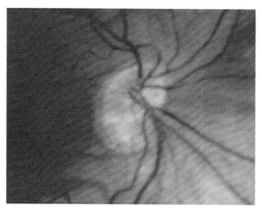

Fig. 11. Tilted optic disc. The temporal edge of the disc is tilted and appears elevated with an inferior nasal tilt. (*Image courtesy* of Kathleen B. Digre, MD. Neuro-Ophthalmology Virtual Education Library (NOVEL) – The Moran Eye Center Neuro-Ophthalmology Collection https://collections.lib.utah.edu/ark:/87278/s6s49q95)

MRI (for any indication) and fundus photography showed an imaging sign associated with IIH in half, most commonly empty sella (33.1%), enlarged Meckel caves (15.9%), and increased perioptic CSF (10.8%).[70] Only 5 patients had papilledema, including 3 with IIH and 2 with a glioblastoma. IIH was misdiagnosed in nearly 20% of case reports.[71]

In addition to subjecting patients to unnecessary testing and procedures, conveying an incorrect diagnosis has psychological implications. Patients seeking an explanation for their headaches and other symptoms often incorporate the misdiagnosis into their self-conception, and it is difficult to convince them later that the disorder is not present.

Retinal Manifestations

Optic neuropathy from papilledema is not the sole contributor to visual loss in IIH. Retinal abnormalities associated with IIH include subretinal fluid, chorioretinal folds, macular exudates, choroidal neovascular membrane, venous stasis retinopathy, choroidal infarction, and branch retinal vein occlusion.[72] Hemorrhages on the optic

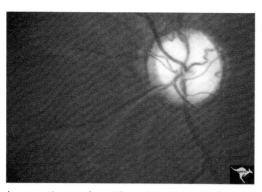

Fig. 12. Postpapilledema optic atrophy with peripapillary gliosis and arteriolar sheathing. (Image courtesy of William F. Hoyt, MD. Neuro-Ophthalmology Virtual Education Library (NOVEL) - The William F. Hoyt Neuro-Ophthalmology Collection https://collections.lib.utah.edu/ark:/87278/s6hq6wf8.)

disc, and cotton wool spots correlate with worse visual acuity and visual field loss at presentation.[73]

Ocular Motility Abnormalities

Unilateral or bilateral abducens nerve palsies are nonlocalizing signs of increased intracranial pressure, resulting in binocular, horizontal diplopia that is most apparent with distance viewing. Mild degrees of ophthalmoparesis and overlapping images that may be misinterpreted as blurred vision; monocular viewing with each eye independently (showing a single, clear image from each eye) reveals an ocular alignment problem. Examination shows an esotropia or esophoria (which may be asymptomatic). Vertical diplopia from a skew deviation, oculomotor (pupil sparing or complete) or trochlear nerve palsy, or multiple ocular motor nerve involvement is uncommon.[70] Complete or partial generalized ophthalmoplegia is rare, requiring exclusion of a secondary cause, such as cerebral venous sinus thrombosis.[74,75] Ocular motor paresis generally resolves with the reduction of CSF pressure.

EVALUATION
Fundus Imaging

Major advances in optic nerve and retinal imaging allow more accurate assessment of ocular structures affected by IIH. Some are widely available, others are emerging and all enhance the clinical database to guide treatment.

Optical coherence tomography

Spectral domain optical coherence tomography (OCT) uses infrared light reflection to image cross-sectional, high-resolution images of the optic nerve head, peripapillary retinal nerve fiber layer (RNFL), and macula[76] (**Fig. 13**). RNFL thickness correlates with LP opening pressure and increases with papilledema and other processes

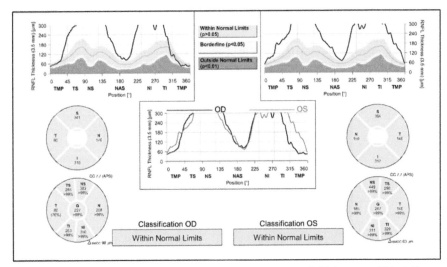

Fig. 13. OCT of bilateral papilledema. The green area is normal thickness and black line on top represents the RNFL thickness in each eye, which is so thick (elevated) that it is off the scale. The software's indication of "within normal limits" is erroneous, as normal average RNFL thickness (indicated in the center of the lower green circles) for individuals aged <70 years is 103.62 ± 8.29 μm.

causing optic disc elevation.[77] RNFL thinning arises from any condition producing optic nerve damage or atrophy. Thus, decreasing RNFL measurements may reflect improvement in optic disc edema and a good visual prognosis but can also indicate axonal loss.[78] OCT is useful for monitoring optic disc edema and differentiating it from pseudopapilledema caused by optic disc drusen. While very sensitive to changes in the optic nerve head geometry and surrounding retinal changes occurring with papilledema, OCT requires consistent technique and expert interpretation to avoid diagnostic errors. It is utilized as an adjunctive measurement with fundoscopy, perimetry, and fundus photography.

Fundus photography
Fundus photography is valuable for documenting the appearance of the optic nerve, vessels, and surrounding retina. Previously only obtainable in ophthalmology offices and performed by trained ophthalmic photographers, fundus photography is more widely available than ever before with the advent of nonmydriatic photography, table-top cameras, handheld cameras, and smart phone-based cameras. Given the challenges of learning fundoscopy, some neurologists and emergency departments have adopted nonmydriatic fundus photography as an alternative to direct ophthalmoscopy.[76] The resolution, field of view, image color, storage capacity, ability to transfer and store images, and cost vary widely.[79] Emerging artificial intelligence deep-learning systems provide a high degree of accuracy in the diagnosis of papilledema and other optic nerve and retinal disorders using photography without requiring input from an eye care specialist.[80]

Orbital ultrasonography
Orbital ultrasonography is a noninvasive technique that measures the optic nerve sheath diameter through a closed eyelid. The technique effectively differentiates true papilledema from optic nerve drusen and may be useful the detection and follow-up evaluation of papilledema in IIH. A meta-analysis assessing the correlation of optic nerve sheath diameter to CSF opening pressure found an overall accuracy of 0.811 to 0.945, but the risk of bias was relatively high with wide 95% CIs.[81]

Fluorescein angiography
Fluorescein angiography demonstrates the circulation of the retina as the intravenous fluorescein dye travels through the retinal choroid, arterioles, and then veins before being excreted by the kidneys. Papilledema produces extravasation of dye from the optic nerve head leading to pooling, leakage, and staining. Allergic reactions to fluorescein uncommonly occur and are fatal in 1 in 200,000 people.[82]

Visual Function Tests

Similar to glaucoma, papilledema preferentially affects the arcuate bundles of the RNFL sparing central acuity. Baseline evaluation in the IIHTT revealed visual acuity of 20/20 or better in 70.9% of the most affected (study) eyes and in 77.0% of fellow eyes.[40] However, visual acuity may deteriorate rapidly in IIH and decreased visual acuity at baseline portends a poor prognosis and reduced quality of life.[35,83]

Perimetry
Perimetry remains the most useful test for evaluating visual function and guiding treatment in PTCS or IIH. As most of the visual field loss is in the periphery, only about one-third of patients notice it.[84] Threshold automated perimetry is most widely used but Goldmann perimetry is helpful in patients with poor vision or slower response times. In addition to the pattern of visual field loss, the perimetric mean deviation (PMD) is

a summary statistic that compares the patient's responses to normal-sighted eyes at all points tested. PMD was the primary outcome measure in the IIHTT and is used to monitor visual status over time in clinical practice. Being a subjective test, perimetry is influenced by many factors, including patient alertness, concentration, and ability to constantly focus on the central fixation target.

The most common visual field defects at baseline in the IIHTT were nerve fiber bundle (arcuate) defects with or without enlargement of the physiologic blind spot, present in 79% of study eyes and 52% of fellow eyes[40] (**Fig. 13**). Central scotomas, paracentral scotomas, peripheral defects, and generalized constriction may occur[85] (**Fig. 14**). It is important to differentiate generalized constriction from functional visual loss.[51]

Imaging

MRI of the brain is the initial imaging test for suspected IIH, both to exclude another cause of intracranial hypertension or optic disc edema and to demonstrate abnormalities consistent with the disorder. Additional venous imaging (MR or computed tomographic [CT] venogram) helps to exclude cerebral venous sinus thrombosis and may reveal venous sinus stenosis related to IIH. Some patients have a normal MRI although imaging findings of increased CSF pressure are generally present. A CT scan with contrast is recommended if MRI is contraindicated or unavailable.[66] A systemic review and meta-analysis of MRI found a pooled sensitivity of ranging from 6.1% to 68.6% and pooled specificity ranging from 84.0% and 99.2%.[86] Transverse sinus stenosis had a pooled sensitivity of 84.4% (95% CI 65.9%–93.9%) and pooled specificity of 94.9% (95% CI 91.7%–96.9%).

Pituitary flattening (empty sella)

As IIH produces skull base and calvarial thinning, the most common brain imaging abnormality is pituitary flattening or "empty sella" (**Fig. 15**), which is most easily seen in the midline sagittal views.[87] The sellar floor is often expanded with an average cross-

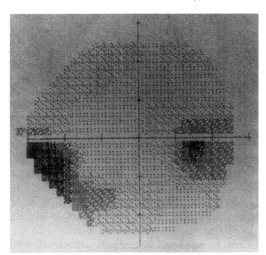

Fig. 14. Automated threshold perimetry (Humphrey Instruments, Allergan-Humphrey, San Leandro, CA, USA) of the central 24 shows an enlarged blind spot and inferonasal depression in a patient with pseudotumor cerebri and mild papilledema. (*From* Friedman DI. Pseudotumor cerebri. Neurosurg Clin North Am 1999;10:612; with permission. *Adapted from* The Pseudotumor Cerebri Syndrome, NCL 32.2, P363–396, MAY 2014, **Fig. 11**)

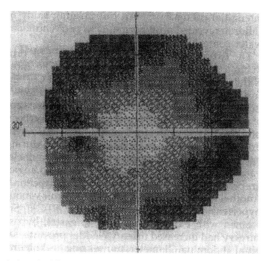

Fig. 15. Automated threshold perimetry (Humphrey Instruments, Allergan-Humphrey, San Leandro, CA, USA) of the central 24 degrees reveals a diffuse reduction in sensitivity with marked generalized constriction of the visual field. Nonphysiological visual field loss may cause a similar pattern of visual field loss and must be excluded. (*From* Friedman DI. Pseudotumor cerebri. Neurosurg Clin North Am 1999;10:613; with permission. *Adapted from* The Pseudotumor Cerebri Syndrome, NCL 32.2, P363–396, MAY 2014, see **Fig. 12**)

sectional area of the sella that is 38% greater than in controls.[88,89] Pituitary flattening is a highly specific finding of IIH (95.3%, P < .0001), and the changes are reversible with successful reduction of CSF pressure in some individuals. However, pituitary flattening is also present in the general population and may be an incidental finding.[70,89] It is more prevalent in female individuals and morbidly obese individuals, with increased age and in individuals with hormonal disturbances, psychiatric conditions, and sensorineural hearing loss.[90–92]

A study of patients with pulsatile tinnitus or IIH undergoing lateral sinus stent placement and a control group found that patients undergoing stent procedures had similar sellar volumes that were significantly higher than in controls (P < .001).[93] The authors postulated that an empty sella is a radiologic sign of lateral sinus stenosis rather than elevated intracranial pressure.

Orbital abnormalities
Orbital changes on MRI are assessed where the optic nerve head meets the globe. Axial brain MR images generally demonstrate the orbital abnormalities of IIH without obtaining special orbital views. The optic nerve head may protrude into the vitreous cavity with papilledema that is more apparent with contrast enhancement.[94] (**Fig. 16**) Other abnormalities include horizontal or vertical tortuosity of the intraorbital optic nerve and expansion of the perioptic subarachnoid space within the optic nerve sheath producing a CSF ring that is greater than 2 mm in width on the coronal images. The changes of the optic nerve sheath complex often improve after treatment but may not return to premorbid size due to altered compliance.[95,96]

Cerebral venous sinus changes
Farb and colleagues first described stenosis of the transverse and sigmoid sinuses on MRV in 2003.[17] They developed a grading system that defined as the highest degree of stenosis occurring from the torcular to the distal sigmoid sinus ranging from

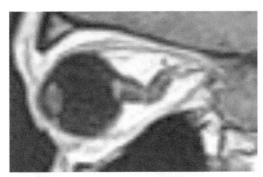

Fig. 16. Sagittal T2-weighted image of the orbit shows a tortuous optic nerve, expanded perioptic subarachnoid space and protrusion of the optic nerve head into the vitreous cavity. There is posterior globe flattening inferior to the optic nerve.

0 (discontinuity or aplastic segment) to 4 (no significant narrowing seen, 75%–100% of luminal diameter present).[17] Stenosis in IIH arises from either extrinsic brain compression producing smooth tapered narrowing or intraluminal obstruction by an enlarged arachnoid granulation. It is identified on postcontrast MR and MRV images. Venous sinus stenosis is the most sensitive and reliable imaging finding in IIH.[97] It is not exclusive to IIH; 33% of the general population has unilateral transverse sinus stenosis, 5% has bilateral stenosis and 1% has unilateral stenosis with contralateral hypoplasia.[98]

Other neuroimaging findings

- Dehiscence or thinning of the bone overlying the semicircular canals[99,100]
- Enlargement of Meckel cave
- Widened foramen ovale[96]
- Meningoceles, that is, protrusions of the meninges through the skull base at Meckel cave or the petrous apex, seen in approximately 10% of patients[101]
- Cerebellar tonsillar descent, present in 10% to 15% of patients, mimicking a Chiari I malformation but more likely to be associated with pituitary flattening and bilateral transverse sinus stenosis in IIH than in a true Chiari I. Clinical correlation in required to prevent unnecessary decompression surgery.[102]
- Skull base and calvarial thinning[87]

Cerebrospinal Fluid Pressure Measurement

An LP is required for the diagnosis of PTCS with the following goals:

- Meet the diagnostic criteria for a definite diagnosis
- Exclude abnormalities in the CSF composition suggestive of a secondary cause
- Transient or permanent symptomatic relief of headache
- Lower CSF pressure to temporize visual function

Several factors affect the CSF pressure measurement during an LP including the following:

- Patient positioning
  - The lateral decubitus position affords the most accurate measurement. When performed in the prone position, using the extension tubing to place the base of the manometer at the level of the right atrium approximates readings in the lateral decubitus with a margin of error of 10 mm CSF.[103]

- ○ Leg positioning (extended or flexed) has no significant effect on the measurement in children.[104]
- ○ Telemetric ICP monitors use a pressure sensor in the brain parenchyma readable by external hand-held equipment. A small study in women with IIH demonstrated increased ICP after prolonged recumbence but no diurnal variation.[105] As the device is implanted in the brain, its utility for routine management of IIH is limited.
- Sedation, respiratory rate
  - ○ Moderate-to-deep sedation may decrease the respiratory rate leading to hypercapnia and falsely elevated CSF pressure readings.[6]
  - ○ Data are conflicting but a randomized trial of ketamine, often used for sedation in children, concluded that it increased CSF pressure.[106]
- Medications
  - ○ Concurrent use of a CSF-lowering medication results in a misleadingly low measurement. The elimination half-life of a single dose of oral acetazolamide is 10 to 15 hours; thus, patients should discontinue the medication 2 to 3 days (5 half-lives) prior to the LP for an accurate assessment.[107]
  - ○ Serum half-lives of other medications used to treat IIH are acetazolamide extended-release capsules (10–15 hours), methazolamide (14 hours), furosemide (2 hours), dexamethasone (36–72 hours), prednisone (3–4 hours), and topiramate (21 hours).[107]
- Valsalva maneuver, crying, and pain
  - ○ Even when performed under fluoroscopic guidance, an LP is often painful and many patients have considerable anxiety regarding the procedure. Crying, muscular tensing, and Valsalva maneuvers increase CSF pressure.
  - ○ Normotensive patients can elevate their LP opening pressure into the abnormal range with voluntary Valsalva maneuver, sometimes doubling the baseline value.[108]
  - ○ Pretreatment with a mild anxiolytic may be helpful in such cases.
- Age
  - ○ A prospective study of 197 children aged up to 18 years showed a mean LP opening pressure of 196 mm CSF and the 10th and 90th percentile were 115 and 280 mm CSF, respectively.[5]
  - ○ Normal pressure in adults ranges from 60 to 250 mm CSF (median 180–190 mm CSF) with considerable variability and some normal individuals having pressures of 300 cm CSF or higher.[109]
- Body mass index
  - ○ The effect of BMI on CSF pressure is debatable but likely negligible.
  - ○ The IIHTT and earlier studies found no correlation between BMI and LP opening pressure.[110,111] Others studies found a linear correlation between BMI and LP opening pressure.[4,112,113]

Recommended CSF studies are glucose, protein, and cell count with differential. Patients with no apparent risk factors for IIH (eg, nonobese men, and young children) or atypical presentations warrant additional testing for malignancy, infectious, and inflammatory causes. CSF contents should be normal. CSF protein is normal (15–45 mg/dL) or in the lower range of normal but increases slightly with higher LP opening pressures.[114]

As patients often have relief of symptoms following an LP, remove enough CSF to achieve a closing pressure in the mid-to-high normal range (approximately 150–180 mm CSF).[115] Relying on volume alone as the endpoint ("high volume LP") has no definite benefit and may result in a post-LP headache requiring emergency visits and blood patches.[116,117]

Occasionally, patients with mild papilledema have long-lasting or permanent resolution of signs and symptoms following an LP. This is likely related to compensatory expansion of the cerebral venous sinuses with CSF removal, allowing greater absorption of CSF into the cerebral veins.

THERAPEUTIC OPTIONS

Multidisciplinary management is recommended with a "team captain" coordinating care, usually a neuro-ophthalmologist or neurologist. Other collaborators may include ophthalmologists, neurosurgeons, interventional radiologists, endocrinologists, weight management specialists, sleep specialists, headache medicine specialists and mental health providers, depending on a patient's needs.[118]

The overall approach to therapy is primarily informed by the patient's visual status, considering visual acuity, perimetry, and papilledema grade. Headache treatment and long-term management to control the disease and prevent recurrence are initiated concurrently.[118,119]

Do All Patients Need Treatment?

IIH is occasionally asymptomatic and incidentally discovered on routine eye examination. Such patients typically have mild disc edema and visual field loss but occasionally have a PMD in the moderate range (worse than 7 dB).[120] Whether this represents a milder form of disease or a presymptomatic phase is uncertain although the papilledema resolves after a short course of acetazolamide in most cases. It is imperative to confirm the diagnosis of IIH, exclude a secondary cause, and initiate treatment if visual field loss is present with adequate follow-up examinations to monitor the visual status.

Medical Therapy

No medication is approved by the Food and Drug Administration (FDA) for IIH treatment. Carbonic anhydrase inhibitors and other diuretics are typically first-line medications.

Acetazolamide and methazolamide. Acetazolamide is the only medication with class I evidence of effectiveness for patients with mild visual field loss based on the IIHTT (see "Headache" section).[29] It reduces the secretion of CSF from the choroid plexus by inhibiting carbonic anhydrase and is also a mild diuretic. Compared to the placebo group in the IIHTT, the acetazolamide group showed statistically significant improvement in PMD (primary outcome) in the more severely affected eye at 6 months (treatment effect 0.71 dB, 95% CI 0–1.54, $P = .050$).[29] Treatment effect in the fellow eye at 6 months also significantly improved. Participants with Frisén papilledema grade of 3 to 5 at baseline had experienced greater improvement in PMD than those with milder papilledema. Acetazolamide was also associated with greater improvement in papilledema grade, general and visual quality of life measures, weight loss, and LP opening pressure compared to placebo. The only metric for which acetazolamide was not superior to placebo was headache disability.

The recommended initial dosage of acetazolamide in adults is 500 mg bid, gradually increasing to a maximum 2000 mg bid as needed and tolerated. If the initial dose is not tolerated, it may be incrementally decreased. Common side effects are paresthesia, nausea, diarrhea, abdominal pain, fatigue, altered taste sensation, polyuria, and metabolic acidosis with low serum CO_2.[121,122] Metabolic acidosis is common and does not require treatment with sodium bicarbonate unless severe or the patient experiences dyspnea. Uncommon but severe reactions are Stevens–Johnson syndrome, aplastic anemia, and renal stones. The addition of other diuretics may cause profound hypokalemia, requiring close monitoring and potassium supplementation. Methazolamide (25–150 mg bid) was not studied in IIH but is generally better tolerated than acetazolamide and used in clinical practice.

Topiramate. Topiramate, which contains a sulfonamide group, also has carbonic anhydrase inhibiting properties with multiple additional actions, including the release of calcitonin gene-related peptide (CGRP) and glutamate from trigeminal nerve endings.[123] A prospective, randomized open-label study of topiramate and acetazolamide in 40 patients with mild visual loss showed improved perimetry in both cohorts with no statistically significant difference between groups.[124] Headaches improved in both groups but the topiramate group achieved greater weight loss. An in vivo study in healthy female rats found that subcutaneous topiramate lowered intracranial pressure at clinical and high doses by 32% ($P = .0009$) and 21% ($P = .15$), respectively, whereas acetazolamide, furosemide, amiloride, and octreotide had no significant effect on CSF pressure.[125]

Topiramate is initiated at 25 mg daily, gradually increasing the dosage to 50 mg bid or more depending on effectiveness and tolerability. Common, reversible, side effects are paresthesia, fatigue, anorexia, weight loss, nausea, diarrhea, cognitive impairment, and calcium phosphate nephrolithiasis.[123] Topiramate rarely precipitates bilateral acute angle closure glaucoma, typically within the first few weeks of treatment and related to choroidal effusion and secondary pupillary block.[126]

Furosemide and other diuretics. Furosemide is loop diuretic that reduces CSF secretion in the choroid plexus. It has never been studied as a single agent for IIH treatment and requires close electrolyte monitoring for hypokalemia and hyponatremia. Bumetanide, thiazide diuretics, ethacrynic acid, spironolactone, and amiloride are also options; the latter 3 do not contain a sulfonamide group.

Sulfa allergy considerations. The carbonic anhydrase inhibitors are sulfur based, in contrast to sulfonamide antibiotics that contain an arylamine side chain.[127] Although patients with "sulfa allergy" to sulfonamide antimicrobials are more likely to have an allergic reaction to sulfonamide nonantimicrobials (9.9% vs 1.6%), penicillin is a greater predictor of sulfonamide nonantimicrobial allergy (OR 3.9% 14.2%).[128] Thus, a previous allergic reaction to a sulfonamide antibiotic is not an absolute contraindication to a carbonic anhydrase inhibitor.

Other medications

- Corticosteroids: Corticosteroids acutely lower intracranial pressure but their withdrawal may precipitate IIH. Long-term usage is associated with weight gain, fluid retention, bone loss, and de novo intracranial hypertension. Corticosteroids are not recommended except for a short course of treatment in patients with fulminant IIH.
- Octreotide: A prospective series (n = 26) of daily subcutaneous octreotide, a somatostatin analog, showed improved symptoms and normalization of papilledema and CSF pressure with no recurrence over a 3 year period.[129]
- Metformin: A study of patients with (n = 23) and without (n = 9) polycystic ovary syndrome on stable conventional IIH treatment (acetazolamide, topiramate, and furosemide) compared adding metformin plus a low-calorie diet alone to the diet alone.[130] Women with PCOS treated with metformin and diet lost more weight (-7.7%, $P = .0015$) than those with PCOS treated with diet alone (n = 9, -3.3%) or women without PCOS but with hyperinsulinemia (n = 6) treated with metformin and diet (-2.4%). The percentage of women with papilledema decreased in all 3 groups with no between-group differences.

- GLP-1 receptor agonists: An open label study showed significantly more weight loss, decrease in headache days, and reduction in acetazolamide dosage with GLP-1 receptor agonists but no effect on visual parameters.[131] Gastrointestinal side effects were common. A small randomized, placebo-controlled trial of exenatide versus placebo showed a significant lowering of intracranial pressure up to 12 weeks.[132] Visual acuity improved slightly in the exenatide group with no change in PMD or RNFL thickness. Headache frequency and disability were unchanged, and there were no significant differences between groups in BMI or quality of life.

Headache treatment. Separate headache treatment is often needed in addition to CSF-lowering strategies. Headache medications are typically selected per the headache phenotype. None of the headache medications are specifically FDA-approved for IIH treatment. Nonsteroidal anti-inflammatory medications, simple analgesics, triptans, dihydroergotamine, lasmiditan, and gepants are options for acute treatment. Topiramate (discussed earlier) is FDA-approved medication for migraine prevention but contraindicated during pregnancy. Other options include low-dose tricyclic antidepressants, antihypertensives, onabotulinumtoxinA (chronic migraine phenotype), zonisamide, and anti-CGRP monoclonal antibodies.[133] Neuromodulation devices are nonpharmacologic options used for acute and preventive treatment. Opioids and preventive medications causing weight gain or fluid retention should be avoided. Careful monitoring and counseling are required to prevent acute medication overuse.

Therapeutic lumbar punctures. Therapeutic lumbar punctures are useful for treating occasional exacerbations, controlling CSF pressure during pregnancy and as a temporizing measure in patients with declining vision or fulminant IIH while awaiting surgery.

Weight management. Most patients with IIH are obese and many indicate a lifelong struggle with their weight. Weight loss improves many aspects of the disease over time, including recurrence.[134] A meta-analysis of bariatric surgery and nonsurgical weight loss published in 2017 concluded that bariatric surgery produced a substantially greater change in BMI (17.5 vs 4.2 kg/m^2) and was more effective than nonsurgical weight loss for improving papilledema and headache symptoms.[135] Previous studies indicated that a 6% to 10% reduction in weight when combined with medical therapy improved papilledema and visual field loss, forming the basis of the recommended initial goal for weight reduction.[136,137]

IIHTT participants incorporated a supervised low-sodium weight reduction diet with lifestyle modification.[29] Enrollees received weekly education and guidance from a weight loss coach with a goal of a 10% reduction in body weight over 6 months. Those assigned to receive acetazolamide experienced a greater reduction in weight (−7.50 kg, from 107.72 to 100.22 kg) than those assigned to placebo (−3.45 kg, from 107.72 kg to 104.27 kg; 95% CI −6.77 to −01.83, $P < .001$).

The IIH-Weight trial randomized 66 female individuals in the United Kingdom with active IIH and a BMI of 35 kg/m^2 or greater to bariatric surgery or community weight loss management program (Weight Watchers).[138] The primary outcome was LP opening pressure at 12 months. The Roux-en-Y procedure was most commonly selected. Overall retention of participants was excellent, but adherence to the Weight Watchers program was fairly low. CSF pressure significantly decreased in the bariatric surgery group compared to community weight loss arm (adjusted mean [SE] difference −6.0 [1.8] cm CSF; 95% CI −9.5 to −2.4 cm CSF, $P = .001$). A 24% loss of weight in the bariatric surgery group correlated with normalization of CSF pressure.[139]

Bariatric surgery is a viable option for motivated patients who can transform their eating habits and commit to postoperative follow-up to prevent nutritional complications. A meta-analysis assessing weight regain in individuals following Roux-en-Y and sleeve gastrectomy found that the incidence of weight-regain of greater than 10% was 17.6% (n = 2314, 95% CI 16.9–18.3).[140]

Neurosurgical and Interventional Techniques

Procedural treatment (CSF diversion and cerebral venous sinus stenting) is incorporated in patients with moderate and severe visual loss. There are no comparative trials to guide clinical decision-making which often depends on local resources and expertise.

Cerebrospinal fluid diversion procedures

The effectiveness of shunts for improving or stabilizing visual parameters is difficult to assess as they are not consistently evaluated and reported. A systematic review and meta-analysis of the shunting literature published from 1988 to 2019 included 15 studies and 372 patients undergoing LP shunting (LPS, 58.6%), ventriculoperitoneal (VP) shunting (VPS, 40.9%), and cisterno-atrial shunting (0.5%).[141] No study used standardized headache assessments. Shunting produced overall "complete" or "significant" improvement in 91% of patients with moderate heterogeneity. Eleven studies reported papilledema outcomes that improved by 95% with high heterogeneity. Overall improvement for visual outcomes (not otherwise specified) was 85% with high heterogeneity. Revisions were required in 155 patients having 436 revisions during the mean follow-up duration of 33.9 months, for an overall revision rate of 42% or 1.2 revisions per patient. Of those, the average number was 2.8 per patient, 4.7 in the LPS group and 1.3 per patient in the VPS group. The most common reason for revision was recurrent symptoms or signs of intracranial hypertension with shunt obstruction which is not always detectable on imaging studies.[142]

Complications reported by others also include meningitis, nerve root injury or radicular pain in the lumbar spine, cauda equina syndrome, flipping of the shunt valve in the peritoneum, wound healing issues, CSF fluid-cutaneous fistula, skin dehiscence, new cardiac arrhythmias, and seizure.[143,144] Shunt dependency may occur.[145] High complication rates of LPS and advances in technology shifted neurosurgical preference to VPS. The BASICS trial showed higher VPS revision rates in patients with IIH (32.9%) compared to participants without IIH (23.6%) with increased use of programmable valves and antisiphon in the cohort with IIH.[145]

Programmable differential control valves incorporate a hand-held programmer that uses a magnetic device to "unlock" the valve and change the setting. The higher the numerical valve setting, the higher the range of opening valve pressure (ie, less fluid is drained). Valves must also compensate for orthostatic changes in hydrostatic pressure, which sometimes require an antisiphon device placed distal to the shunt valve. Serious complications include intraventricular hemorrhage, infection, postoperative seizures, bowel perforation, and infection.[145] Most commonly used valves are MRI compatible up to 3Tesla.

Optic nerve sheath fenestration. Optic nerve sheath fenestration (ONSF) involves cutting incisions or windows into the optic nerve sheath to release the perineural subarachnoid CSF into the orbit.[146] Surgical approaches include orbitotomy and endonasal transsphenoid endoscopy.[147,148] The mechanism of improved papilledema is uncertain but may be related to fenestration itself, providing CSF egress or from secondary scarring between the optic nerve and the sheath, compartmentalizing the optic nerve from intracranial hypertension. ONSF is indicated for visual loss in the setting of papilledema and has several advantages over shunting.

- There is no indwelling hardware.
- It can be performed in the outpatient setting.
- A unilateral procedure may result in bilateral visual improvement.[149]

A systematic review from 1985 to 2014 included 525 procedures in 341 patients with a mean duration of follow-up of 42.3 months.[150] Visual acuity improved in 67%, visual field improved in 64%, and improvements in headache and papilledema were not reported.[150] Worsening of either visual field or papilledema occurred in 15.9% with an overall revision rate of 8%. Smaller studies in the pediatric population indicate ONSF successfully improves vision and papilledema.[151] A systematic review of 34 patients undergoing endonasal endoscopic ONSF found improvements in visual field (93.8%), visual acuity (85.3%), papilledema (81.4%), and headache (81.8%).[152] A small study found that 2 or 3 revisions can be successfully performed without an increased complication rates.[153]

Postoperative diplopia is typically transient but occasionally requires corrective strabismus surgery.[154] Less common complications are pupillary dysfunction, transient ocular discomfort, progressive visual decline, intrasheath hemorrhage, ischemic optic neuropathy, and localized peripheral corneal thinning.[149]

Cerebral venous sinus stenting. The postulated mechanism of efficacy of venous sinus stenting in IIH is alleviation of focal extramural compression.[155] Stenting increases the diameter and decreases the pressure in the narrowed cerebral venous sinus, restoring CSF absorption into the venous system (see **Fig.1**). Failure of or intolerance to medical treatment is generally a prerequisite for stenting; it has also been successfully used to treat fulminant IIH.[156] Stenting is only rarely considered for treating IIH without papilledema for headache alone.[157]

Cerebral venous angiography and manometry are performed after identifying a venous sinus stenosis on neuroimaging to identify potential candidates for stenting. A microcatheter or pressure guidewire is advanced into the stenotic dural venous sinus to measure the pressure differential proximal and distal to the stenosis (gradient).[158] The minimal gradient required for stenting is not standardized, but most centers require at least 8 to 10 mm Hg.[159] Several studies confirm that the larger the gradient, the greater the likelihood of success, and a systematic review concluded that a gradient of 21 mm Hg was more likely to result in favorable outcomes.[160,161] Follow-up angiography and manometry are performed after stent deployment. Patients take dual antiplatelet therapy prior to and for 3 to 6 months postprocedure.

A meta-analysis of stenting for IIH identified 49 studies of stenting reporting 1626 (83% female) individuals.[157] Although data were incomplete, and duration of follow-up varied between studies, improvements in presenting features were as follows: mean CSF pressure (average decrease 13.3 cm CSF, n = 250), TVOs (79.6%, n = 160), pulsatile tinnitus (84.7%, n = 515), diplopia (93%, n = 86), and nonspecific visual symptoms (eg, "blurred vision," 76.2%, n = 537). Papilledema resolved in 40.8% and improved in 38.2% (n = 1116). Headache resolved in 36.7% and improved in 40.7% (n = 1105). Perimetry (n = 386) improved in 239 patients, 125 were unchanged, and 17 worsened. Mean PMD improved from −7.35 to −4.72 dB. Nine percent required a secondary surgical or restenting procedure, which the authors believe is an underestimate related to limited follow-up time. The most common complications were headache (11.38%), stent thrombosis

(0.92%), stent-adjacent stenosis (2.46%), in-stent stenosis (1.48%), and femoral pseudoaneurysm (0.55%).

Uncommon complications included retroperitoneal or minor neck hematoma; 22.3% experienced persistence, and worsening and/or recurrence of their initial symptoms.[157] A large database study also found overall improvement after shunting and most patients were able to reduce oral medications.[162]

Other reported complications include hearing loss, dural intracranial fistula, occlusion of the contralateral sinus, and complications of antiplatelet therapy.[158] Serious adverse events occur less than 3% of cases, including stent thrombosis, subdural hematoma, subarachnoid hemorrhage, obstructive hydrocephalus, and death.[150]

Special Circumstances

Idiopathic intracranial hypertension and pregnancy. Although pregnant women are no more likely to develop IIH than age and parity-matched peers, IIH occurs during or just prior to pregnancy in 5% to 8% of cases, producing angst in patients and obstetricians alike.[163,164] It is imperative to exclude cerebral venous sinus thrombosis when IIH develops either during pregnancy or the postpartum period. IIH during pregnancy is managed similarly to the nongravid state, and there is no contraindication to women with IIH becoming pregnant. However, a study in the United Kingdom found that women with IIH had a lower live birth rates (54.1%) compared to women with PCOS (67.9%, $P < .0001$) and the general population (57.7%, $P < .0001$).[165] Concerningly, pre-eclampsia was 5.3 fold higher, gestational diabetes risk was higher, and elective cesarean section rates were more than twice that of the general population (OR 2.4) or with pregnancies prior to a diagnosis of IIH (OR 2.2).[165] The contribution of obesity to these findings is uncertain but likely relevant.

Acetazolamide is the first-line medical treatment. Furosemide, chlorthalidone, and hydrochlorothiazide have been successfully used but topiramate is contraindicated due to risk of teratogenicity.[166] Short courses of corticosteroids, such as dexamethasone, prednisone, prednisolone, and methylprednisolone, are employed in cases of visual deterioration. Avoiding excessive weight gain during gestation is recommended by employing dietary management without producing ketosis, which may harm the fetus.[166] Sequential LPs, shunting, and ONSF have sparse data for guidance although shunting carries the potential complications of infection and catheter perforation of the enlarging uterus or other organs in the peritoneal cavity. There are no reports of venous sinus stenting during pregnancy and the required antiplatelet therapy prior to and after stenting is contraindicated. The patient's visual status should be monitored throughout gestation.

IIH does not affect fetal outcomes, the method of delivery, or choice of anesthesia. Pregnancy termination is not needed although there are rare reports of improvement following termination of pregnancy, inducing early delivery or planned caesarean section in cases of fulminant IIH.[166]

Pediatric idiopathic intracranial hypertension. Many aspects of IIH are similar in adults and children, but some differences exist including the diagnostic LP opening pressure (see earlier discussion). Children may experience nausea or vomiting, are less likely than adults to have headaches and are more likely to be asymptomatic.[167]

Children should be carefully evaluated for secondary causes of the PTCS, including venous obstruction secondary to otitis media, mastoiditis, iron deficiency, and other hypercoagulable states.[168] Medications, such as tetracyclines, retinoids, vitamin A toxicity, corticosteroid withdrawal, and growth hormone replacement, are commonly implicated, particularly in teens undergoing acne treatment. Other symptoms and associated conditions are similar to those in adults.

Evaluation and treatment are the same as in adults. Children aged as young as 4 years can perform automated perimetry.[169] OCT is helpful as it is noninvasive and does not require pupillary dilation.[168] All of the surgical and interventional procedures used in adults have been incorporated in pediatric management, although not widely reported.

Fulminant idiopathic intracranial hypertension. Fulminant IIH is diagnosed when fewer than 4 weeks elapse between symptom onset and severe visual loss or when vision rapidly worsens over days.[170] Most patients are overweight female individuals of childbearing age although it has also been reported in children and men.[156] Patients with fulminant IIH are at high risk for profound visual loss and require inpatient treatment incorporating aggressive medical and surgical management strategies. Initiation of high-dose acetazolamide (oral or intravenous [IV]) with or without IV methylprednisolone is temporized with a lumbar drain, serial LPs, or extraventricular drainage if an interventional procedure is not readily available.[156] Shunting, ONSF, and stenting are employed as soon as possible, and more than 1 procedure is often required. After the initial management, patients should be followed closely to monitor for recurrence. Despite heroic efforts, devastating visual loss may occur.

Prognosis. Although most patients with IIH have very good outcomes regarding visual function,[171] relapse is possible. Risk factors identified for poor prognosis in the IIHTT were[83,172,173]

- Male sex
- Decreased visual acuity at baseline
- High-grade papilledema
- Randomization to placebo
- Optic disc hemorrhages at baseline.

Real-world evidence prospectively collected from 490 patients over a 9 year period showed that two-thirds of patients were in ocular remission at first visit.[174] Relapse occurred in 3.7%. The most predictive factor was papilledema as measured by OCT. Increases in BMI after diagnosis and disease duration were also impactful. A personal history of migraine and daily headaches at the initial visit portended a poor prognosis for ongoing headache.

Optic disc hemorrhages at baseline were a risk for poor visual outcome in the IIHTT.[173] Studies agree that the extent of transverse venous sinus stenosis on MRV does not predict visual outcome.[175,176]

A retrospective study in children (n = 103) seen between 2012 and 2020 found no relationship between age or LP opening pressure at presentation and long-term prognosis.[177] However, in a smaller pediatric study, the rate of recurrence was higher in prepubertal children than in adults, and 55.6% of children achieved complete clinical resolution.[178]

Other factors associated with poor prognosis are

- Anemia
- Renal failure
- Systemic hypertension
- Fulminant IIH
- Macular retinal ganglion cell-inner plexiform layer complex thickness on OCT at presentation[179]
- Generalized visual field constriction at presentation[180]
- Delay in treatment.[180]

SUMMARY

The diagnosis of PTCS and IIH is straightforward in most cases but underdiagnosis and misdiagnosis are still common, related to omission of fundoscopy, inaccurate interpretation of the optic disc appearance, and diagnosing IIH based on neuroimaging findings. Adherence to the diagnostic criteria helps to prevent these occurrences. IIH without papilledema is likely overdiagnosed owing to reliance on imaging findings or LP opening pressure, neither of which is specific for IIH.

Advances in technology allow neurologists to perform office-based fundus imaging. However, a multidisciplinary approach is still required to address the entire scope of management and ongoing monitoring is imperative. Medical and procedural interventions are incorporated in the early stages to preserve vision. Bariatric surgery and GLP-1 agonists have promise for producing adequate weight loss for disease remission. Additional headache treatment is warranted in many cases. Ongoing monitoring of visual function, headache, and weight is needed to prevent progression or relapse. Treatment failure is suspected when symptoms and signs worsen following any of the medical surgical or interventional procedures.

The prognosis is generally good, although ongoing headaches and reduced quality of life may persist. Some patients experience permanent visual field loss or blindness. IIH research is robust and progressing rapidly. Ambulatory telemetric ICP monitoring using an implanted sensor is evolving to provide measurements in real-world situations.[181] Emerging insights into the pathophysiology of IIH will hopefully translate into more effective and better-tolerated treatments.

CLINICS CARE POINTS

Major challenges faced by clinicians are

- Prompt and accurate diagnosis
- Excluding a secondary cause
- Accurate assessment of visual function and optic discs
- Effective therapy to reduce of CSF pressure
- Headache management
- Addressing relevant, contributory coexisting conditions
- Ongoing monitoring and preventing recurrence

DISCLOSURE

Dr D.I. Friedman served on advisory boards for Abbvie, Collegium, Eli Lilly, Impel NeuroPharma, Lundbeck, Pfizer, and Zosano Pharmaand and as a speaker for Abbvie and Impel Neuropharma. She is a consultant for Pfizer. She is on the editorial board of Neurology Reviews and the Journal of Neuro-Ophthalmology, medical advisor to the Spinal CSF Leak Foundation and HealthyWomen, and on the Board of Directors of the Southern Headache Society.

REFERENCES

1. Friedman DI, Liu GT, Digre KB. Revised diagnostic criteria for the pseudotumor cerebri syndrome in adults and children. Neurology 2013;81:1159–65.

2. Corbett JJ, Mehta MP. Cerebrospinal fluid pressure in normal obese subjects and patients with pseudotumor cerebri. Neurology 1983;33:1386–8.

3. Bateman DE, Wingrove B. Comparison of the range of lumbar cerebrospinal flid pressure in adults with normal cerebrospinal fluid pressure and in idiopathic intracranial hypertension. J Neuroophthlamol 2022;42:502–4.

4. Bo SH, Lundqvist C. Cerebrospinal fluid opening pressure in clinical practice – a prospective study. J Neurol 2020;267:3696–701.

5. Avery RA, Shah SS, Licht DJ, et al. Reference range for cerebrospinal fluid opening pressure in children. N Engl J Med 2010;363(9):891–3.

6. Avery RA. Reference range of cerebrospinal fluid opening pressure in children: historical overview and current data. Neuropediatrics 2014;45(4):206–11.

7. Radhakrishnan K, Ahlskog JE, Garrity JA, et al. Idiopathic intracranial hypertension. Mayo Clin Proc 1994;69:169–80.

8. McClusky G, Doherty-Allan R, McCarron P, et al. Meta-analysis and systemic review of population based epidemiological studies in idiopathic intracranial hypertension. Eur J Neurol 2018;25(10):1218–27.

9. Brahma V, Snow J, Tam V, et al. Socioeconomic and geographic disparities in idiopathic intracranial hypertension. Neurology 2021;96(23):e2854–60.

10. Hamdallah IN, Shamseddeen HN, Zelada Getty JL, et al. Greater than expected prevalence of pseudotumor cerebri: a prospective study. Surg Obes Relat Dis 2013;9(1):77–82.

11. Sheldon CA, Paley GL, Xiao R, et al. Pediatric idiopathic intracranial hypertension: age, gender, and anthropometric features at diagnosis in a large, retrospective, multisite cohort. Ophthalmology 2016;123(11):2424–31.

12. Kamboj A, Brown MM, Abel AS. Intracranial hypertension associated with testosterone therapy in female-to-male trangender patients: A case report and literature review. Semin Ophthalmol 2023;38(6):559–64.

13. Nayman T, Hébert M, Ospina LH. Idiopathic intracranial hypertension in a pediatric transgender patient. Am J Ophthalmol Case Rep 2021;24:10128.

14. Gutkind NE, Tse DT, Johnson TE, et al. Idiopathic intracranial hypertension in female-to-male transgender patients on exogenous testosterone therapy. Ophthalmic Plast Reconstr Surg 2023;39(5):449–53.

15. Hornby C, Mollan SP, Mitchell J, et al. What do transgender patients teach us about idiopathic intracranial hypertension? Neuro Ophthalmol 2017;41(6):326–9.

16. Dandy WE. Intracranial pressure without brain tumor: Diagnosis and treatment. Ann Surg 1937;106:492–513.

17. Farb RI, Vanek I, Scott JN, et al. Idiopathic intracranial hypertension: the prevalence and morphology of sinovenous stenosis. Neurology 2003;60:1418–24.

18. Westgate CSJ, Markey K, Mitchell JL, et al. Increased systemic and adipose 11β-HSD1 activity in idiopathic intracranial hypertension. Eur J Endocrinol 2022;187(2):323–33.

19. Botfield HF, Uldall MS, Westgate CSJ, et al. A glucagon-like peptide-1 receptor agonist reduces intracranial pressure in a rat model of hydrocephalus. Sci Transl Med 2017;9(404):eaan0972.

20. A trial to determine the efficacy and safety of Presendin in IIH. ClinicalTrials.gov Identifier NCT05347147 (accessed 12/21/23).

21. Ahrén B. Paradigm shift in the management of metabolic diseases- next generation incretin therapy. Endocrinology 2023;164(12). bquad166.

22. Digre KB, Corbett JJ. Idiopathic intracranial hypertension (pseudotumor cerebri): A reappraisal. Neurol 2001;7:2–67.

23. Friedman DI, Streeten DH. Idiopathic intracranial hypertension and orthostatic edema may share a common pathogenesis. Neurology 1998;50:1099–104.

24. Wall M, George D. Idiopathic intracranial hypertension: A prospective study of 50 patients. Brain 1991;114:155–80.

25. Mukharesh L, Mouffard MA, Fortin E, et al. Pseudotumor cerebri syndrome with COVID-19: A case series. J Neuro Ophthalmol 2022;42(3):e545–7.

26. Balendra R, North M, Kumar G, et al. Raised intracranial pressure (pseudotumor cerebri) associated with severe acute respiratory syndrome Coronavirus 2. J Neuroophthalmology 2022;42(2):e459–62.

27. Dinkin M, Sathi S. Neuro-ophthalmic visual impairment in the setting of COVID-19. Semin Neurol 2023;43(2):268–85.

28. Rabaji MT, Rafizadel SM, Aghajani AH, et al. Idiopathic intracranial hypertension as a neurological manifestation of COVID-19: A case report. J Fr Ophthalmol 2022;45(7):e303–5.

29. NORDIC Idiopathic Intracranial Hypertension Study Group Writing Committee, Wall M, McDermott MP, Kieburtz KD, et al. Effect of acetazolamide on visual function in patients with idiopathic intracranial hypertension and mild visual loss: the idiopathic intracranial hypertension treatment trial. JAMA 2014; 311(16):1641–51.

30. Friedman DI, McDermott MP, Kieburtz K, et al. The Idiopathic Intracranial Hypertension Treatment Trial: Design consideration and methods. J Neuro Ophthalmol 2014;34:107–17.

31. Friedman DI, Quiros PA, Subramanian PS, et al. Headache in idiopathic intracranial hypertension: Findings from the Idiopathic Intracranial Hypertension Treatment Trial. Headache 2017;57(8):1195–205.

32. The International Classification of Headache Disorders, 3rd edition (beta version). Cephalalgia 2013;33:644–82.

33. Mollen SP, Grech O, Sinclair AJ. Headache attributed to idiopathic intracranial hypertension and persistent post-idiopathic intracranial hypertension: A narrative review. Headache 2021;61(6):808–16.

34. Mulla Y, Markey KA, Wooley RL, et al. Headache determines quality of life in idiopathic intracranial hypertension. J Headache Pain 2015;16:521.

35. Digre KB, Bruce BB, McDermott MP, et al. Quality of life in idiopathic intracranial hypertension at diagnosis: IIH Treatment Trial results. Neurology 2015;84(24): 2449–56.

36. Adderley NJ, Subramanian A, Perrins M, et al. Headache, opiate use, and prescribing trends in women with idiopathic intracranial hypertension: A population-based matched cohort study. Neurology 2022;99(18):e1968–78.

37. Friedman DI, Rausch EA. Headache diagnoses in patients with treated idiopathic intracranial hypertension. Neurology 2002;58:1551–3.

38. Yri HM, Rönnbäck C, Wegener M, et al. The course of headache in idiopathic intracranial hypertension: a 12- month prospective follow-up study. Eur J Neurol 2014;21(12):1458–64.

39. Su M, Yu S. Chronic migraine: A process of dysmodulation and sensitization. Mol Pain 2018;14. 1744806918767697.

40. Wall W, Kupersmith MJ, Kieburtz KD, et al. The Idiopathic Intracranial Hypertension Trial. Clinical profiles at baseline. JAMA Neurol 2014;71(6):693–701.

41. Sadun AA, Wang MY. Abnormalities of the optic disc. Handb Clin Neurol 2011; 102:115–57.

42. Smith ER, Caton MT, Villanueva-Meyer JE, et al. Brain herniation (encephalocele) into arachnoid granulations: prevalence and association with pulsatile

tinnitus and idiopathic intracranial hypertension. Neuroradiology 2022;64(9): 1747–54.

43. Essibayi MA, Oushy SH, Lanzino G, et al. Venous causes of pulsatile tinnitus: clinical presentation, clinical and radiographic evaluation, pathogenesis, and endovascular treatments: A literature review. Neurosurgery 2021;89(5):760–8.

44. Kline NL, Angster K, Archer E, et al. Association of pulse synchronous tinnitus and sigmoid sinus wall abnormalities in patients with idiopathic intracranial hypertension. Am J Otolaryngol 2020;41(6):102675.

45. Widmeyer JR, Sismanis A, Felton W, et al. Magnetic resonance imaging findings in idiopathic intracranial hypertension with and without pulsatile tinnitus: An age-matched cohort study. Otol Neurotol 2023;44(5):525–8.

46. Shim T, Chillakuru Y, Moncada P, et al. Sensorineural hearing loss and tinnitus characteristics in patients with idiopathic intracranial hypertension. Otol Neurotol 2021;42(9):1323–8.

47. Yri HM, Fagerlund B, Forchhammer HB, et al. Cognitive function in idiopathic intracranial hypertension: a prospective case-control study. BMJ Open 2014; 4(4):e004376.

48. Zur D, Naftaliev E, Kesler A. Evidence of multidomain mild cognitive impairment in idiopathic intracranial hypertension. J Neuro Ophthalmol 2015;35(1):26–30.

49. Giuseffi V, Wall M, Siegel PZ, et al. Symptoms and disease associations in idiopathic intracranial hypertension (pseudotumor cerebri). Neurology 1991;41: 239–44.

50. Al-Hashel JY, Ismail II, Ibrahim M, et al. Demographics, clinical characteristics and management of idiopathic intracranial hypertension in Kuwait: A single-center experience. Front Neurol 2020;11:672.

51. Ney JJ, Volpe N, Liu GT, et al. Functional visual loss in idiopathic intracranial hypertension. Ophthalmology 2009;116:1808–13.

52. Matthews Y-Y, Dean F, Lim MJ, et al. Pseudotumor cerebri in childhood: incidence, clinical profile and risk factors in a national prospective population-based cohort study. Arch Dis Child 2017;1-2:715–21.

53. Chen BS, Newman NJ, Biousse V. Atypical presentations of idiopathic intracranial hypertension. Taiwan J Ophthalmol 2021;11(1):25–8.

54. Bidot S, Levy JM, Saindane AM, et al. Spontaneous skull base cerebrospinal fluid leaks and their relationship to idiopathic intracranial hypertension? Am J Rhinol Allergy 2021;35(1):36–43.

55. Sulioti G, Gray T, Amrhein TJ. Popping the balloon: Abrupt onset of a spinal CSF leak and spontaneous intracranial hypotension in idiopathic intracranial hypotension, a case report. Headache 2022;62(2):208–11.

56. Bassan H, Berkner L, Stolovitch C, et al. Asymptomatic idiopathic intracranial hypertension in children. Acta Neurol Scand 2008;118(4):251–5.

57. Lyons HS, Mollan SP, Liu GT, et al. Different characteristics or pre-pubertal and post-pubertal idiopathic intracranial hypertension: A narrative review. Neuro Ophthalmol 2022;47(2):62–74.

58. Vosoughi AR, Margolin EA, Miceli JA. Idiopathic intracranial hypertension: Incidental discovery versus symptomatic presentation. J Neuro Ophthalmol 2022; 42(2):187–91.

59. Frisén L. Swelling of the optic nerve head: a staging scheme. J Neurol Neurosurg Psychiatry 1982;45:13–8.

60. Friedman DI, Digre KB. Headache medicine meets neuro-ophthalmology: Exam techniques and challenging cases. Headache 2013;53(4):703–16.

61. Genizi J, Meiselles D, Arnowitz E, et al. Optic nerve drusen is highly prevalent among children with pseudotumor cerebri syndrome. Front Neurol 2021;12: 789673.

62. Jacks AS, Miller NR. Spontaneous venous pulsations: aetiology and significance. J Neurol Neurosurg Psychiatr 2003;7491:7–9.

63. Shariflou S, Agar A, Rose K, et al. Objective quantification of spontaneous retinal venous pulsations using a novel tablet-based ophthalmoscope. Transl Vis Sci Technol 2020;9(4):10.

64. Panahi A, Rezaee A, Jaajati F, et al. Autonomous assessment of spontaneous retinal venous pulsations in fundus videos using a deep learning framework. Sci Rep 2023;13(1):14445.

65. Mallery RM, Rehmani OF, Woo JH, et al. Utility of magnetic resonance imaging features for improving the diagnosis of idiopathic intracranial pressure without papilledema. J Neuro Ophthalmol 2019;39(3):299–307.

66. Wang MTM, Prime ZJ, Xu W, et al. Diagnostic performance of neuroimaging in suspected idiopathic intracranial hypertension. J Clin Neurosci 2022;96:56–60.

67. Korsbæk JJ, Jensen RH, Høgedal L, et al. Diagnosis of idiopathic intracranial hypertension: A proposal for evidence-based diagnostic criteria. Cephalalgia 2023;43(4). 333102431152795.

68. Digre KB, Nakamoto BK, Warner JEA, et al. A comparison of idiopathic intracranial hypertension with and without papilledema. Headache 2009;49(2):185–93.

69. Fisayo A, Bruce BB, Newman NJ, et al. Overdiagnosis of idiopathic intracranial hypertension. Neurology 2016;86(4):341–50.

70. Chen BS, Meyer BI, Saindane AM, et al. Prevalence of incidentally detected signs of intracranial hypertension on magnetic resonance imaging and their association with papilledema. JAMA Neurol 2021;78(6):718–25.

71. Eshtaighi A, Zaslavsky K, Nicholson P, et al. Extent of transverse sinus stenosis does not predict visual outcomes in idiopathic intracranial hypertension. Eye 2022;36:1390–5.

72. Nichani P, Micieli JA. Retinal manifestations of idiopathic intracranial hypertension. Ophthalmol Retina 2021;5(5):429–37.

73. Micieli JA, Bruce BB, Vasseneix C, et al. Optic nerve appearance as a predictor of visual outcome in patients with idiopathic intracranial hypertension. Br J Ophthalmol 2019;103(10):1429–35.

74. Mathkour M, Scullen T, Kilgore M, et al. Complete ophthalmoplegia secondary to idiopathic intracranial hypertension managed successfully by dural sinus stenting: A case report and systematic review. Clin Neurol Neurosurg 2021;209: 106910.

75. Friedman DI, Forman S, Levi L, et al. Unusual ocular motility disturbances with increased intracranial pressure. Neurology 1998;50:1893–6.

76. Biousse V, Danesh-Meyer HV, Saindane AM, et al. Imaging of the optic nerve: technological advances and future prospects. Lancet Neurol 2022;21(12): 1135–50.

77. Vijay V, Mollan SP, Mitchell JL, et al. Using optical coherence tomography as a surrogate of measurements of intracranial pressure in idiopathic intracranial hypertension. JAMA Ophthalmol 2020;138:1264–71.

78. Huang-Link Y, Eleftheriou A, Yang G, et al. Optical coherence tomography represents a sensitive and reliable tool for routine monitoring of idiopathic intracranial hypertension with and without papilledema. Eur J Neurol 2019;26:808-e57.

79. Mishra C, Tripathy K. Fundus camera. In: StatPearls. Treasure Island (FL): StatPearls Publishing; 2023.

80. Biousse V, Newman NJ, Najjar RP, et al. Optic disc classification by deep learning vs expert neuro-ophthalmologists. Ann Neurol 2020;88:785–95.
81. Robba C, Santori G, Czosnyka M, et al. Optic nerve sheath diameter measured sonographically as non-invasive estimator of intracranial pressure: a systematic review and meta-analysis. Intensive Care Med 2018;44:1284–94.
82. Baddam DO, Ragi SD, Tsang SH, et al. Ophthalmic fluorescein angiography. Methods Mol Bio 2023;2560:153–60.
83. Wall M, Falardeau J, Fletcher WA, et al. Risk factors for poor visual outcome in patients with idiopathic intracranial hypertension. Neurology 2015;85(9): 799–805.
84. Wall M. The importance of visual field testing in idiopathic intracranial hypertension. Continuum 2014;20:1067–74.
85. Wall M, Subramani A, Chong LX, et al. Threshold static automated perimetry of the full visual field in idiopathic hypertension. Invest Ophthalmol Vis Sci 2019; 60(6):1895–905.
86. Kwee RM, Kwee TC. Systemic review and meta-analysis of MRI signs for diagnosis of idiopathic intracranial hypertension. Eur J Radiol 2019;116:106–15.
87. Barke M, Muniz Castro H, Adesina O-OO, et al. Thinning of the skull base and calvarial thickness in patients with idiopathic intracranial hypertension. J Neuro Ophthalmol 2022;42(2):192–8.
88. Kyung SE, Botelho JV, Horton JC. Enlargement of the sella turcica in pseudotumor cerebri. J Neurosurg 2014;120(2):538–42.
89. Barkatullah AF, Leishangthem L, Moss HE. MRI findings as markers of idiopathic intracranial hypertension. Curr Opin Neurol 2021;34:75–823.
90. Hardjasudarma M, White KE, Nandy I, et al. Sellar emptiness on routine magnetic resonance imaging. South Med J 1994;87(3):340–3.
91. Schmill L-PA, Peters S, Juhasz J, et al. MRI signs of intracranial hypertension in morbidly obese and normal-weight individuals. Röfo 2024;196(2):176–85.
92. Debnath J, Ravikumar R, Sharma V, et al. 'Empty sella' on routine MRI studies: An incidental finding or otherwise? Med J Armed Forces India 2016;72(1):33–7.
93. Zetchi A, Labeyrie M-A, Nicolini E, et al. Empty sella is a sign of symptomatic lateral sinus stenosis and not intracranial hypertension. Am J Neuroradiol 2019;40(10):1694–700.
94. Passi N, Degnan A, Levy L. MR imaging of papilledema and visual pathways: Effects of increased intracranial pressure and pathophysiologic mechanisms. Am J Neuroradiol 2012;34(5):919–24.
95. Batur Caglayan H, Ucar M, Hasanreisoglu M, et al. Magnetic resonance imaging of idiopathic intracranial hypertension. J Neuro Ophthalmol 2019;39(3):324–9.
96. Butros SR, Goncalves LF, Thompson AD, et al. Imaging features of idiopathic intracranial hypertension, including a new finding: widening of the foramen ovale. Acta Radiol 2012;53(6):682–8.
97. Zhao K, Gu W, Liu C, et al. Advances in the understanding of the complex role of venous sinus stenosis in idiopathic intracranial hypertension. J Magn Reson Imag 2022;56(3):545–54.
98. Durst CR, Ornan DA, Reardon MA, et al. Prevalence of dural venous sinus stenosis and hypoplasia in a generalized population. J Neurointerventional Surg 2016;8(11):1173–7.
99. Lansley JA, Tucker W, Eriksen MR, et al. Sigmoid sinus diverticulum, dehiscence, and venous sinus stenosis: Potential causes of pulsatile tinnitus in patients with idiopathic intracranial hypertension? AJNR 2017;38:1783–8.

100. Berkiten G, Gürbüz D, Akan O, et al. Dehiscence or thinning or bone overlying the superior semicircular canal in idiopathic intracranial hypertension. Eur Arch Oto-Rhino-Laryngol 2022;279(6):2899–904.

101. Bialer OY, Rueda MP, Bruce BB, et al. Meningoceles in idiopathic intracranial hypertension. Am J Roentgenol 2014;202(3):608–13.

102. Ebrahimzadeh SA, Du E, Chang Y-M, et al. MRI findings differentiating tonsillar herniation caused by idiopathic intracranial hypertension from Chiari I malformation. Neuroradiology 2022;64(12):2307–14.

103. Abel AS, Brace JR, McKinney AM, et al. Effect of patient positioning on cerebrospinal opening pressure. J Neuro Ophthalmol 2014;3493:218–22.

104. Avery RA, Mistry RD, Shah SS, et al. Patient positioning during lumbar puncture has no meaningful effect on cerebrospinal fluid opening pressure in children. J Child Neurol 2010;25:616–9.

105. Mitchell JL, Buckham R, Lyons H, et al. Evaluation of diurnal and postural intracranial pressure employing telemetric monitoring in idiopathic intracranial hypertension. Fluids Barriers CNS 2022;19:85.

106. Michalczyk K, Sullivan JE, Berkenbosch JW. Pretreatment with midazolam blunts the rise in intracranial pressure associated with ketamine sedation for lumbar puncture in children. Pediatr Crit Care Med 2013;14:e149–55.

107. Available at: https://www.PDR.net. Accessed December 15, 2023.

108. Neville L, Egan RA. Frequency and amplitude of elevation of cerebrospinal fluid resting pressure by the Valsalva maneuver. Can J Ophthlamol 2005;40(6):775–7.

109. Lee SCM, Lueck CJ. Cerebrospinal fluid pressure in adults. J Neuro Ophthalmol 2014;34(3):278–83.

110. Bono F, Lupdao MR, Sera P, et al. Obesity does not induce abnormal CSF pressure in patients with normal MR venography. Neurology 2002;59:1641–3.

111. Whitely W, Al-Shahi R, Warlow CP, et al. CSF opening pressure: reference interval and the effect of body mass index. Neurology 2006;67:1690–1.

112. Wakerley BR, Warner R, Cole M, et al. Clin Neurol Neurosurg 2020;188:105597.

113. Berdahl JP, Fleischman D, Zaydlarova J, et al. Body mass index has a linear relationship with cerebrospinal fluid pressure. Invest Ophthalmol Vis Sci 2012;53(3):1422–7.

114. Berezovsky E, Bruce BB, Vasseneix C, et al. Cerebrospinal total protein in idiopathic intracranial hypertension. J Neurol Sci 2017;381-226:9.

115. Perloff MD, Parikh SK, Fiorito-Torres F, et al. Cerebrospinal fluid removal for idiopathic intracranial hypertension: Less cerebrospinal fluid is best. J Neuro Ophthalmol 2019;39(3):330–2.

116. Lu P, Goyal M, Huecker J, et al. Identifying incidence of and risk factors for fluoroscopy-guided lumbar puncture and subsequent persistent low-pressure syndrome in patients with idiopathic intracranial hypertension. J Neuro Ophthalmol 2019;39(2):161–4.

117. Didier-Laurent A, De Gaalon S, Ferhat S, et al. Does post-dural puncture headache exist in idiopathic intracranial hypertension? A pilot study. Rev Neurol (Paris) 2021;177(6):676–82.

118. Mollan SP, Davies B, Silver NC, et al. Idiopathic intracranial hypertension: consensus guidelines on management. J Neurol Neurosurg Psychiatry 2018;89(10):1088–100.

119. Hoffmann J, Mollan SP, Paemeleire K, et al. European Headache Federation guidelines on intracranial hypertension. J Headache Pain 2018;19(1):93.

120. Rohani N, Foroozan R. Clinical course of asymptomatic patients with papilledema from idiopathic intracranial hypertension. Can J Ophthalmol 2023;58(4): 324–7.
121. Schmickl CN, Owens RL, Orr JE, et al. Side effects of acetazolamide: a systemic review and meta-analysis assessing overall risk and dose dependence. BMJ Open Respir Res 2020;7(1):e000557.
122. ten Hove MW, Friedman DI, Patel AD, et al. Safety and tolerability of acetazolamide in the Idiopathic Intracranial Hypertension Trial. J Neuro Ophthalmol 2016;36(1):13–9.
123. Hu C, Zhang Y, Tan G. Advances in topiramate as prophylactic treatment for migraine. Brain Behav 2021;11(10):e2290.
124. Çelebisoy N, Gökçay F, Şirin H, et al. Treatment of idiopathic intracranial hypertension; topiramate vs. acetazolamide, an open-label study. Acta Neurol Scand 2007;116:322–7.
125. Scotton WJ, Botfield HF, Westgate CSJ, et al. Topiramate is more effective than acetazolamide at lowering intracranial pressure. Cephalalgia 2019;39(2): 209–18.
126. Al Owaifeer AM, AlSultan ZM, Badawi AH. Topiramate-induced angle closure: A systematic review of case reports and case series. Indian J Ophthalmol 2022; 70(5):1491–501.
127. Shah TJ, Moshirfar M, Hoopes PC Sr. "Doctor, I have a sulfa allergy." Clarifying the myths of cross reactivity. Ophthlamol Ther 2018;7(2):211–5.
128. Strom BL, Schinnar R, Apter AJ, et al. Absence of cross-reactivity between sulfonamide antibiotics and sulfonamide non-antibiotics. N Engl J Med 2003; 349(17):1628–35.
129. Panagopoulos GN, Deftereos SN, Tagaris GA, et al. Octreotide: a therapeutic option for idiopathic intracranial hypertension. Neurol Neurophysiol Neurosci 2007;10:1.
130. Glueck CJ, Golnik KC, Aregawi D, et al. Changes in weight, papilledema, headache, visual field, and life status in response to diet and metformin in women with idiopathic intracranial hypertension with and without concurrent polycystic ovary syndrome or hyperinsulinemia. Transl Res 2006;148(5):215–22.
131. Krajnc N, Itariu B, Macher S, et al. Treatment with GLP-1 receptor agonists is associated with significant weight loss and headache outcomes in idiopathic intracranial hypertension. J Headache Pain 2023;24(1):89.
132. Mitchell JL, Lyons HS, Walker JW, et al. the effect of GLP-1RA exenatide on idiopathic intracranial hypertension: a randomized controlled trial. Brain 2023; 146(5):1821–30.
133. Yiangyou A, Mitchell JL, Fisher C, et al. Erenumab for headaches in idiopathic intracranial hypertension. Headache 2021;61(1):157–69.
134. Ko MW, Chang SC, Ridha MA, et al. Weight gain and recurrence in idiopathic intracranial hypertension: a case-control study. Neurology 2011;76(18):1564–7.
135. Manfield JH, Yu K-H, Efthimiou E, et al. Bariatric surgery or non-surgical weight loss for idiopathic intracranial hypertension? A systematic review and comparison meta-analysis. Obes Surg 2017;27(2):513–21.
136. Kupersmith MJ, Gamell L, Turbin R, et al. Effect of weight loss on the course of idiopathic intracranial hypertension in women. Neurology 1998;50:1094–8.
137. Johnson LN, Krohel GB, Madsen RW, et al. The role of weight loss and acetazolamide in the treatment of idiopathic intracranial hypertension (pseudotumor cerebri). Ophthalmology 1998;105:2313–7.

138. Mollan SP, Mitchell JL, Ottridge RS, et al. Effectiveness of bariatric surgery vs community weight management intervention for the treatment of idiopathic intracranial hypertension: a randomized clinical trial. JAMA Neurol 2021;78(6): 678–86.

139. Mollan SP, Mitchell JL, Yiangou A, et al. Association of amount of weight lost after bariatric surgery with intracranial pressure in women with idiopathic intracranial hypertension. Neurology 2022;99(11):e1090–9.

140. Athanasiadis DI, Martin A, Kapsampelis P, et al. Factors associated with weight regain post-bariatric surgery: a systematic review. Surg Endosc 2021;35: 2069–84.

141. Salih M, Enriquez-Marulanda A, Khorasanizedeh M, et al. Cerebrospinal fluid shunting for idiopathic intracranial hypertension: A systematic review, meta-analysis, and implications for a modern management protocol. Neurosurgery 2022;91:529–40.

142. Liu A, Elder BD, Sankey EW, et al. Are shunt series and shunt patency studies useful in patients with shunted idiopathic intracranial hypertension? Clin Neurol Neurosurg 2015;138:899–993.

143. Brune A, Girgla T, Trobe JD. Complications of ventriculoperitoneal shunt for idiopathic intracranial hypertension: A single-institution study of 32 patients. J Neuro Ophthalmol 2021;41(2):224–32.

144. Azad TD, Shang Y, Varshneya K, et al. Lumboperitoneal and ventriculoperitoneal shunting for idiopathic intracranial hypertension demonstrate comparable failure and complication rates. Neurosurgery 2020;86(2):272–80.

145. Sunderland GJ, Jenkinson MD, Conroy EJ, et al. Neurosurgical CSF diversion in idiopathic intracranial hypertension: A narrative review. Life 2021;11:393.

146. Chen H, Zhang Q, Tan S, et al. Update on the application of optic nerve sheath fenestration. Restor Neurol Neurosci 2017;35(3):275–86.

147. Blessing NW, Tse DT. Optic nerve sheath fenestration: A revised lateral approach for nerve access. Orbit 2019;38(2):137–43.

148. Santos RC, Gupta B, Santiago RB, et al. Endoscopic endonasal optic nerve sheath decompression (EONSD) for idiopathic intracranial hypertension: Technical details and meta-analysis. Clin Neurol Neurosurg 2023;229:107750.

149. El-Masri S, Wilson M, Goh J, et al. A 20-year multicentre retrospective review of optic nerve sheath fenestration outcomes. Ther Adv Neurol Disord 2023;16. 17562864231197994.

150. Kalyvas AV, Hughes M, Koutsarmakis C, et al. Efficacy, complications and cost of surgical interventions for idiopathic intracranial hypertension: a systemic review of the literature. Acta Neurochir 2017;158(1):33–49.

151. Bersani TA, Meeker AR, Sismanis DN, et al. Pediatric and adult vision restoration after optic nerve sheath decompression for idiopathic intracranial hypertension. Orbit 2016;35(3):132–9.

152. Tarrats L, Hernández G, Busquets JM, et al. Outcomes of endoscopic optic nerve sheath decompression in patients with idiopathic intracranial hypertension. Int Forum Allergy Rhinol 2017;7(6):615–23.

153. Anzeljc AJ, Fias P, Hayak BR, et al. A 15-year review of secondary and tertiary optic nerve sheath fenestration for idiopathic intracranial hypertension. Orbit 2018;37(4):266–72.

154. Gilbert AL, Chwalisz B, Mallery R. Complications of optic nerve sheath fenestration as a treatment for idiopathic intracranial hypertension. Semin Ophthalmol 2018;33(1):36–41.

155. Lim J, Monteiro A, Kuo CC, et al. Stenting for venous sinus stenosis in patients with idiopathic intracranial hypertension: An updated systematic review and meta-analysis of the literature. Neurosurgery 2023. https://doi.org/10.1227/neu.0000000000002718. Online ahead of print.

156. Bouffard MC. Fulminant idiopathic intracranial hypertension. Curr Neurol Neurosci Rep 2020;20(4):8.

157. Dinkin MJ, Patsalides A. Idiopathic intracranial venous hypertension: toward a better understanding of venous sinus stenosis and the role of stenting in idiopathic intracranial hypertension. J Neuroophthalmology 2023;45:451–63.

158. Kabanovski A, Kisilevsky E, Yang Y, et al. Dural venous sinus stenting in the treatment of idiopathic intracranial hypertension: A systemic review and critique of the literature. Surv Ophthalmol 2022;65(1):271–87.

159. Akhter A, Schulz L, Inger HE, et al. Current indications for management options in pseudotumor cerebri. Neurol Clin 2022;40(2):391–404.

160. McDougall CM, Ban VS, Beecher J, et al. Fifty shades of gradients: does pressure gradient in venous sinus stenting for idiopathic intracranial hypertension matter? A systematic review. J Neurosurg 2018;130(3):999–1005.

161. Wang S, Tong X, Li X, et al. Association of post-intervention pressure gradient with symptom-free at 6 months in idiopathic intracranial hypertension with venous sinus stenosis treated by stenting. Intervent Neuroradiol 2023;29(4):413–8.

162. Nia AM, Srinivasan VM, Lall R, et al. Dural venous sinus stenting in idiopathic intracranial hypertension: A national database study of 541 patients. World Neurosurg 2022;167:e451–5.

163. Digre KB, Varner MW, Corbett JJ. Pseudotumor cerebri and pregnancy. Neurology 1984;34(6):721–9.

164. Sundholm A, Burkill S, Walendlind E, et al. A national Swedish case-control study investigating incidence and factors associated with idiopathic intracranial hypertension. Cephalalgia 2021;41(14):1427–36.

165. Thaller M, Mytton J, Wakerley BR, et al. Idiopathic intracranial hypertension: Evaluation of births and fertility through the Hospital Episode Statistics dataset. BJOG 2022;129(12):2019–27.

166. Scott C, Kaliaperumal C. Idiopathic intracranial hypertension and pregnancy: A comprehensive review of management. Clin Neurol Neurosurg 2022;217:107240.

167. Gaier ED, Heidary G. Pediatric idiopathic intracranial hypertension. Semin Neurol 2019;39(06):704–10.

168. Cleves-Bayon C. Idiopathic intracranial hypertension in children and adolescents: An update. Headache 2018;58(3):485–93.

169. Stiebel-Kalish H, Lusky M, Yassur Y, et al. Swedish interactive thresholding algorithm fast for following visual fields in prepubertal idiopathic intracranial hypertension. Ophthalmology 2004;111(9):1673–5.

170. Thambisetty M, Lavin PJ, Newman NJ, et al. Fulminant idiopathic intracranial hypertension. Neurology 2007;68:229–32.

171. Xu W, Prime Z, Papchenko T, et al. Long term outcomes of idiopathic intracranial hypertension: Observational study and literature review. Clin Neurol Neurosurg 2021;205:106463.

172. Behbehani R, Ali A, Al-Moosa A. Course and predictors of visual outcome of idiopathic intracranial hypertension. Neuro Ophthalmol 2021;46(2):80–4.

173. Wall M, Thurtell MJ, NORDIC Idiopathic Intracranial hypertension Study Group. Optic disc haemorrhages at baseline as a risk factor for poor outcome in the

Idiopathic Intracranial Hypertension Treatment Trial. Br J Ophthalmol 2017; 101(9):1256–60.

174. Thaller M, Homer V, Hyder Y, et al. The idiopathic intracranial hypertension prospective cohort study: evaluation of prognostic factors and outcomes. J Neurol 2023;270(2):851–63.

175. Eshtaighi A, Zaslavshy K, Nicholson P, et al. Extent of transverse stenosis does not predict visual outcomes in idiopathic intracranial hypertension. Eye (Lond) 2022;36(7):1390–5.

176. Riggeal BD, Bruce BB, Saindane AM, et al. Clinical course of idiopathic intracranial hypertension with transverse sinus stenosis. Neurology 2013;80(3):289–95.

177. Ozturk G, Turkdogan D, Unver O, et al. How do presentation age and CSF opening pressure affect long-term prognosis of pseudotumor cerebri in children? Experience of a single tertiary clinic. Childs Nerv Sys 2022;3891:95–102.

178. Ávarez FL, Fernández-Ramos JA, León RC, et al. Pseudotumor cerebri in the paediatric population: clinical features, treatment and prognosis. Neurologia 2021;S0213-4853(21):00085–92.

179. Chen JJ, Thurtell MJ, Longmuir R, et al. Causes and prognosis of visual acuity at the time of initial presentation in idiopathic intracranial hypertension. Invest Ophthalmol Vis Sci 2015;56(6):3850–9.

180. KesKin AO, Idiman F, Kaya D, et al. Idiopathic intracranial hypertension: Etiological factors, clinical features, and prognosis. Noro Psikiyatr Ars 2018;57(1):23–6.

181. Mitchell JL, Mollan SP, Vijay V, et al. Novel advances in monitoring and therapeutic approaches in idiopathic intracranial hypertension. Curr Opin Neurol 2019; 32(3):422–31.

Spontaneous Intracranial Hypotension

Clinical Presentation, Diagnosis, and Treatment Strategies

Jr-Wei Wu, MD[a,b,c], Shuu-Jiun Wang, MD[a,c,d],*

KEYWORDS

- Spontaneous intracranial hypotension • Spinal CSF leaks • Low-pressure headache
- Epidural blood patch • MR myelography • CT myelography

KEY POINTS

- SIH is not always present as an orthostatic headache; orthostatic headache could not always be attributed to SIH.
- MR myelography is an accurate and non-invasive approach for identifying and localizing spinal CSF leaks.
- The duration of the symptoms is an important factor when using brain MRI findings alone for diagnosing SIH.
- Epidural blood patch with large blood volume (>22.5 mL) is the preferred treatment for SIH.
- We reserved surgical repair for patients not responsive to 3 or 4 EBPs.

INTRODUCTION

Spontaneous intracranial hypotension (SIH) is a group of clinical conditions caused by spinal cerebrospinal fluid (CSF) leaks from dural ruptures, leaking meningeal diverticulum, or CSF-venous fistula.[1–3] The annual incidence of SIH is estimated at 3.7 per 100,000 individuals.[4] SIH exhibits a female predominance with a female/male ratio of approximately 2:1, predominantly in individuals from their mid-30s to mid-50s.[5] The most common symptom of SIH is acute orthostatic headaches, which are

[a] Department of Neurology, Neurological Institute, Taipei Veterans General Hospital, No. 201, Sec. 2, Shi-Pai Road, Taipei, 11217, Taiwan; [b] Center for Quality Management, Taipei Veterans General Hospital, No. 201, Sec. 2, Shi-Pai Road, Taipei, 11217, Taiwan; [c] College of Medicine, National Yang Ming Chiao Tung University, No. 155, Sec. 2, Shi-Pai Road, Taipei, 11217, Taiwan; [d] Brain Research Center, National Yang Ming Chiao Tung University, No. 155, Sec. 2, Shi-Pai Road, Taipei, 11217, Taiwan
* Corresponding author. Neurological Institute, Taipei Veterans General Hospital, No. 201, Sec. 2, Shi-Pai Road, Taipei 11217, Taiwan.
E-mail addresses: sjwang@vghtpe.gov.tw; k123.wang@msa.hinet.net

Neurol Clin 42 (2024) 473–486
https://doi.org/10.1016/j.ncl.2024.02.002
0733-8619/24/© 2024 Elsevier Inc. All rights reserved.

generally similar to symptoms of low-pressure headaches secondary to dural puncture, trauma, or other surgical procedures,[5] but more severe and protracted. Currently, the International Classification of Headache Disorders, 3rd edition (ICHD-3), states that an SIH diagnosis (code 7.2.3) involves low CSF pressure (<60 mm CSF) and/or a CSF leak suggestive via imaging. Of note, the SIH might manifest even without a CSF pressure less than 60 mm CSF, implying that CSF volume reduction or CSF hypovolemia might be more relevant than pressure reduction in its pathophysiology.[6] Also, despite the term "spontaneous" in its diagnostic entity, many patients have trivial injuries or intense activities before SIH.[2] There are several spinal neuroimaging findings in SIH, which could directly or indirectly identify the spinal CSF leaks.[7,8] In the past decade, CSF-venous fistulas has been proposed as a novel cause of SIH.[9] Also, a wide variety of brain MRI abnormalities have been described, along with the development of a scoring system based on these findings, providing valuable diagnostic assistance.[10]

CLINICAL PRESENTATIONS

The clinical presentation of SIH is classified into classical and nonclassical symptoms.[1] The classical symptom of SIH is acute orthostatic headache that typically worsens on sitting or standing and alleviates when lying down.[3] One myth is that all patients with SIH have an orthostatic headache.[11] However, previous studies showed that typical orthostatic headache accounts for 75% to 93% of patients with SIH.[5,12] Conversely, orthostatic headaches might have several differential diagnoses.[11,13] For example, postural orthostatic tachycardia syndrome is an autonomic dysfunction characterized by orthostatic intolerance and abnormally increased heart rates when shifting to an upright posture, commonly accompanied by fatigue, nausea, and headache.[2] Other conditions, such as persistent postural-perceptual dizziness or vasovagal syncope, should be considered in patients with orthostatic headaches.[13]

The nonclassical symptoms could be further divided into headache and nonheadache atypical symptoms.[2] Among nonclassical headache symptoms, headache in SIH might mimic migraine or tension-type headache without an obvious orthostatic component.[14] Also, some patients might present with thunderclap headaches, cough headaches, exercise headaches, or even sex-induced headaches.[14–16] In some situations, patients might report a daily headache that resembles a new daily persistent headache.[13] Therefore, a detailed history taking for the initial clinical presentations and evidence of trivial trauma before the new-onset headache is crucial for making a tentative diagnosis of SIH. However, patients with SIH may exhibit a spectrum of nonheadache symptoms, which can occur with or without the presence of headaches.[1] Previous reports showed SIH might present as conscious disturbance, frontotemporal-like dementia, abducens nerve palsies, oculomotor or trochlear nerve palsies, parkinsonian features, and even chorea.[2] The pathophysiology behind these symptoms might be linked to brain descent resulting from a decreased CSF volume and reduced buoyant effect.[2] The sinking brain with tension or compression on various cranial or brainstem structures leads to the crowding of the posterior fossa and traction of brain structures, and results in these neurologic symptoms.[2] Another group of nonheadache atypical symptoms is cochleovestibular manifestations, including hyperacusis, tinnitus, or dizziness.[2] The underlying mechanism of cochleovestibular symptoms in SIH is changes in perilymph pressure.[17] These atypical clinical presentations of SIH are also important in daily practice because this group of patients is easily misdiagnosed as other disorders and the treatment of spinal CSF leaks might be delayed.

DIAGNOSIS

The criteria for diagnosing SIH, as defined in the ICHD-3, encompass the demonstration of characteristic signs on head MRI, the detection of CSF leakage via spinal imaging, or the confirmation of reduced CSF pressure through lumbar puncture (**Box 1**).[6] In the subsequent paragraphs, we provide an in-depth overview of each diagnostic procedure.

LUMBAR PUNCTURE

Confirming low CSF pressure (<60 mm CSF) by lumbar puncture was previously considered a required examination for SIH. Nonetheless, it is noteworthy that not all individuals with SIH consistently have a low CSF pressure lower than the diagnostic threshold (ie, <60 mm CSF).[11] One study found that only 34% of confirmed SIH cases exhibited CSF pressures less than 60 mm CSF, and 21% of patients had pressures exceeding 120 mm CSF.[18] The same study showed that 5% of patients have an open pressure exceeding 200 mm CSF.[18] Also, a large meta-analysis that included 738 patients from 21 papers found that 32% of confirmed patients with SIH had normal open pressure, 67% had low pressure (<6 mm CSF), and 3% had high pressure (>200 mm CSF).[5] In fact, the actual percentage of SIH with normal CSF pressure might be higher than the published cases because some patients might not receive a definite diagnosis of SIH or have not been published. Given that normal CSF pressure does not exclude the possibility of SIH, and the lumbar puncture *per se* causes or worsens spinal CSF leaks, the diagnostic value of lumbar puncture for SIH is debatable.[11] In our experience, we usually perform gadolinium-enhanced brain MRI and spinal neuroimaging at the same time to make the diagnosis and the spinal leaking sites of SIH.

SPINAL NEUROIMAGING

Currently, several spinal neuroimaging methods have been developed for the diagnosis of SIH, localization of the leaks, or determining the cause.[7] The spinal neuroimaging

---

Box 1
The ICHD-3 diagnostic criteria of low-pressure headache and SIH

7.2 Headache attributed to low CSF pressure
A. Any headache fulfilling criterion C.
B. Either or both of the following:
    1. Low CSF pressure (<60 mm CSF).
    2. Evidence of CSF leakage on imaging.
C. Headache has developed in temporal relation to the low CSF pressure or CSF leakage, or led to its discovery.
D. Not better accounted for by another ICHD-3 diagnosis.

7.2.3 Headache attributed to spontaneous intracranial hypotension
A. Headache fulfilling criteria for 7.2 Headache attributed to low CSF pressure, and criterion C below.
B. Absence of a procedure or trauma known to be able to cause CSF leakage.
C. Headache has developed in temporal relation to occurrence of low CSF pressure or CSF leakage, or has led to its discovery.
D. Not better accounted for by another ICHD-3 diagnosis.

Note:
1. 7.2.3 *Headache attributed to spontaneous intracranial hypotension* cannot be diagnosed in a patient who has had a dural puncture within the prior month.
2. Dural puncture to measure CSF pressure directly is not necessary in patients with positive MRI signs of leakage, such as dural enhancement with contrast.

methods include spinal MRI, computed tomography myelography (CTM), radionuclide cisternography, magnetic resonance myelography (MRM; with and without intrathecal gadolinium), and digital subtraction myelography (DSM).[7] In this review, the strengths and limitation of these examinations are described next.

Computed Tomography Myelography

CTM is widely used for localizing the leak sites, which could directly demonstrate the spinal CSF leaks and confirm the diagnosis.[7] The CTM relies on dural puncture and injection of the iodinated contrast into the thecal sac, followed by a whole spine computed tomography (CT) scan.[19] In SIH, patients may show extravasation of contrast outside of the dura.[19] Nonetheless, in instances of high-flow CSF leaks, the contrast material may spread quickly within the epidural space, potentially dispersing before the CT scan.[7] Consequently, CTM may not effectively detect the leak site in patients with high-flow CSF leaks.[7] To solve this problem, some institutions introduced ultrafast dynamic CTM, capturing images immediately after the intrathecal contrast injection. For better neuroimaging acquisition, patients need to rapidly change their postures, including lateral decubitus position, prone, and supine positions.[20] Another strength of dynamic CTM is that it could help identify CSF-venous fistula, a newly described cause for SIH in 2014.[9,21] In CTM, the contrast material could be found in the spinal segmental vein, intercostal vein, or vertebral epidural venous plexus.[9] The shortcomings of CTM include its invasive nature and the associated radiation risk. Moreover, the necessity of lumbar puncture for the contrast injection might aggravate CSF leakage.

Magnetic Resonance Myelography (With and Without Intrathecal Gadolinium)

Spinal MRI is frequently used in the detection of CSF leaks in cases of SIH.[7] The protocols for detecting SIH include conventional T2-weighted MRI, noncontrast MRM, and intrathecal gadolinium-enhanced MRM (Gd-MRM).[7] Using conventional T2-weighted spinal MRI, spinal CSF leaks are often indicated by a T2 hyperintense fluid signal in the extradural space. Nonetheless, in the absence of fat suppression, fat and fluid can appear hyperintense in T2-weighted images. To differentiate fluid and fat, T1-weighted imaging is helpful, because leaked fluid typically exhibits a decreased T1 signal, aiding in its identification. However, the heavily T2-weighted MRM, a noninvasive technique that has no need for intravenous or intrathecal contrast, offers a better visualization of spinal CSF leaks.[22] This method uses the fast spin echo method to further enhance the CSF high signal intensity and has shown efficacy comparable with CTM.[22] This imaging method can categorize spinal CSF leaks into three distinct types: (1) high-cervical retrospinal CSF collections, (2) CSF leaks along the nerve root sleeve, and (3) epidural CSF collections (**Fig. 1**).[22] A high-cervical retrospinal CSF collection is a known false localization indicator, because it does not indicate the site of CSF leaks.[23] Following a dural tear, the leaked CSF spreads into the epidural space or exits the spinal canal through the neuroforamina, leading to the epidural CSF collections and CSF leaks around the nerve root sleeve.[7] Moreover, the extent of this epidural CSF collection had prognostic significance; patients with a longer anterior (or ventral) epidural CSF collection usually require more epidural blood patches (EBPs) for treating the spinal CSF leaks.[24] One recent study confirms that MRM is not inferior to CTM for the detection of SIH.[25]

Intrathecal Gd-MRM is a novel imaging approach that enables the direct observation of spinal CSF leaks.[7] The Gd-MRI involves the intrathecal injection of gadolinium, followed by T1-weighted spinal MRI. This technique seeks to take advantage of direct observation of CSF leaks with contrast of CTM and the better contrast resolution of

MRI. Studies comparing the diagnostic efficacy of Gd-MRM and CTM have found that Gd-MRM can identify an additional 21% to 23% of patients with SIH who tested negative with CTM.[26,27] This suggests that Gd-MRM might be more effective in detecting leaks associated with meningeal diverticula.[26,27] However, intrathecal gadolinium is not currently approved by the Food and Drug Administration and remains an off-label use.[7,28]

Digital Subtraction Myelography

DSM has a good temporal resolution and is effective in pinpointing the leaked site.[29] The DSM involves a fluoroscopy-guided lumbar puncture followed by the intrathecal administration of a contrast agent.[7] Subsequent to contrast injection, the procedure table is inclined head-downward, allowing for real-time visualization of the contrast medium's leakage through dural defects.[7] DSM works better in identifying the leaks on the dependent part of the thecal sac, with a restricted coverage area. Moreover, this invasive diagnostic procedure requires patient cooperation or even general anesthesia in some cases.[7] The strength of DSM is to identify high-flow leaks, but the use of DSM is limited by its invasive nature and, thus, not the first choice of spinal work-up for SIH.[7]

Radionuclide Cisternography

Radionuclide cisternography, first developed by Di Chiro in 1964[30] and once a regular method for detecting spinal CSF leaks, is no longer included in the ICHD-3 recommendations.[6,31] This technique involves intrathecal administration of radiotracer through lumbar puncture. There are two kinds of tracer: indium 111 diethylenetriaminepenta-acetic acid (^{111}InDTPA) and technetium-99m-diethylene-triamine-pentaacetate (^{99m}Tc-DTPA), but only ^{111}InDTPA was approved by the European Medicines Agency.[32] After the intrathecal injection, patients receive sequential scans immediately after injection, then 1, 2, 4, 24, or 48 hours postinjection.[32] The image findings for spinal CSF leakage could be categorized into direct and indirect (or surrogate) signs.[32] The direct sign is the accumulation of radiotracer in parathecal areas adjacent to the leak sites. However, because of its limited resolution, direct identification of the CSF leak sites is rarely observed in radionuclide cisternography.[33] Indirect signs encompass a reduced radiotracer activity over cerebral convexities, and activity usually does not extend beyond the basal cisterns.[32] Additionally, early tracer presence in the kidneys and bladder indicates indirect evidence of CSF leakage, although this may be confounded by systemic absorption of the tracer at the lumbar puncture site.[32] A significant limitation of this method is its poor spatial and temporal resolution. However, radionuclide cisternography allows sequential scanning with an extended duration, which offers a unique advantage, particularly in detecting CSF leaks with extremely slow flow rates.[7]

BRAIN NEUROIMAGING

In real-world practice, some patients might not have classic orthostatic headaches as their initial presentation, and these patients with neurologic manifestations more often receive a head MRI instead of spinal imaging as their first neuroimaging study. Hence, it is important to recognize typical MRI findings of SIH. To date, several brain MRI findings for SIH have been reported, and the main brain MRI findings are shown in **Fig. 1**.[2,34,35] According to their underlying mechanism, these brain morphologic changes could be classified as cerebral venous dilation-related and brain descent-related MRI findings.[10,34]

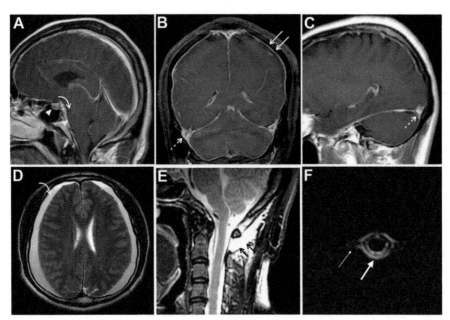

Fig. 1. (*A*) Sagittal T1-weighted image (T1WI) C + MR shows narrowed midbrain-pons angle (*curved arrow*), pituitary hyperemia (*white arrowhead*), flattening of pons or effacement of the prepontine cistern (*yellow arrowhead*), and narrowed angle between the vein of Galen and straight sinus (*red lines*). (*B*) Sagittal T1WI C + MR shows pachymeningeal enhancement (*arrows*) and engorgement of venous sinus (*dotted arrow*). (*C*) Sagittal T1WI C + MR shows venous distention sign of transverse sinus (*dotted arrow*). (*D*) Axial T2WI MR shows bilateral subdural effusion (*curved arrow*). (*E*) Sagittal T2WI MR shows high-cervical retrospinal CSF collections (*arrows*), which is a false indicator of CSF leak site. (*F*) MRM shows epidural CSF collections (*thick arrow*) and periradicular leaks along the nerve root sleeve (*thin arrow*).

Cerebral Venous Dilation–Related MRI Findings

The cerebral venous dilation–related findings can be explained by the Monro-Kellie doctrine.[10,36] The Monro-Kellie doctrine posits that the total volume of brain tissue, blood vessels, and CSF within the cranial cavity is fixed.[3] During CSF hypovolemia, a compensatory expansion of the vascular components may occur.[3] Because of the superior elasticity of venous walls relative to arterial walls, the cerebral venous system is more likely to dilate as a compensation for decreased CSF volume.[10] The brain MRI signs that link to this mechanism include diffuse pachymeningeal enhancement, the venous distention sign, and pituitary hyperemia (or pituitary enlargement).[10] Diffuse pachymeningeal enhancement might be the most well-known brain MRI finding of SIH.[3] However, some conditions might mimic the pachymeningeal enhancement in SIH, such as metastasis, lymphoma, or pachymeningitis of granulomatous disease. These conditions usually have a heterogeneous pattern and thus could be used for differential diagnosis.[37] MRI findings associated with dilation of cerebral sinuses are also important cues for the neuroimaging diagnosis, which could be observed in the transverse sinus or superior sagittal sinus.[35] Among them, the convex of the dominant transverse sinus in sagittal view, namely the venous distention sign, is helpful for diagnosing SIH (sensitivity, 94%; specificity, 94%).[38] Pituitary hyperemia or enlarged pituitary gland has been reported in SIH and frequently misinterpreted as a tumor or adenoma.[39] However, several factors, such as gender and age, are associated with the diameter of the pituitary gland and hamper its diagnostic value for SIH.[40]

Brain Descent–Related MRI Findings

In addition to cerebral venous dilation, the depletion of CSF causes a negative pressure and a reduced buoyancy of these intracranial structures and results in a downward shift of brain structures in SIH.[10] Several brain descent–related MRI findings have been described, including the narrowed midbrain-pons angle (or pontomesencephalic angle),[24] narrowed prepontine cisternal space thickness,[35] narrowed angle between the vein of Galen and straight sinus,[41] flattening of pons,[42] tonsillar descent, and posterior fossa crowdedness.[11] In patients with brain descent–related MRI findings, it is important to differentiate SIH from Chiari malformation type 1 because both conditions might have a displacement of the cerebellar tonsils.[43] Compared with Chiari malformation type 1, patients with SIH are more likely to have a narrow midbrain-pons angle (<45°) and a narrower slope of the third ventricular floor (<−15°).[43] Of note, the midbrain-pons angle could be used as a predictor for treatment outcome; patients with a midbrain-pons angle greater than or equal to 40° are generally associated with a better response to EBP.[24]

Time Sequence of Different MRI Findings

The presence of brain MRI findings of SIH is associated with the duration from disease onset. For example, the diffuse pachymeningeal enhancement might not be present in some patients with a short interval (∼6.5 days) after symptom onset.[44] Also, the presence cerebral venous dilation–related findings is generally earlier than brain descent–related MRI findings.[34] Therefore, it is dangerous to exclude the possibility of SIH simply based on the absence of brain MRI abnormalities.[34] In recent years, a scoring system based on six brain MRI findings, namely the Bern score, had been proposed for the diagnostic purpose of SIH.[35] According to this scoring system, a score less than two points indicates low probability, a score between three and four points suggests intermediate probability, and a score of greater than or equal to five points is high probability for SIH.[35] However, our recent study found that patients with SIH with a shorter disease duration (<17 days) are less likely to have a score of greater than or equal to five points.[45] In patients with less than 17 days of symptom onset, it is better to arrange further work-ups for spinal CSF leaks in those with score greater than or equal to three points.[45] Therefore, the duration of the symptoms is an important factor when using brain MRI findings alone for diagnosing SIH.[34]

TREATMENT

The treatment of SIH includes conservative treatment, EBP, and surgical repair. Recently, an early EBP has been the mainstream treatment strategy.[46] The following paragraph details the current therapeutic options.

Conservative Treatments

Conservative approaches for SIH typically encompass such measures as strictly bed rest, sufficient hydration (2.0–2.5 L daily), analgesics, steroid, and caffeine.[46] To date, the effectiveness of these conservative treatments has not been evaluated in controlled studies. A recent meta-analysis examined 748 patients from 17 articles, which found only 28% of patients response to conservative treatment.[5] Given the potentially devastating complications of SIH, such as subdural hematoma, more aggressive interventions should be considered earlier.[45] In our practice, a targeted

EBP is often used at an early stage, sometimes even bypassing initial conservative treatments.

The conservative treatments also include medication options, namely caffeine, steroids, and theophylline. In a double-blind placebo-controlled study, caffeine 300 mg/day just temporarily alleviated the intensity of postdural puncture headache (PDPH), yet patients ultimately required an EBP.[47] Another option is theophylline, with a randomized controlled trial demonstrating that patients who received 250 mg of intravenous aminophylline experienced a reduction in headache intensity 8 hours after treatment compared with those in the placebo group.[48] Although case reports have suggested the efficacy of corticosteroids in this context, a controlled study found no significant therapeutic advantage of corticosteroids in the treatment of PDPH.[49] It is important to note that although SIH and PDPH are characterized by spinal CSF leaks, differences exist in the location and volume of these leaks. Consequently, the findings from studies on treatment of PDPH may not be directly applicable to SIH cases.

Epidural Blood Patch

EBP is the treatment of choice for SIH with good effectiveness and acceptable side effects.[3] It could be performed by an experienced anesthesiologist or neuroradiologist, with local anesthesia.[46] The effectiveness of EBP stems from two mechanisms: the immediate and late effect.[3] The immediate effect is direct compression of the dural sac and filling of the epidural space with the injected blood, and the late effect is fibrosis and healing of the dural tears.[3] In our experience, patients typically have improvement immediately or within 1 day of the procedure, regardless of the location of the EBP. However, close monitoring, including the use of a headache diary, is essential to confirm the effective treatment of CSF leaks.[46] Patients with residual symptoms or without any improvement need a repeat EBP.[46] The EBP used has a wide variety of protocols, including differences in injection techniques, volumes of blood used, and the recommended duration of bed rest posttreatment. Nowadays, several studies have identified factors associated with a better response to EBP in SIH.

Currently, EBPs could be classified by their location (targeted or nontargeted) or the injected blood volume (large or small volume).[5] A nontarget EBP is uniformly administered at the lumbar level. Some specialists recommend the Trendelenburg position after injection to promote the cranial migration of the injected blood.[50] However, a targeted EBP requires precise blood injection at the site of the CSF leak, necessitating accurate spinal neuroimaging conducted by a skilled neuroradiologist for leak localization. One study found that targeted EBP has a higher success rate compared with the nontargeted approach,[51] but recent meta-analysis did not show differences between the two methods.[5] The 2023 United Kingdom multidisciplinary consensus guideline recommend the nontargeted EBP for all patients with SIH after 2 weeks of conservative treatment,[46] and reserved the targeted EBP for those not responsive to nontargeted EBPs. In our experience, the targeted EBP had a better efficacy if the leak sites had been accurately localized and performed by experienced hands. Another important factor is the volume of injected blood. We reported that a greater volume of blood ($\geq$22.5 mL) injected during the initial EBP correlates with a more favorable outcome.[24] The same study also identified certain neuroimaging markers, such as the longer ventral epidural CSF collection and a narrowing midbrain-pons angle (<40°), predict less optimal treatment efficacy.[24] The finding of favorable outcome of large-volume EBPs (>20 mL) had been further proved by the meta-analysis.[5] EBPs usually have minor and transient side effects, including numbness, paraesthesia, or radicular pain corresponding to the injection site.[5]

Surgical Repair

Surgical interventions for spinal CSF leaks typically involve either partial or bilateral laminectomy.[52] Patients with widespread leaks require multilevel laminectomies, and this approach is associated with an increased risk of postoperative instability.[52] In our experience, four EBPs could have a 99% success rate; therefore, surgical repair is generally considered after the failure of at least three or four EBPs because of its invasive nature.[2,53] In patients with CSF-venous fistula, the endovascular treatment is recommended as the first-line treatment, followed by EBP or a surgical intervention with nerve root ligation.[46,54] The total recovery rate of nerve root ligation for CSF-venous fistula is 69%.[55] The surgical repair of dural tears involves suturing the defect directly, optionally reinforced with muscle or fat grafting.[56] Meningeal diverticula that are leaking may be suture-ligated or supported with muscle patches or absorbable gelatin sponge.[57]

COMPLICATIONS AND MANAGEMENTS
Subdural Hematoma or Effusion

Subdural hematoma is the most common complication in cases of SIH, which affects approximately 20% to 25% of patients with SIH.[2] Those with a subdural hematoma/effusion may present with neurologic deficits or headaches, and a significant subdural hematoma can lead to herniation or even death. For patients with SIH with subdural hematoma, burr hole evacuation is recommended when the hematoma's thickness is greater than or equal to 10 mm or there is impaired cognitive function.[58] In patients who require surgical intervention for their subdural hematoma/effusion, the spinal CSF leak should be treated with EBP or direct surgical repair at the same time as the surgical intervention for subdural hematoma.[58]

Cerebral Venous Thrombosis

Cerebral venous thrombosis (CVT) is an uncommon complication observed in approximately 2% of individuals with SIH.[59] There are two explanations for CVT in SIH. The first explanation is that SIH causes enlargement of cerebral veins in accordance with the Monro-Kellie doctrine.[59] This dilation results in reduced blood flow velocities within the cerebral veins, consequently facilitating thrombus formation. This hypothesis is bolstered by a study that quantified alterations in blood flow velocity subsequent to lumbar intervention, revealing a 50% decrease in blood flow velocity within the straight sinus as measured by transcranial Doppler ultrasound.[60] The second explanation is the strangulation of cerebral veins that occurs because of brain sagging, which may also cause the development of a thrombus.[59] In patients with complicated CVT, a detailed diagnostic evaluation is essential, using MR or CT venography.[46] EBP is recommended to cease the spinal CSF leaks that contribute to the pathogenesis of venous thrombosis.[46] Expert opinions recommend the usage of anticoagulation for CVT for 3 to 6 months for SIH or PDPH headache.[46,61,62] Also, patients with a higher risk of recurrent seizure (ie, supratentorial lesions or seizures at presentation) require antiepileptics.[61,63] Patients with SIH complicated by CVT generally have a good prognosis.[61]

Superficial Siderosis

Superficial siderosis is a rare complication of SIH, characterized by depositions of hemosiderin in the leptomeninges and subpial layer, which could be identified in the surface of the cerebral and cerebellar cortex, brainstem, and spinal cord.[64] The clinical presentation includes tremors, nystagmus, dysarthria, hearing loss, ataxia, and myelopathy.[64] The cause of superficial siderosis is the chronic intermittent or continuous bleeding into the CSF-containing subarachnoid space.[64] Consequently, diagnostic imaging for patients with SIH should incorporate sequences sensitive to blood products, such as susceptibility-weighted imaging or gradient echo sequences.[46] It is important to highlight that the occurrence of superficial siderosis escalated from 0% at the 2-year mark to 10.5% at 8 years, 32.7% after 12 years, and 57.9% at the 16-year follow-up.[65] Because of its chronic nature, management strategies for superficial siderosis in SIH should prioritize resolving the underlying spinal CSF leak.

SUMMARY

SIH is typically presented as an acute orthostatic headache, but other atypical headaches or neurologic symptoms are also possible. The diagnosis of SIH relies on brain MRI or spinal neuroimaging, and MRM provides a noninvasive approach for identifying and localizing spinal leak sites. The latest consensus suggests a prompt application of EBP with a large blood volume, and conservative treatments have limited benefits. For patients with persistent symptoms after repeated EBP, surgical intervention to repair the CSF leak may be necessary.

CLINICS CARE POINTS

- SIH does not invariably manifest as orthostatic headache, and not every case of orthostatic headache is indicative of spinal CSF leaks.
- MRM provides a noninvasive approach for identifying and localizing spinal leak sites.
- The duration of symptoms should be considered when interpreting brain MRI abnormalities for the diagnosis of SIH.
- EBP with large blood volume (>22.5 mL) is the preferred treatment of SIH; we recommend performing EBP earlier in all patients diagnosed with SIH.
- Surgical repair is reserved for patients not responsive to three or four EBPs.

DISCLOSURE

The authors declare no competing interests.

REFERENCES

1. Schievink WI. Spontaneous intracranial hypotension. N Engl J Med 2021;385(23): 2173–8.
2. Wang S-J. Spontaneous intracranial hypotension 2021;27(3):746–66. https://doi.org/10.1212/con.0000000000000979. Continuum (Minneap Minn).
3. Mokri B. Spontaneous low pressure, low CSF volume headaches: spontaneous CSF leaks. Headache 2013;53(7):1034–53.
4. Schievink WI, Maya MM, Moser FG, et al. Incidence of spontaneous intracranial hypotension in a community: Beverly Hills, California, 2006-2020. Cephalalgia : an International Journal of Headache 2022;42(4–5):312–6.
5. D'Antona L, Jaime Merchan MA, Vassiliou A, et al. Clinical presentation, investigation findings, and treatment outcomes of spontaneous intracranial hypotension syndrome: a systematic review and meta-analysis. JAMA Neurol 2021;78(3): 329–37.

6. Headache Classification Committee of the International Headache Society (IHS). The international classification of headache disorders, 3rd edition. Cephalalgia : an international journal of headache 2018;38(1):1–211. https://doi.org/10.1177/0333102417738202.

7. Kranz PG, Luetmer PH, Diehn FE, et al. Myelographic techniques for the detection of spinal CSF leaks in spontaneous intracranial hypotension. AJR American journal of Roentgenology 2016;206(1):8–19.

8. Dobrocky T, Nicholson P, Häni L, et al. Spontaneous intracranial hypotension: searching for the CSF leak. Lancet Neurol 2022;21(4):369–80.

9. Kranz PG, Gray L, Malinzak MD, et al. CSF–venous fistulas: anatomy and diagnostic imaging. Am J Roentgenol 2021;217(6):1418–29.

10. Wu JW, Wang YF, Fuh JL, et al. Correlations among brain and spinal MRI findings in spontaneous intracranial hypotension. Cephalalgia: an international journal of headache 2018;38(14):1998–2005.

11. Kranz PG, Gray L, Amrhein TJ. Spontaneous intracranial hypotension: 10 myths and misperceptions. Headache 2018;58(7):948–59.

12. Mea E, Chiapparini L, Savoiardo M, et al. Application of IHS criteria to headache attributed to spontaneous intracranial hypotension in a large population. Cephalalgia : an International Journal of Headache 2009;29(4):418–22.

13. D'Amico D, Usai S, Chiapparini L, et al. Headache in spontaneous intracranial hypotension: an overview with indications for differential diagnosis in the clinical practice. Neurol Sci 2020;41(Suppl 2):423–7.

14. Schievink WI. Misdiagnosis of spontaneous intracranial hypotension. Arch Neurol 2003;60(12):1713–8.

15. Paulson GW, Klawans HL Jr. Benign orgasmic cephalgia. Headache 1974;13(4):181–7.

16. Antonescu-Ghelmez D, Butnariu I, Antonescu F, et al. Thunderclap headache revealing dural tears with symptomatic intracranial hypotension: report of two cases. Case Report. Frontiers in Neurology 2023;14. https://doi.org/10.3389/fneur.2023.1132793.

17. Portier F, de Minteguiaga C, Racy E, et al. Spontaneous intracranial hypotension: a rare cause of labyrinthine hydrops. Ann Otol Rhinol Laryngol 2002;111(9):817–20.

18. Kranz PG, Tanpitukpongse TP, Choudhury KR, et al. How common is normal cerebrospinal fluid pressure in spontaneous intracranial hypotension? Cephalalgia : an International Journal of Headache 2016;36(13):1209–17.

19. Wendl CM, Schambach F, Zimmer C, et al. CT myelography for the planning and guidance of targeted epidural blood patches in patients with persistent spinal CSF leakage. AJNR American Journal of Neuroradiology 2012;33(3):541–4.

20. Luetmer PH, Mokri B. Dynamic CT myelography: a technique for localizing high-flow spinal cerebrospinal fluid leaks. AJNR American journal of Neuroradiology 2003;24(8):1711–4.

21. Schievink WI, Moser FG, Maya MM. CSF-venous fistula in spontaneous intracranial hypotension. Neurology 2014;83(5):472–3.

22. Wang YF, Lirng JF, Fuh JL, et al. Heavily T2-weighted MR myelography vs CT myelography in spontaneous intracranial hypotension. Neurology 2009;73(22):1892–8.

23. Medina JH, Abrams K, Falcone S, et al. Spinal imaging findings in spontaneous intracranial hypotension. AJR Am J Roentgenol 2010;195(2):459–64.

24. Wu JW, Hseu SS, Fuh JL, et al. Factors predicting response to the first epidural blood patch in spontaneous intracranial hypotension. Brain 2017;140(2):344–52.

25. Tay ASS, Maya M, Moser FG, et al. Computed tomography vs heavily T2-weighted magnetic resonance myelography for the initial evaluation of patients with spontaneous intracranial hypotension. JAMA Neurol 2021;78(10):1275–6.

26. Chazen JL, Talbott JF, Lantos JE, et al. MR myelography for identification of spinal CSF leak in spontaneous intracranial hypotension. AJNR American Journal of Neuroradiology 2014;35(10):2007–12.

27. Akbar JJ, Luetmer PH, Schwartz KM, et al. The role of MR myelography with intrathecal gadolinium in localization of spinal CSF leaks in patients with spontaneous intracranial hypotension. AJNR American Journal Of Neuroradiology 2012;33(3):535–40.

28. Ringstad G, Valnes LM, Vatnehol SAS, et al. Prospective T1 mapping to assess gadolinium retention in brain after intrathecal gadobutrol. Neuroradiology 2023;65(9):1321–31.

29. Hoxworth JM, Patel AC, Bosch EP, et al. Localization of a rapid CSF leak with digital subtraction myelography. AJNR American Journal of Neuroradiology 2009;30(3):516–9.

30. Di Chiro G. New radiographic and isotopic procedures in neurological diagnosis: useful new diagnostic tools are a refinement of pneumoencephalography, a new tracer for radioactive brain scanning, and the use of radio-iodinated serum albumin injected into the cerebrospinal fluid cavities for head scanning purposes. JAMA 1964;188(6):524–9.

31. Hyun SH, Lee K-H, Lee SJ, et al. Potential value of radionuclide cisternography in diagnosis and management planning of spontaneous intracranial hypotension. Clin Neurol Neurosurg 2008;110(7):657–61.

32. Greiser J, Groeber S, Weisheit T, et al. Radionuclide cisternography with [64Cu] Cu-DOTA. Pharmaceuticals 2023;16(9):1269.

33. Mokri B. Radioisotope cisternography in spontaneous CSF leaks: interpretations and misinterpretations. Headache J Head Face Pain 2014;54(8):1358–68.

34. Wu J-W, Wang Y-F, Hseu S-S, et al. The time sequences of brain mri findings in spontaneous intracranial hypotension (S20.004) 2019;92(15 Supplement):S20.004.

35. Dobrocky T, Grunder L, Breiding PS, et al. Assessing spinal cerebrospinal fluid leaks in spontaneous intracranial hypotension with a scoring system based on brain magnetic resonance imaging findings. JAMA Neurol 2019;76(5):580–7.

36. Wu J-W, Wang Y-F, Hseu S-S, et al. Brain volume changes in spontaneous intracranial hypotension: revisiting the Monro-Kellie doctrine. Cephalalgia : an International Journal of Headache 2021/01/01 2020;41(1):58–68.

37. Smirniotopoulos JG, Murphy FM, Rushing EJ, et al. Patterns of contrast enhancement in the brain and meninges. Radiographics 2007;27(2):525–51.

38. Farb RI, Forghani R, Lee SK, et al. The venous distension sign: a diagnostic sign of intracranial hypotension at MR imaging of the brain. AJNR American Journal of Neuroradiology 2007;28(8):1489–93.

39. Schievink WI. Spontaneous spinal cerebrospinal fluid leaks and intracranial hypotension. JAMA 2006;295(19):2286–96.

40. Grams AE, Gempt J, Stahl A, et al. Female pituitary size in relation to age and hormonal factors. Neuroendocrinology 2010;92(2):128–32.

41. Savoiardo M, Minati L, Farina L, et al. Spontaneous intracranial hypotension with deep brain swelling. Brain:Journal of Neurology 2007;130(Pt 7):1884–93.

42. Ahn AH, Berman BD, Dillon WP. Spontaneous intracranial hypotension-hypovolemia associated with tacrolimus. Headache 2010;50(8):1386–9.

43. Houk JL, Amrhein TJ, Gray L, et al. Differentiation of Chiari malformation type 1 and spontaneous intracranial hypotension using objective measurements of midbrain sagging. J Neurosurg 2022;136(6):1796–803.

44. Fuh JL, Wang SJ, Lai TH, et al. The timing of MRI determines the presence or absence of diffuse pachymeningeal enhancement in patients with spontaneous intracranial hypotension. Cephalalgia : an International Journal of Headache 2008;28(4):318–22.

45. Chen ST, Wu JW, Wang YF, et al. The time sequence of brain MRI findings in spontaneous intracranial hypotension. Cephalalgia : an International Journal of Headache 2022;42(1):12–9.

46. Cheema S, Anderson J, Angus-Leppan H, et al. Multidisciplinary consensus guideline for the diagnosis and management of spontaneous intracranial hypotension. Journal of Neurology, Neurosurgery, and Psychiatry 2023;94(10):835–43.

47. Camann WR, Murray RS, Mushlin PS, et al. Effects of oral caffeine on postdural puncture headache. A double-blind, placebo-controlled trial. Anesth Analg 1990;70(2):181–4.

48. Wu C, Guan D, Ren M, et al. Aminophylline for treatment of postdural puncture headache: a randomized clinical trial. Neurology 2018;90(17):e1523–9.

49. Najafi A, Emami S, Khajavi M, et al. Is epidural dexamethasone effective in preventing postdural puncture headache? Acta Anaesthesiol Taiwanica 2014;52(3): 95–100.

50. Ferrante E, Arpino I, Citterio A, et al. Epidural blood patch in Trendelenburg position pre-medicated with acetazolamide to treat spontaneous intracranial hypotension. Eur J Neurol 2010;17(5):715–9.

51. Cho K-I, Moon H-S, Jeon H-J, et al. Spontaneous intracranial hypotension. Neurology 2011;76(13):1139–44.

52. Beck J, Hubbe U, Klingler J-H, et al. Minimally invasive surgery for spinal cerebrospinal fluid leaks in spontaneous intracranial hypotension. J Neurosurg Spine 2023;38(1):147–52.

53. Lin P-T, Wang Y-F, Hseu S-S, et al. The SIH-EBP Score: a grading scale to predict the response to the first epidural blood patch in spontaneous intracranial hypotension. Cephalalgia : an International Journal of Headache 2023;43(3). https://doi.org/10.1177/03331024221147488. 03331024221147488.

54. Brinjikji W, Savastano LE, Atkinson JLD, et al. A novel endovascular therapy for CSF hypotension secondary to CSF-venous fistulas. AJNR American Journal of Neuroradiology 2021;42(5):882–7.

55. Konovalov A, Gadzhiagaev V, Vinogradov E, et al. Surgical treatment efficacy of CSF-venous fistulas: systematic review. World Neurosurgery 2022; 161:91–6.

56. Matsuhashi A, Takai K, Taniguchi M. Microsurgical anatomy and treatment of dural defects in spontaneous spinal cerebrospinal fluid leaks. J Neurosurg Spine 2020;34(3):522–30.

57. Schievink WI, Morreale VM, Atkinson JLD, et al. Surgical treatment of spontaneous spinal cerebrospinal fluid leaks. J Neurosurg 1998;88(2):243–6.

58. Chen YC, Wang YF, Li JY, et al. Treatment and prognosis of subdural hematoma in patients with spontaneous intracranial hypotension. Cephalalgia 2016;36(3): 225–31.

59. Schievink WI, Maya MM. Cerebral venous thrombosis in spontaneous intracranial hypotension. Headache 2008;48(10):1511–9.

60. Canhão P, Batista P, Falcão F. Lumbar puncture and dural sinus thrombosis: a causal or casual association? Cerebrovasc Dis 2005;19(1):53–6.

61. Ferro JM, Bousser MG, Canhão P, et al. European Stroke Organization guideline for the diagnosis and treatment of cerebral venous thrombosis: endorsed by the European Academy of Neurology. Eur J Neurol 2017;24(10):1203–13.

62. Saposnik G, Barinagarrementeria F, Brown RD Jr, et al. Diagnosis and management of cerebral venous thrombosis: a statement for healthcare professionals from the American Heart Association/American Stroke Association. Stroke 2011;42(4):1158–92.

63. Field TS, Hill MD. Cerebral venous thrombosis. Stroke 2019;50(6):1598–604.

64. Schievink WI, Maya MM, Harris J, et al. Infratentorial superficial siderosis and spontaneous intracranial hypotension. Ann Neurol 2023;93(1):64–75.

65. Schievink WI, Maya M, Moser F, et al. Long-term risks of persistent ventral spinal CSF leaks in SIH: superficial siderosis and bibrachial amyotrophy. Neurology 2021;97(19):e1964–70.

Headache in Brain Tumors

Soomi Cho, MD, Min Kyung Chu, MD, PhD*

KEYWORDS

- Brain tumor • Cancer • Diagnosis • Headache • Intracranial neoplasm
- Pathophysiology • Treatment

KEY POINTS

- Headache is a cardinal symptom of brain tumors.
- Clinical presentation of headache in brain tumors varies across cases.
- Diverse mechanisms are involved in the pathogenesis of headache in brain tumors.
- If findings are suggestive of a brain tumor, a comprehensive evaluation including neuro-imaging should be conducted.

INTRODUCTION

Headache is a common condition in the general population. According to epidemiologic studies, 50% to 60% of individuals in the general population experience headaches annually.[1] Although most headaches are caused by primary headache disorders, some of them develop owing to serious causes and may result in death or severe disability.[2] Headache is a cardinal symptom of brain tumors, and brain tumors are important causes of secondary headache disorders, which can be life-threatening. Nevertheless, early detection and accurate diagnosis can be challenging because of the low prevalence of brain tumors and its various clinical manifestations.

In this review, the epidemiologic details, clinical manifestations, mechanisms, diagnostic approaches, and management of headaches in patients with brain tumors are discussed. In addition, the authors describe rare syndromes presenting as headache and treatment-related headache in patients with brain tumors.

EPIDEMIOLOGY
Overview

The 1-year prevalence of brain tumors in individuals with undifferentiated headache without known malignancy is 0.15%. The prevalence of brain tumors in individuals with headache fulfilling criteria of primary headache disorder is even lower (0.05%).[3] In contrast, headache is reported in 48% to 71% of patients with brain tumors.[4–8]

Department of Neurology, Yonsei University College of Medicine, Republic of Korea
* Corresponding author. 50-1 Yonsei-ro, Seodaemoon-gu, Seoul 03722, Republic of Korea.
E-mail address: chumk@yonsei.ac.kr

Neurol Clin 42 (2024) 487–496
https://doi.org/10.1016/j.ncl.2023.12.004
0733-8619/24/© 2023 Elsevier Inc. All rights reserved.

The prevalence of headache differs according to the location and type of brain tumor, history of headache, and age of the patient. The prevalence of headache is the highest in intraventricular and midline tumors (92%–95%), followed by infratentorial tumors (70%–84%), and supratentorial tumors (55%–60%), which has the lowest prevalence.[6,9,10] Intracranial pressure, degree of midline shift, and brain edema also affect the prevalence of headache.[5,6] A previous headache history and change in headache pattern may predict the risk of headache in brain tumors.[5,8] Alteration in headache pattern was noted in 82.5% of patients with preexisting headache.[7] Further, only 38% of patients with brain tumors without preexisting headaches developed headache. Age also influences the prevalence of headache, which ranges from 48% to 71% in adults with brain tumors,[4–8] with children having a lower prevalence (33%).[10] Both older adults and young individuals with brain tumors are less likely to have headache. Only 8% of patients aged greater than 75 years experienced headache, as per a previous study.[11] Among patients aged less than 1 year, only 8% of them had a headache.[9]

New Headache or Change in Headache in Brain Tumors

Appearance of a new headache or change in headache in a patient with a known malignancy suggests brain metastasis and should be investigated. Intracranial metastasis was noted in 32% of patients with cancer with new or changed headache.[12] Emesis, headache lasting less than 10 weeks, and non-tension-type headache (TTH) were significant factors indicating intracranial metastasis. Another study reported that 54% of patients with intracranial metastasis had new or changed headache.[13]

Headache in Leptomeningeal Metastasis

Headache has been reported in 30% to 40% of patients with leptomeningeal metastasis.[14–16] Breast cancer, lung cancer, melanoma, leukemia, and lymphoma are common tumors causing leptomeningeal metastasis. Patients with leptomeningeal metastasis may present with increased intracranial pressure and diffuse encephalopathy without focal neurologic signs or symptoms.

CLINICAL MANIFESTATIONS
Overview of Presentation and Course

The classical manifestation of brain tumors has been described as severe, early morning, or nocturnal headache usually accompanying nausea or vomiting, which is aggravated during Valsalva maneuver.[17] Nevertheless, various clinical features of headache have been reported in patients with brain tumors.[5–8]

In brain tumors, headache is mostly intermittent and progressive. In a previous study, headache was a pressing/tightening quality in 60.2% and pulsating quality in 33.7% of patients.[8] Headache was more often moderate, with severe headache in 35.7% of the patients. Its duration was 30 minutes to 4 hours in 41.8% and 4 to 72 hours in 35.7% of patients. Morning or evening headache presented in only one-third of patients.[5,6,8] Headache aggravation by Valsalva maneuver was noted in 10% to 20% of patients. Nausea and vomiting accompanied headache in 17% to 60% of patients. Other headache types include migraine-like headache with visual aura, exercise headache, stabbing headache, and orthostatic headache.[18–21] Headache in brain tumors mostly presents with other neurologic symptoms and signs such as nausea/emesis, speech disturbance, personality change, papilledema, blurred vision, motor weakness, gait disturbance, seizures, and other focal neurologic deficits.[12,22]

Headaches with Typical Features of Primary Headache Disorders

Headaches in patients with brain tumors are mostly atypical, that is, progressive in nature, middle, or old age and nocturnal or evening onset, associated with nausea or vomiting, and unresponsive to analgesics. Headaches presenting with typical features of primary headache disorders are found in the minority of patients. Typical migraine and TTH-like headaches are reported in 5% to 30% of patients with tumors who experience headache.[6,8] Further, migraine-type headache was reported in 5% of patients and TTH-like headache in 30% to 40% of patients.[6–8]

Isolated Headache in Brain Tumor

Isolated headache without other neurologic symptoms may occur as an initial symptom in patients with brain tumor. Only 2% to 8% of adults with brain tumors reported isolated headache without other symptoms, and most of them developed other neurologic symptoms within 10 weeks.[7,8,23] Therefore, isolated headache lasting greater than 10 weeks will only be exceptionally secondarily attributed to brain tumors. The low prevalence of isolated headache was also observed in children with brain tumors. An American registry study including 3291 children with brain tumors demonstrated that less than 1% of children had headache as their sole symptom and less than 3% had no neurologic abnormality on examination.[9]

Lateralization of Headache

Headache lateralization does not always predict the location of brain tumor. Among 115 patients with brain tumors presenting with headache, lateralization of the tumor and headache coincided in only one-third of these patients.[6] In contrast, in another study, all patients with unilateral headache had tumors on the ipsilateral side.[5] Laterality of headache was predictive of tumor location in 82.8% of side-locked headache associated with ipsilateral tumors. Among patients with strict bilateral headache, 53.3% had bi-hemispheric tumors and 25% had midline tumors.[8] Most of the patients with infratentorial tumors have supratentorial headache.

Tumor Types

Tumor types may influence the presentation of headache. The occurrence of headache in primary and metastatic brain tumors is equal.[5,7,8,23,24] In general, slow-growing supratentorial tumors are less likely to cause headache than rapid-growing tumors.[22,25] Meningiomas are usually slow progressing and cause headache significantly less often than gliomas. Headache occurs in approximately one-third of patients with supratentorial meningiomas.[26]

Headache Characteristics According to the Special Locations of Brain Tumors

Skull base
Headache, head pain, or sensory change may occur in patients with tumors in the skull base. Clinical presentation varies according to the location of the skull base tumors (**Table 1**).

Pituitary tumors
Headache is reported in 70% of patients with pituitary tumor.[27] Trigeminal autonomic cephalalgia (TAC)-like headache is known to be a typical feature of headache caused by pituitary tumors. However, migraine-type headache is more common than TAC-like headache in patients with pituitary tumors. Moreover, 76% of patients with pituitary tumors had migraine-like headaches, 5% had short-lasting unilateral neuralgiform headache attacks with conjunctival injection and tearing-like headaches, 4% had

Table 1
Clinical presentation of skull base tumors according to location

Location	Clinical Presentation
Orbital syndrome	Dull unilateral supraorbital headache, blurred vision followed by proptosis, diplopia, and external ophthalmoplegia
Parasellar syndrome	Unilateral frontal headache, diplopia, and ocular paresis without proptosis
Middle fossa or Gasserian ganglion syndrome	Pain, diplopia, and sensory change in the maxillary or mandibular division of the trigeminal nerve. Motor symptoms are not common
Jugular foramen syndrome	Glossopharyngeal neuralgia; dysarthria and dysphasia; hoarseness and vocal cord palsy; and palatal, tongue, or ipsilateral sternocleidomastoid or trapezius weakness
Occipital condyle syndrome	Severe, localized, unilateral occipital pain or dysarthria or dysphagia due to unilateral 12th cranial nerve palsy.

cluster-like headaches, 1% had hemicrania continua-like headaches, and 27% had primary stabbing headaches.[28] Secondary TAC-like headache is also observed in conditions other than pituitary tumors, including neurovascular and other lesions. Some of the secondary TACs are responsive to medications used to treat primary TACs such as verapamil, lithium, and indomethacin. Pituitary apoplexy caused by infarction or hemorrhage into a pituitary tumor demonstrates acute onset of intense headache associated with visual loss, facial numbness, or somnolence.[29]

Cerebrospinal fluid obstruction and cystic nature

Intraventricular cystic lesions, such as colloid cyst, may cause severe paroxysmal headache due to positional change. Apart from headache, these tumors may be asymptomatic.[30] Patients still die from colloid cysts when they present with catastrophic acute deterioration due to blockage of the foramen of Munroe by the pedunculated tumor.[31] Nevertheless, classical presentation of intraventricular colloid cysts is not common, with 92% of patients reporting generalized intermittent headache and only 2% reporting a postural component. Papilledema was observed in 72% of patients. Ataxia, diminished vision, and urinary incontinency were observed in 26%, 20%, and 17% of patients, respectively. Rupture of tumor cyst into the cerebrospinal fluid (CSF) may occur, which causes severe headache due to inflammatory reactions by irritating cystic contents.[32]

MECHANISMS

The mechanisms involved in the pathogenesis of headache in brain tumors are as follows:[17,25]

- Local and distant traction on pain-sensitive structures
- Mass effect caused by enlarging tumor mass and cerebral edema
- Infarction
- Hemorrhage
- Venous thrombosis
- Hydrocephalus
- Tumor secretion

Pain structures are veins draining into the large venous sinuses, middle meningeal arteries, major arteries at the skull base, cranial nerves with afferent pain fibers from the head, and intracranial and extracranial arteries.

Headache Related to Treatment of Brain Tumors

Treatment-related causes of headache in brain tumors include post-craniotomy, radiotherapy, chemotherapeutic agents, antiemetics and steroid withdrawal, and surgical procedures other than craniotomy.[33,34] Possible mechanisms of headache are post-craniotomy pain, posterior reversible encephalopathy syndrome, intracranial hypertension, cerebral venous thrombosis, chemical meningitis, and biological agent-related headache (**Table 2**).[17] Intrathecal chemotherapy induces headache in 25% of patients.[34,35] Common anticancer drugs that cause headache are asparaginase, etoposide, fludarabine, hexamethylamine, ixabepilone, methotrexate, nelarabine, retinoic acids, tamoxifen, temozolomide, and intrathecal chemotherapeutic agents.[36]

Persistent post-craniotomy headache can occur in patients treated with supratentorial craniotomy.[37,38] Among 126 consecutive patients who underwent craniotomy, 15.7% of them had persistent headache for greater than 2 months.[38] Suboccipital craniotomy was associated with a higher prevalence of post-craniotomy headache. Among 1657 patients who underwent surgery for acoustic neuroma, one-third of the patients had postoperative headache.[39] In another study including 192 patients who underwent acoustic neuroma surgery, 64% of patients reported post-craniotomy headache, and 86% of them had persistent headache for greater than 3 months.[40]

Stroke-like migraine attacks after radiation therapy (SMART) syndrome is a rare condition that involves migraine-like headache with focal neurologic deficits in patients undergoing cranial radiotherapy.[41] The episodes of SMART syndrome start many years after radiotherapy. These patients have prolonged reversible episodes of migraine-type headache and focal neurologic deficits including seizures. Recovery occurs over several days to weeks. Brain MRI of SMART syndrome often reveals ribbon-like cortical enhancement of the involved hemisphere.

DIAGNOSTIC APPROACH TOWARD HEADACHE IN PATIENTS WITH CANCER

Diagnosis of headache attributed to space-occupying intracranial neoplasms is based on the International Classification of Headache Disorders, 3rd edition (ICHD-3; code 7.4.1; **Box 1**). ICHD-3 also recommends the diagnostic criteria for headache attributed directly to neoplasm (code 7.4.2), headache attributed to carcinomatous meningitis (code 7.4.3), and headache attributed to hypothalamic or pituitary hyper- or hyposecretion (code 7.4.4). For headache attributed to colloid cyst of the third ventricle, ICHD-3 recommends additional criteria (code 7.4.1.1).[42]

All cancer patients with new or change in headache should be suspected to have brain metastasis unless otherwise evaluated. In addition to metastasis, hemorrhage into tumors, infarction, and infection could cause headache in patients with brain

Table 2	
Clinical syndromes of central nervous system caused by anticancer drugs	
Clinical Syndromes	**Causative Anticancer Drugs**
Posterior reversible encephalopathy syndrome	Cyclophosphamide, ifosfamide, gemcitabine, bevacizumab, or sorafenib
Intracranial hypertension	Retinoids
Cerebral venous thrombosis	L-asparaginase
Aseptic meningitis	Methotrexate; ara-C
Biological agents	Blinatumomab, chimeric antigen receptor T-cell infusion, interferon-α, interleukin-2, ipilimumab, rituximab, or tamoxifen

---

Box 1
Diagnostic criteria of headache attributed to intracranial neoplasia in the International Classification of Headache Disorders, 3rd edition

7.4.1. Headache attributed to intracranial neoplasm
    A. Any headache fulfilling criterion C
    B. A space-occupying intracranial neoplasm has been demonstrated
    C. Evidence of causation demonstrated by at least two of the following:
        1. Headache has developed in temporal relation to development of the neoplasm or led to its discovery
        2. Either or both of the following:
            a. Headache has significantly worsened in parallel with worsening of the neoplasm
            b. Headache has significantly improved in temporal relation to successful treatment of the neoplasm
        3. Headache has at least one of the following four characteristics:
            a. Progressive
            b. Worse in the morning and/or when lying down
            c. Aggravated by Valsalva-like maneuvers
            d. Accompanied by nausea and/or vomiting
    D. Not better accounted for by another ICHD-3 diagnosis.

7.4.2. Headache attributed to carcinomatous meningitis
    A. Any headache fulfilling criterion C
    B. Carcinomatous meningitis has been demonstrated
    C. Evidence of causation demonstrated by at least two of the following:
        1. Headache has developed in temporal relation to development of the carcinomatous meningitis
        2. Either or both of the following:
            a. Headache has significantly worsened in parallel with worsening of the carcinomatous meningitis
            b. Headache has significantly improved in parallel with improvement in the carcinomatous meningitis
        3. Headache is associated with cranial nerve palsies and/or encephalopathy

7.4.3. Headache attributed to hypothalamic or pituitary hyper- or hyposecretion
    A. Any headache fulfilling criterion C
    B. Hypothalamic or pituitary hyper- or hyposecretion associated with pituitary adenoma has been demonstrated
    C. Evidence of causation demonstrated by at least two of the following:
        1. Headache has developed in temporal relation to onset of hypothalamic or pituitary hyper or hyposecretion
        2. Either or both of the following:
            a. Headache has significantly worsened in parallel with worsening of the hypothalamic or pituitary hyper- or hyposecretion
            b. Headache has significantly improved in parallel with improvement in the hypothalamic or pituitary hyper- or hyposecretion
    D. Not better accounted for by another ICHD-3 diagnosis.

---

tumors. Older patients with progressive headache, emesis, meningismus, nocturnal or early morning headache, and worsening of headache by Valsalva maneuver should be suspected for secondary headache caused by brain tumors.[6,43] New-onset TAC in patients should be evaluated as the secondary cause for pituitary or cavernous sinus pathologies.[17]

Diagnostic Workup

There are many causes of new headache in patients with cancer other than primary brain tumors and metastasis, such as side effects of cancer therapy, hemorrhage, infarction, infection, and metabolic causes.[17,44] After careful history taking and neurologic examination, neuroimaging studies are an essential process in the evaluation of suspected brain tumors in most cases. MRI with gadolinium enhancement is superior to computed tomography (CT) in detecting parenchymal and leptomeningeal metastasis, and magnetic resonance venogram is superior to CT in detecting venous sinus thrombosis.[45–47] If clinical symptoms and signs are compatible but neuroimaging studies reveal negative findings, CSF study including cytology should be considered. As a significantly high rate (25%–50%) of false-negative CSF study findings exists, a repeat of the study is required if clinical conditions are suggestive of tumors, but the initial result is negative.

MANAGEMENT

Considering that headaches observed in brain tumors are mostly secondary headaches, the optimized treatment of brain tumors can lead to effective management of headaches in most patients. The treatments of primary and secondary brain tumors are beyond the scope of this review. In general, the management of headache in patients with brain tumors depends on tumor type and location, associated symptoms, functional status of the patient, and disease progression.[17,22] However, life expectancy is limited and treatment is palliative in many patients with metastatic brain tumors. Therefore, headache should be managed aggressively with analgesics and narcotics.

If the headache is attributed to increased intracranial pressure caused by mass effect secondary to tumor-associated edema, corticosteroids can provide a good symptomatic relief for the headache before other definitive treatments. Headache caused by radiation necrosis may also respond to corticosteroids.[48] Potential complications of corticosteroids include avascular necrosis of the hip and exacerbation of diabetes. Headache in metastatic brain tumors can be managed by whole-brain radiation therapy.[49,50] Surgical resection or stereotactic radiosurgery can be helpful in limited numbers of patient with metastatic brain tumors.[48,51]

For headache in patients with pituitary tumors, surgical resection and drug therapies including somatostatin analogs and dopamine agonists can relieve headache. However, the response is variable.[28,52]

SUMMARY

Headache in patients with brain tumors can have many presentations. When a new headache or alteration in headache occurs in patients with a known malignancy, a high level of suspicion is warranted. If brain tumors are suspected, a comprehensive evaluation should be conducted using appropriate methods such as brain imaging and CSF study. To avoid patient anxiety and unnecessary evaluations, it is important to acknowledge that the treatment of brain tumors may cause headaches. Given that the life expectancy of many patients with brain tumors is limited, prompt management of headaches is essential to improve their quality of life.

CLINICS CARE POINTS

- Clinical presentation of headache in patients with brain tumor varies according to age; tumor location, type, and progression; intracranial pressure; headache history; and treatment.

- If new headache or change in headache occurs in patients with known malignancy, brain tumor should be highly suspected.
- Considering many patients with brain tumors and headache have limited life expectancy, prompt management of headache should be performed to improve their quality of life.

FUNDING

This research was supported by a grant from the Korea Health Technology R&D Project through the Korea Health Industry Development Institute (KHIDI), funded by the Ministry of Health & Welfare, Republic of Korea (Grant No.: HV22C0106) and a National Research Foundation of Korea (NRF) grant from the Korean government (MSIT) (2022R1A2C1091767). The funders had no role in study design, data collection and analysis, decision to publish, or preparation of the manuscript.

DISCLOSURE

M.K. Chu was a site investigator for a multicenter trial sponsored by Biohaven Pharmaceuticals, Allergan Korea, and Ildong Pharmaceutical Company. He has received lecture honoraria from Eli Lilly and Company, Handok-Teva, and Ildong Pharmaceutical Company over the past 24 months. He has received grants from the Yonsei University College of Medicine (6–2021–0229), the Korea Health Industry Development Institute (KHIDI) (HVC22CO106), and the National Research Foundation of Korea grant from the Korean Government (MSIT) (2022R1A2C1091767).

REFERENCES

1. Stovner LJ, Hagen K, Linde M, et al. The global prevalence of headache: an update, with analysis of the influences of methodological factors on prevalence estimates. J Headache Pain 2022;23(1):34.
2. Robbins MS. Diagnosis and Management of Headache: A Review. JAMA 2021; 325(18):1874–85.
3. Kernick D, Stapley S, Goadsby PJ, et al. What happens to new-onset headache presented to primary care? A case-cohort study using electronic primary care records. Cephalalgia 2008;28(11):1188–95.
4. Davies E, Clarke C. Early symptoms of brain tumours. J Neurol Neurosurg Psychiatry 2004;75(8):1205–6.
5. Forsyth PA, Posner JB. Headaches in patients with brain tumors: a study of 111 patients. Neurology 1993;43(9):1678–83.
6. Pfund Z, Szapáry L, Jászberényi O, et al. Headache in intracranial tumors. Cephalalgia 1999;19(9):787–90 [discussion: 765].
7. Schankin CJ, Ferrari U, Reinisch VM, et al. Characteristics of brain tumour-associated headache. Cephalalgia 2007;27(8):904–11.
8. Valentinis L, Tuniz F, Valent F, et al. Headache attributed to intracranial tumours: a prospective cohort study. Cephalalgia 2010;30(4):389–98.
9. The epidemiology of headache among children with brain tumor. Headache in children with brain tumors. The Childhood Brain Tumor Consortium. J Neuro Oncol 1991;10(1):31–46.
10. Wilne S, Collier J, Kennedy C, et al. Presentation of childhood CNS tumours: a systematic review and meta-analysis. Lancet Oncol 2007;8(8):685–95.
11. Lowry JK, Snyder JJ, Lowry PW. Brain tumors in the elderly: recent trends in a Minnesota cohort study. Arch Neurol 1998;55(7):922–8.

12. Christiaans MH, Kelder JC, Arnoldus EP, et al. Prediction of intracranial metastases in cancer patients with headache. Cancer 2002;94(7):2063–8.

13. Argyriou AA, Chroni E, Polychronopoulos P, et al. Headache characteristics and brain metastases prediction in cancer patients. Eur J Cancer Care 2006; 15(1):90–5.

14. Balm M, Hammack J. Leptomeningeal carcinomatosis. Presenting features and prognostic factors. Arch Neurol 1996;53(7):626–32.

15. Jayson GC, Howell A. Carcinomatous meningitis in solid tumours. Ann Oncol 1996;7(8):773–86.

16. Wasserstrom WR, Glass JP, Posner JB. Diagnosis and treatment of leptomeningeal metastases from solid tumors: experience with 90 patients. Cancer 1982; 49(4):759–72.

17. Kirby S, Purdy RA. Headaches and brain tumors. Neurol Clin 2014;32(2):423–32.

18. Rooke ED. Benign exertional headache. Med Clin North Am 1968;52(4):801–8.

19. Pepin EP. Cerebral metastasis presenting as migraine with aura. Lancet 1990; 336(8707):127–8.

20. Smith RM, Robertson CE, Garza I. Orthostatic headache from supratentorial meningioma. Cephalalgia 2015;35(13):1214.

21. Mascellino AM, Lay CL, Newman LC. Stabbing headache as the presenting manifestation of intracranial meningioma: a report of two patients. Headache 2001;41(6):599–601.

22. Loghin M, Levin VA. Headache related to brain tumors. Curr Treat Options Neurol 2006;8(1):21–32.

23. Vázquez-Barquero A, Ibáñez FJ, Herrera S, et al. Isolated headache as the presenting clinical manifestation of intracranial tumors: a prospective study. Cephalalgia 1994;14(4):270–2.

24. Suwanwela N, Phanthumchinda K, Kaoropthum S. Headache in brain tumor: a cross-sectional study. Headache 1994;34(7):435–8.

25. Kunkle EC, Ray BS, Wolff HG. Studies on Headache: The Mechanisms and Significance of the Headache Associated with Brain Tumor. Bull N Y Acad Med 1942; 18(6):400–22.

26. Englot DJ, Magill ST, Han SJ, et al. Seizures in supratentorial meningioma: a systematic review and meta-analysis. J Neurosurg 2016;124(6):1552–61.

27. Levy MJ, Jäger HR, Powell M, et al. Pituitary volume and headache: size is not everything. Arch Neurol 2004;61(5):721–5.

28. Levy MJ, Matharu MS, Meeran K, et al. The clinical characteristics of headache in patients with pituitary tumours. Brain 2005;128(Pt 8):1921–30.

29. Turgut M, Ozsunar Y, Başak S, et al. Pituitary apoplexy: an overview of 186 cases published during the last century. Acta Neurochir 2010;152(5):749–61.

30. de Witt Hamer PC, Verstegen MJ, De Haan RJ, et al. High risk of acute deterioration in patients harboring symptomatic colloid cysts of the third ventricle. J Neurosurg 2002;96(6):1041–5.

31. Desai KI, Nadkarni TD, Muzumdar DP, et al. Surgical management of colloid cyst of the third ventricle–a study of 105 cases. Surg Neurol 2002;57(5):295–302 [discussion 302-294].

32. Stendel R, Pietilä TA, Lehmann K, et al. Ruptured intracranial dermoid cysts. Surg Neurol 2002;57(6):391–8 [discussion 398].

33. Flexman AM, Ng JL, Gelb AW. Acute and chronic pain following craniotomy. Curr Opin Anaesthesiol 2010;23(5):551–7.

34. Soffietti R, Trevisan E, Rudà R. Neurologic complications of chemotherapy and other newer and experimental approaches. Handb Clin Neurol 2014;121: 1199–218.
35. Glantz MJ, Jaeckle KA, Chamberlain MC, et al. A randomized controlled trial comparing intrathecal sustained-release cytarabine (DepoCyt) to intrathecal methotrexate in patients with neoplastic meningitis from solid tumors. Clin Cancer Res 1999;5(11):3394–402.
36. Stone JB, DeAngelis LM. Cancer-treatment-induced neurotoxicity–focus on newer treatments. Nat Rev Clin Oncol 2016;13(2):92–105.
37. Gee JR, Ishaq Y, Vijayan N. Postcraniotomy headache. Headache 2003;43(3): 276–8.
38. Kaur A, Selwa L, Fromes G, et al. Persistent headache after supratentorial craniotomy. Neurosurgery 2000;47(3):633–6.
39. Ryzenman JM, Pensak ML, Tew JM Jr. Headache: a quality of life analysis in a cohort of 1,657 patients undergoing acoustic neuroma surgery, results from the acoustic neuroma association. Laryngoscope 2005;115(4):703–11.
40. Rimaaja T, Haanpää M, Blomstedt G, et al. Headaches after acoustic neuroma surgery. Cephalalgia 2007;27(10):1128–35.
41. Armstrong AE, Gillan E, DiMario FJ Jr. SMART syndrome (stroke-like migraine attacks after radiation therapy) in adult and pediatric patients. J Child Neurol 2014; 29(3):336–41.
42. Headache Classification Committee of the International Headache Society (IHS) The International Classification of Headache Disorders, 3rd edition. Cephalalgia. 2018;38(1):1-211.
43. Pladdet I, Boven E, Nauta J, et al. Palliative care for brain metastases of solid tumour types. Neth J Med 1989;34(1–2):10–21.
44. Kahn K, Finkel A. It IS a tumor – current review of headache and brain tumor. Curr Pain Headache Rep 2014;18(6):421.
45. Fink KR, Fink JR. Imaging of brain metastases. Surg Neurol Int 2013;4(Suppl 4): S209–19.
46. Khandelwal N, Agarwal A, Kochhar R, et al. Comparison of CT venography with MR venography in cerebral sinovenous thrombosis. AJR Am J Roentgenol 2006; 187(6):1637–43.
47. Chamberlain MC, Sandy AD, Press GA. Leptomeningeal metastasis: a comparison of gadolinium-enhanced MR and contrast-enhanced CT of the brain. Neurology 1990;40(3 Pt 1):435–8.
48. Sayan M, Mustafayev TZ, Balmuk A, et al. Management of symptomatic radiation necrosis after stereotactic radiosurgery and clinical factors for treatment response. Radiat Oncol J 2020;38(3):176–80.
49. Borgelt B, Gelber R, Kramer S, et al. The palliation of brain metastases: final results of the first two studies by the Radiation Therapy Oncology Group. Int J Radiat Oncol Biol Phys 1980;6(1):1–9.
50. Wong J, Hird A, Zhang L, et al. Symptoms and quality of life in cancer patients with brain metastases following palliative radiotherapy. Int J Radiat Oncol Biol Phys 2009;75(4):1125–31.
51. Kondziolka D, Patel A, Lunsford LD, et al. Stereotactic radiosurgery plus whole brain radiotherapy versus radiotherapy alone for patients with multiple brain metastases. Int J Radiat Oncol Biol Phys 1999;45(2):427–34.
52. Abe T, Matsumoto K, Kuwazawa J, et al. Headache associated with pituitary adenomas. Headache 1998;38(10):782–6.

Headache Attributed to a Substance or Its Withdrawal

Mark Obermann, MD, PhD, MHBA[a,b,*],
Zaza Katsarava, MD, PhD, MSc[b,c,d]

KEYWORDS

- Medication-overuse headache • Secondary headache • Substance • Exposure
- Withdrawal

KEY POINTS

- Despite the current headache classification, there is no certainty of a causal relationship between the use of any substance and the development of headache.
- Medication-overuse headache is a common headache disorder and a serious public health problem all over the world.
- Drug withdrawal is the key element in the treatment of medication-overuse headache.

INTRODUCTION

Headache is classified as secondary when it first appears in close temporal proximity to another illness that is known to cause headaches or meets other criteria for causation by the disorder, according to the International Classification of Headache Disorders, Third Edition (ICHD-3, Tab.1).[1] Put differently, a secondary headache is a headache that happens to be associated with another illness that is known to have the potential to cause headaches. There are two conceivable scenarios. First, a recognized headache-causing condition is associated with new-onset headaches. Second, there is a significant temporal correlation between the worsening of a preexisting primary headache and another disorder that is known to be able to cause headache.

These beliefs also apply to headaches attributed to a substance or its withdrawal.[1] According to Chapter eight of the ICHD-3, the diagnosis requires (1) scientific proof (clinical experience and pathophysiological notion) that the substance causes headaches and (2) a temporal correlation between the substance's use and the headache's

ᵃ Department of Neurology, Hospital Weser-Egge, Brenkhaeuser Str. 71, Hoexter 37671, Germany; ᵇ Department of Neurology, University of Duisburg-Essen, Hufelandstr. 55, Essen 45147, Germany; ᶜ Evangelical Hospital Unna, Holbeinstr. 10, Unna 59423, Germany; ᵈ EVEX Medical Corporation, 3 Vekua Street, Tiblisi, Republic of Georgia
* Corresponding author. Department of Neurology, Hospital Weser-Egge, Brenkhaeuser Str. 71, Hoexter 37671, Germany
E-mail address: mark.obermann@uni-due.de

Neurol Clin 42 (2024) 497–506
https://doi.org/10.1016/j.ncl.2023.12.005
0733-8619/24/© 2023 Elsevier Inc. All rights reserved.

beginning. The drug must cause the headache to occur or get worse, and if exposure stops, the headache must considerably lessen or resolve.[2] Chapter eight is divided into three subsections consisting of headache attributed to use of or exposure to a substance, medication-overuse headache (MOH), and headache attributed to substance withdrawal.

The problem is that the association with headache does not prove of a direct causation and with very common conditions such as tension-type headache or migraine; there is always the chance of mere coincidence of occurring headache when taking or withdrawing certain substances or medications.

Headache as a mere symptom of systemic disease should always be kept in mind while evaluating the following conditions to prevent misdiagnosis and inadequate treatment consecutively.[1]

MEDICATION-OVERUSE HEADACHE
History

Peters and Horton first recognized MOH in the 1950s when describing chronic intractable headache in patients with migraine who used ergotamine frequently.[3,4] In the 1980s, clinical case series were published that described the new phenomenon of daily headache in patients with tension-type headache and migraine using analgesics or ergots frequently. Later, triptans were described as causing headache as well.[5] Most importantly, they underlined the fact that this chronic headache resolved after discontinuation of regular drug intake in the majority of patients.[6–9]

Definition

The ICHD-3 defined MOH as headache occurring on 15 or more days per month in patients with a preexisting primary headache disorder and developing as a consequence of regular use of acute or symptomatic headache medications for more than three consecutive months.[1]

There is an ongoing discussion whether MOH is a distinct disease entity or simply a complication of the underlying primary headache disorder. This is based on the fact that MOH was never described to have developed without the patient suffering either from migraine or tension-type headache or both. Even though this argument cannot be dismissed completely, the chronification of a primary headache disorder does not require medication overuse, the response to withdrawal in the majority of patients is measurable, and the significant disease burden on global health associated with MOH seems to justify the implementation of clearly defined and unique diagnostic criteria to empower clinicians to recognize and treat these patients sufficiently[10–12] (**Box 1**).

Epidemiology

Most patients with MOH are women between the age of 40 and 45 years. Most have migraine, and some have tension-type headache or a combination of both. Their average disease duration of their primary headache is 20 years and that of their medication overuse is 5 years. Anti-headache drugs are widely overused all over the world. Epidemiologic studies demonstrated that about 0.5% to 2% of the general population suffer from chronic headache associated with the overuse of headache medication.[13–19] Typical risk factors for the development of MOH are low socioeconomic status, personal, or family history of migraine or tension-type headache as underlying biological trait, overuse of any kind of headache medication, preexisting musculoskeletal pain, depression, and family history of substance abuse. Anxiety, obsessive-

---

Box 1
General diagnostic criteria for headache attributed to a substance or its withdrawal

A. Headache fulfilling criterion C

B. Use of, exposure to, or withdrawal from a substance known to be able to cause headache has occurred

C. Evidence of causation demonstrated by at least two of the following:
   1. Headache has developed in temporal relation to use of, exposure to, or withdrawal from the substance
   2. Either of the following:
      a. Headache has significantly improved or resolved in close temporal relation to cessation of use of or exposure to the substance
      b. Headache has significantly improved or resolved within a defined period after withdrawal from the substance
   3. Headache has characteristics typical for use of, exposure to, or withdrawal from the substance
   4. Other evidence exists of causation

D. Not better accounted for by another ICHD-3 diagnosis.

---

compulsive disorder, obesity, and difficulties to sleep further increase the risk to develop MOH.[20]

PATHOPHYSIOLOGY

The understanding of MOH pathophysiology is still incomplete. Genetic studies showed polymorphic variants in genes associated with the dopaminergic system (DRD2, DRD4, SLC6A3), as well as genes related to drug-dependence pathways (ACE, BDNF, HDAC3, WSF1) that may be responsible for an increased susceptibility to develop MOH in certain headache patients.[21] Abnormal modulation of the serotoninergic system,[22,23] sensitization of certain nociceptive pathways,[24–26] and structural changes in the ventromedial prefrontal cortex, nucleus accumbens, and the ventral tegmental area/substantia nigra following frequent administration of triptans or analgesics were described as potential pathophysiological mechanisms associated with the development of MOH.[27,28] Some of these mechanisms are comparable to changes seen in dependence and addictive behavior usually seen in psychiatric disorders.[28] Changes in these higher level processing networks are complex, highly interdependent, and most likely express a very different degree of influence in each individual patient, despite a common phenotypic presentation. Most of these changes were reversible after drug discontinuation.[26,28] No laboratory or neuroimaging biomarkers are available to distinguish MOH from other chronic headache disorders, so that it remains a purely clinical diagnosis.

Treatment

Discontinuation of the overused medication is the hallmark of MOH treatment.[29–31] The choice between outpatient and inpatient setting depends on the type of overused drugs, the patient's motivation, duration of overuse, previous detoxification attempts, and comorbidities. Inpatient withdrawal should be considered for patients overusing opioids, tranquilizers, or barbiturates, with a long duration of overuse, psychiatric comorbidities, and previous withdrawal failure. Outpatient treatment may be successful in highly motivated patients, with supportive familial environment, short duration of overuse of triptans or analgesics.[32,33] In some patients with MOH, advice alone or information material to take home was demonstrated to be treatment enough.[34–36]

Abrupt discontinuation of analgesics and triptans is the preferred treatment strategy in most centers, whereas benzodiazepines and opioids should be gradually reduced to avoid withdrawal symptoms. Complete discontinuation of acute headache drugs was superior to a restricted drug intake approach but may be difficult to bear for some patients.[37–39]

Prophylactic treatment of the underlying primary headache disorder should be started in parallel to the withdrawal, to maximize treatment success. The prophylactic treatment may need to be adjusted after successful withdrawal to adapt to the resulting headache frequency (ie, chronic or episodic migraine). Some experts prefer to use drugs that may be used throughout such as topiramate or calcitonin gene-related peptide (CGRP) antibodies. A recent treatment trial of MOH demonstrated no additional benefit of botulinum neurotoxin A in addition to withdrawal compared with withdrawal alone.[37] The treatment of psychiatric comorbidities is important in MOH as they considerably worsen the overall outcome, disease burden, and quality of life.[40] A multiprofessional treatment approach including withdrawal, prophylactic medication, supportive psychological therapy, and lifestyle modifications such as weight loss and physical exercise promises to be the most successful treatment strategy for patients with MOH.[41]

The general outcome of patients with MOH is favorable with about 50% to 70% of patients improving. The continuation of overuse of acute treatment leads to a poor prognosis and the persistence of chronic headache with lower quality of life. A considerable number of patients relapse within 5 years after withdrawal, with the majority of patients experience this relapse within the first year. Thus, the first year should be closely monitored with special emphasis on patient education and proactive inquiry of the patients' medication usage. Patients with the combination of migraine and tension-type headache as well as opioid overuse were most at risk to relapse.[8,42,43]

HEADACHE ATTRIBUTED TO USE OF OR EXPOSURE TO A SUBSTANCE
Definition

The headache attributed to use of or exposure to a substance requires the headache onset to occur immediately or within hours after the exposure. The resulting headache is classified according to the substance used to induce it. This principle also applies when the new headache has the characteristics of any primary headache disorder classified in ICHD-3.[1] Most common substances known to induce headache are nitric oxide, phosphodiesterase, cocaine, alcohol, histamine, carbon oxide, and CGRP.[1] In case, a patient has a pre-known primary headache disorder (eg, migraine or tension-type headache) both headache types (primary and secondary) can be classified, as long as the primary headache also occurs without application of the causing substance.[1]

The mere association with the headache does not prove causation. The prevalence of headache in the general population is very high. It may be simple coincidence, symptom of an underlying systemic disease, or a sensitization/predisposition to the development of headache by other factors (drugs, environmental factors) that by itself would not have caused headache.[1]

Pathophysiology

Several substances have been used extensively to induce headache for scientific experiments (eg, nitric oxide [NO], phosphodiesterase inhibitors, and CGRP).[44–47] For example, NO was shown to provoke a delayed migraine attack as well as immediate headache following its application in patients with migraine but also in healthy subjects.[48] The mechanisms induced by NO that lead to headache are complex and include neuronal as well as vascular aspects. NO causes vasodilation through the cyclic guanosine monophosphate cascade and promotes dural vasodilation.[46] NO also releases CGRP from dural afferents, which leads to an increase in meningeal blood flow.[49] It is also involved in the neuroinflammatory cascade of migraine attacks and seems to be involved in central nociception and the central increase of pain responses.[44]

Treatment

The primary treatment option is the immediate cessation of substance exposure that is deemed responsible for causing headache.[2] Delayed onset headache should be treated symptomatic and according to its presenting headache phenotype (ie, migraine or tension-type headache). The glyceryl trinitrate model has been used extensively in humans and animal models to investigate the response to different treatment substances. NO-induced migraine was resolved successfully using triptans, prednisolone, and sodium valproate.[50] NO synthase inhibitors and CGRP antagonists were thoroughly studied in similar models as potential anti-migraine drugs.[50]

Headache Attributed to Substance Withdrawal

The substances best described to cause headache after substance withdrawal are caffeine, estrogens, and opioids.[1] Scientific evidence about these very common conditions is slim, whereas pathophysiological mechanisms were proposed for most of them.[51–53] Headache following the discontinuation after chronic use of other substances was also suggested for corticosteroids, tricyclic antidepressants, selective serotonin reuptake inhibitors, and nonsteroidal anti-inflammatory drugs.[1] There may be many more that have not been formally recognized yet.

A caffeine-withdrawal headache usually develops within 24 hours after the last regular consumption of caffeine with at least 200 mg/day over at least the last 2 weeks.[1] This corresponds to approximately one to two cups of regular coffee or two to three cups of black tea. Red Bull contains 80 mg and Cola between 35 and 70 mg caffeine per serving.[54] The headache should resolve within 7 days after consumption stopped. As caffeine is probably the most frequently consumed psychoactive compound in the world, there is a huge overlap of common primary headache disorders and caffeine consumption, so that there is a considerable chance of having headache while not consuming caffeine without causal relationship.[55]

Possible mechanisms of caffeine in pain regulation were suggested as caffeine being an antagonist of adenosine A1, A2A, and A2B receptors,[56] which are localized at multiple sites such as the thalamus, the spinal cord, and other supraspinal sites.[55] Its analgesic properties seem to be mainly based on interaction with these receptors.[57] In higher concentration not normally reachable by normal dietary intake, further pharmacologic actions can be triggered such as block of GABAA receptors, Ca2+ release, and inhibition of phosphodiesterase.[56] The discontinuation of nurturing these analgesic mechanisms may in consequence lead to the development of headache.[58]

The headache following opioid withdrawal also sets in within 24 hours after the daily consumption of opioids for at least 3 months discontinued. The headache usually resolves within 7 days.[1] There is a multitude of publications regarding mechanisms of opioid actions, overuse and withdrawal in the light of the current opioid epidemic, which would deflect the scope of this article.[59,60] Special pathophysiological focus on the development of headache is rare and mostly regards MOH.

Estrogen withdrawal is usually associated with the pill-free interval of oral contraceptives and should develop within 5 days of discontinuation. Daily consumption of estrogen prior should have been at least 3 weeks. It usually resolves within 3 days.[1] The distinction between estrogen-withdrawal headache and migraine related to the menstrual cycle can be very difficult, especially in those patients with frequent perimenstrual migraine or migraine phenotype of their withdrawal headache.[61]

SUMMARY

The ICHD-3 lists secondary headache attributed to a substance or its withdrawal in Chapter eight. It is divided into three subsections consisting of headache attributed to use of or exposure to a substance, MOH, and headache attributed to substance withdrawal. MOH is widely recognized as the most burdensome in this article and is responsible for approximately 1% of all chronic headache forms. Identified risk factors for the development of MOH are low socioeconomic status, personal or family history of migraine or tension-type headache, overuse of any kind of pain medication, preexisting musculoskeletal pain, depression, and family history of substance abuse. Anxiety, obsessive-compulsive disorder, obesity, and difficulties to sleep further increase the risk to develop MOH. The underlying pathophysiological mechanisms remain insufficiently understood. The most important treatment is withdrawal of the causative drug, as well as implementation of prophylactic medication where necessary. The psychological aspects of chronic headache, patient education, and physical exercise should be implemented in the individual treatment strategy. Most of the patients have a good outcome with considerable relapse rates over time, which should be kept in mind. The other forms of headache attributed to exposure or overuse of a substance are usually benign and treatment is restricted to short-term symptomatic support. Substances most commonly known to induce headache are nitric oxide, phosphodiesterase, cocaine, and carbon oxide. The withdrawal of caffeine, estrogens, and opioids is most often associated with the development of headache, even though many other substances were described in individual patients to may be responsible for their headache. Sometimes, causation is difficult to establish, especially in those patients that suffer from primary headache disorders frequently.

CLINICS CARE POINTS

- In a vast majority of instances, headache attributed to use of or exposure to a substance is rather easily diagnosed based on the history and clearly belongs to a subgroup of secondary headaches.
- Medication-overuse headache (MOH) is considered to be a secondary headache, which develops as a result of regular intake of acute or symptomatic medication(s) used to treat an underlying—usually chronic—primary headache.
- Most common substances known to induce secondary headache are nitric oxide, phosphodiesterase, cocaine, and carbon oxide.
- Withdrawal of caffeine, estrogens, and opioids is most often associated with the development of secondary headache.

DISCLOSURE

None.

REFERENCES

1. Headache Classification Committee of the International Headache Society (IHS) The International Classification of Headache Disorders, 3rd edition. Cephalalgia. 2018;38(1):1-211. doi:10.1177/0333102417738202.
2. Toom K, Braschinsky M, Obermann M, et al. Secondary headache attributed to exposure to or overuse of a substance. Cephalalgia 2021;41(4):443–52.
3. Peters GA, Horton BT. Headache: with special reference to the excessive use of ergotamine preparations and withdrawal effects. Proc Staff Meet Mayo Clin 1951; 26(9):153–61.
4. Horton BT, Peters GA. Clinical manifestations of excessive use of ergotamine preparations and management of withdrawal effect: report of 52 cases. Headache 1963;2:214–27.
5. Limmroth V, Katsarava Z, Fritsche G, et al. Features of medication overuse headache following overuse of different acute headache drugs. Neurology 2002;59(7): 1011–4.
6. Evers S, Suhr B, Bauer B, et al. A retrospective long-term analysis of the epidemiology and features of drug-induced headache. J Neurol 1999;246(9):802–9.
7. Fritsche G, Eberl A, Katsarava Z, et al. Drug-induced headache: long-term follow-up of withdrawal therapy and persistence of drug misuse. Eur Neurol 2001;45(4): 229–35.
8. Katsarava Z, Muessig M, Dzagnidze A, et al. Medication overuse headache: rates and predictors for relapse in a 4-year prospective study. Cephalalgia 2005;25(1):12–5.
9. Pini LA, Cicero AF, Sandrini M. Long-term follow-up of patients treated for chronic headache with analgesic overuse. Cephalalgia 2001;21(9):878–83.
10. Zwart JA, Dyb G, Hagen K, et al. Analgesic use: a predictor of chronic pain and medication overuse headache: the Head-HUNT Study. Neurology 2003;61(2): 160–4.
11. Lance F, Parkes C, Wilkinson M. Does analgesic abuse cause headaches de novo? Headache 1988;28(1):61–2.
12. Steiner TJ, Birbeck GL, Jensen R, et al. Lifting the burden: the first 7 years. J Headache Pain 2010;11(6):451–5.
13. Queiroz LP, Peres MFP, Kowacs F, et al. Chronic daily headache in Brazil: a nationwide population-based study. Cephalalgia 2008;28(12):1264–9.
14. Ayzenberg I, Katsarava Z, Sborowski A, et al. The prevalence of primary headache disorders in Russia: a countrywide survey. Cephalalgia 2012;32(5):373–81.
15. Muzina DJ, Chen W, Bowlin SJ. A large pharmacy claims-based descriptive analysis of patients with migraine and associated pharmacologic treatment patterns. Neuropsychiatric Dis Treat 2011;7:663–72.
16. Jonsson P, Linde M, Hensing G, et al. Sociodemographic differences in medication use, health-care contacts and sickness absence among individuals with medication-overuse headache. J Headache Pain 2012;13(4):281–90.
17. Mehuys E, Paemeleire K, Van Hees T, et al. Self-medication of regular headache: a community pharmacy-based survey. Eur J Neurol 2012;19(8):1093–9.
18. Lucas C, Auray JP, Gaudin AF, et al. Use and misuse of triptans in France: data from the GRIM2000 population survey. Cephalalgia 2004;24(3):197–205.
19. Meskunas CA, Tepper SJ, Rapoport AM, et al. Medications associated with probable medication overuse headache reported in a tertiary care headache center over a 15-year period. Headache 2006;46(5):766–72.

20. Hagen K, Linde M, Steiner TJ, et al. Risk factors for medication-overuse head-ache: an 11-year follow-up study. The Nord-Trøndelag Health Studies. Pain 2012;153(1):56–61.
21. Cargnin S, Viana M, Sances G, et al. A systematic review and critical appraisal of gene polymorphism association studies in medication-overuse headache. Cephalalgia 2018;38(7):1361–73.
22. Potewiratnanond P, le Grand SM, Srikiatkhachorn A, et al. Altered activity in the nucleus raphe magnus underlies cortical hyperexcitability and facilitates trigeminal nociception in a rat model of medication overuse headache. BMC Neurosci 2019;20(1):54.
23. Srikiatkhachorn A, le Grand SM, Supornsilpchai W, et al. Pathophysiology of medication overuse headache–an update. Headache 2014;54(1):204–10.
24. De Felice M, Ossipov MH, Wang R, et al. Triptan-induced latent sensitization: a possible basis for medication overuse headache. Ann Neurol 2010;67(3):325–37.
25. Green AL, Gu P, De Felice M, et al. Increased susceptibility to cortical spreading depression in an animal model of medication-overuse headache. Cephalalgia 2014;34(8):594–604.
26. Ayzenberg I, Obermann M, Nyhuis P, et al. Central sensitization of the trigeminal and somatic nociceptive systems in medication overuse headache mainly involves cerebral supraspinal structures. Cephalalgia 2006;26(9):1106–14.
27. Lai TH, Wang SJ. Neuroimaging Findings in Patients with Medication Overuse Headache. Curr Pain Headache Rep 2018;22(1):1.
28. Schwedt TJ, Chong CD. Medication Overuse Headache: Pathophysiological Insights from Structural and Functional Brain MRI Research. Headache 2017; 57(7):1173–8.
29. Olesen J. Detoxification for medication overuse headache is the primary task. Cephalalgia 2012;32(5):420–2.
30. Engelstoft IMS, Carlsen LN, Munksgaard SB, et al. Complete withdrawal is the most feasible treatment for medication-overuse headache: A randomized controlled open-label trial. Eur J Pain 2019;23(6):1162–70.
31. Nielsen M, Carlsen LN, Munksgaard SB, et al. Complete withdrawal is the most effective approach to reduce disability in patients with medication-overuse head-ache: A randomized controlled open-label trial. Cephalalgia 2019;39(7):863–72.
32. Evers S, Jensen R. European Federation of Neurological Societies. Treatment of medication overuse headache–guideline of the EFNS headache panel. Eur J Neurol 2011;18(9):1115–21.
33. Diener HC, Dodick D, Evers S, et al. Pathophysiology, prevention, and treatment of medication overuse headache. Lancet Neurol 2019;18(9):891–902.
34. Grande RB, Aaseth K, Benth JŠ, et al. Reduction in medication-overuse head-ache after short information. The Akershus study of chronic headache. Eur J Neurol 2011;18(1):129–37.
35. Rossi P, Faroni JV, Tassorelli C, et al. Advice alone versus structured detoxification programmes for complicated medication overuse headache (MOH): a prospective, randomized, open-label trial. J Headache Pain 2013;14(1):10.
36. Kristoffersen ES, Straand J, Vetvik KG, et al. Brief intervention for medication-overuse headache in primary care. The BIMOH study: a double-blind pragmatic cluster randomised parallel controlled trial. J Neurol Neurosurg Psychiatry 2015; 86(5):505–12.
37. Pijpers JA, Kies DA, Louter MA, et al. Acute withdrawal and botulinum toxin A in chronic migraine with medication overuse: a double-blind randomized controlled trial. Brain 2019;142(5):1203–14.

38. Chiang CC, Schwedt TJ, Wang SJ, et al. Treatment of medication-overuse headache: A systematic review. Cephalalgia 2016;36(4):371–86.

39. Grazzi L, Andrasik F. Medication-overuse headache: description, treatment, and relapse prevention. Curr Pain Headache Rep 2006;10(1):71–7.

40. Gaul C, Liesering-Latta E, Schäfer B, et al. Integrated multidisciplinary care of headache disorders: A narrative review. Cephalalgia 2016;36(12):1181–91.

41. Diener HC, Holle D, Solbach K, et al. Medication-overuse headache: risk factors, pathophysiology and management. Nat Rev Neurol 2016;12(10):575–83.

42. Rossi P, Faroni JV, Nappi G. Medication overuse headache: predictors and rates of relapse in migraine patients with low medical needs. A 1-year prospective study. Cephalalgia 2008;28(11):1196–200.

43. Yuan X, Jiang W, Ren X, et al. Predictors of relapse in patients with medication overuse headache in Shanghai: A retrospective study with a 6-month follow-up. J Clin Neurosci 2019;70:33–6.

44. Iversen HK, Olesen J, Tfelt-Hansen P. Intravenous nitroglycerin as an experimental model of vascular headache. Basic characteristics. Pain 1989;38(1):17–24.

45. Kruuse C, Thomsen LL, Jacobsen TB, et al. The phosphodiesterase 5 inhibitor sildenafil has no effect on cerebral blood flow or blood velocity, but nevertheless induces headache in healthy subjects. J Cereb Blood Flow Metabol 2002;22(9):1124–31.

46. Ashina M, Bendtsen L, Jensen R, et al. Nitric oxide-induced headache in patients with chronic tension-type headache. Brain 2000;123(Pt 9):1830–7.

47. Kruuse C, Thomsen LL, Birk S, et al. Migraine can be induced by sildenafil without changes in middle cerebral artery diameter. Brain 2003;126(Pt 1):241–7.

48. Thomsen LL, Kruuse C, Iversen HK, et al. A nitric oxide donor (nitroglycerin) triggers genuine migraine attacks. Eur J Neurol 1994;1(1):73–80.

49. Ashina M, Bendtsen L, Jensen R, et al. Calcitonin gene-related peptide levels during nitric oxide-induced headache in patients with chronic tension-type headache. Eur J Neurol 2001;8(2):173–8.

50. Messlinger K, Lennerz JK, Eberhardt M, et al. CGRP and NO in the trigeminal system: mechanisms and role in headache generation. Headache 2012;52(9):1411–27.

51. Freynhagen R, Elling C, Radic T, et al. Safety of tapentadol compared with other opioids in chronic pain treatment: network meta-analysis of randomized controlled and withdrawal trials. Curr Med Res Opin 2021;37(1):89–100.

52. Somerville BW. Estrogen-withdrawal migraine. I. Duration of exposure required and attempted prophylaxis by premenstrual estrogen administration. Neurology 1975;25(3):239–44.

53. Silverman K, Evans SM, Strain EC, et al. Withdrawal syndrome after the double-blind cessation of caffeine consumption. N Engl J Med 1992;327(16):1109–14.

54. Holle D, Obermann M. Hypnic headache and caffeine. Expert Rev Neurother 2012;12(9):1125–32.

55. Laska EM, Sunshine A, Mueller F, et al. Caffeine as an analgesic adjuvant. JAMA 1984;251(13):1711–8.

56. Fredholm BB, Bättig K, Holmén J, et al. Actions of caffeine in the brain with special reference to factors that contribute to its widespread use. Pharmacol Rev 1999;51(1):83–133.

57. Sawynok J, Yaksh TL. Caffeine as an analgesic adjuvant: a review of pharmacology and mechanisms of action. Pharmacol Rev 1993;45(1):43–85.

58. van Dusseldorp M, Katan MB. Headache caused by caffeine withdrawal among moderate coffee drinkers switched from ordinary to decaffeinated coffee: a 12 week double blind trial. BMJ 1990;300(6739):1558–9.

59. Levin M. Opioids in headache. Headache 2014;54(1):12–21.

60. Ziegler DK. Opiate and opioid use in patients with refractory headache. Cephalalgia 1994;14(1):5–10.

61. Epstein MT, Hockaday JM, Hockaday TD. Migraine and reproductive hormones throughout the menstrual cycle. Lancet 1975;1(7906):543–8.

Headache Associated with Coronavirus Disease 2019

Pedro Augusto Sampaio Rocha-Filho, MD, PhD[a,b],*

KEYWORDS

- COVID-19 • Headache • Headache disorders • Secondary
- Post-acute COVID-19 syndrome • Physiopathology • Disease management
- New daily persistent headache

KEY POINTS

- The headache that occurs in the acute phase of COVID-19 affects around half of patients and is more common in younger people and those with primary headaches, particularly those with migraines.
- The headache that occurs in the acute phase of COVID-19 generally occurs at the beginning of the symptomatic phase, with insidious onset, is bilateral, of moderate to severe intensity, and may be treated with common analgesics and nonhormonal anti-inflammatory drugs.
- Complications brought on by COVID-19 such as cerebrovascular diseases, rhinosinusitis, meningitis, meningoencephalitis, and intracranial hypertension may cause headaches.
- In 10% to 20% of patients with COVID-19, the headache may persist beyond the acute phase, and in general, this headache improves over time.
- Although there are no clinical trials that have assessed the treatment of post-COVID-19 headache, amitriptyline has provided the best evidence for the treatment of this headache.

INTRODUCTION

Neurologic symptoms are common in the acute phase of coronavirus disease 2019 (COVID-19). Around one-fifth of patients consider these to be the symptoms that bother them the most during this phase.[1] As the COVID-19 pandemic progressed, it was discovered that many of these symptoms may persist beyond the acute phase.[2]

Among the most frequent neurologic symptoms in the acute phase of the disease are headache, anosmia, ageusia, and myalgia.[1,3–6] These symptoms are more

[a] Division of Neuropsychiatry, Centro de Ciências Médicas, Universidade Federal de Pernambuco (UFPE), Recife, Brazil; [b] Headache Clinic, Hospital Universitario Oswaldo Cruz, Universidade de Pernambuco, Recife, Brazil
* Rua General Joaquim Inacio, 830, Sala 1412 - Edf The Plaza Business Center, Recife, Pernambuco CEP: 50070-495, Brazil.
E-mail addresses: pedro.rochafilho@ufpe.br; pedroasampaio@gmail.com

Neurol Clin 42 (2024) 507–520
https://doi.org/10.1016/j.ncl.2023.12.006
0733-8619/24/© 2023 Elsevier Inc. All rights reserved.

neurologic.theclinics.com

frequent in patients with mild to moderate conditions.[7–11] The headache[12] and the anosmia[6,12] are considered markers for a better prognosis. With an increase in the vaccinated population and consequently, with an increase in milder cases, understanding and managing the symptoms of the acute phase have gained greater importance.

Similarly, with a drop in postvaccination mortality, persistent symptoms have become a public health problem. Headache is one of the most common persistent neurologic symptoms,[2] thereby bringing a negative impact on the lives of patients.[13,14] A better understanding and management of this headache favor a reduction in the global impact of the disease.

Despite an improvement in the global outlook on COVID-19 over recent years, the disease continues to exhibit neurologic complications, some of which present headaches as a symptom.

This article aims to review the literature on acute and persistent headache and headaches associated with complications of COVID-19. The author reviewed its epidemiology, pathophysiological aspects, and clinical characteristics and considerations were made regarding its management. Greater emphasis has been placed on persistent headache.

HEADACHE IN THE ACUTE PHASE OF COVID-19

The prevalence of headache in the acute phase of COVID-19 is estimated at 47.1% (95% CI: 35.8%–58.6%).[15] Younger people,[9,10,16–19] those with previous headache[17,20] and those with previous migraine,[18,21] present a greater chance of having a headache. There is a divergence in the literature as to whether women are more likely to have headaches[1,9,17,19,20] or whether there is no difference between the sexes.[7,16,18] Although headache is a common symptom in pregnant women with COVID-19, this frequency does not differ from nonpregnant women.[22]

Several mechanisms participate in the pathophysiology of headache. None of them completely explains all cases of headache and not all of them occur in the same patient. Among these mechanisms are direct viral injury, systemic and local inflammatory process, hypoxemia, coagulopathy and endotheliopathy, dehydration, increased intracranial pressure and activation of the trigeminovascular system with release of calcitonin gene-related peptide (CGRP).[23,24]

According to the third edition of the International Classification of Headaches Disorders, headaches that occur in the acute phase of COVID-19 should be classified as acute headache attributed to systemic viral infection. The diagnostic criteria are presented in **Table 1**.[25] Around 94% of those with headache in the acute phase of COVID-19 meet these criteria.[26] Around 60% of patients who presented with headache during other viral infections consider the acute phase headache of COVID-19 as being similar to previous headaches.[27]

Most patients who report a previous primary headache consider the headache in the acute phase of COVID-19 to be different from their previous headaches.[1,16,18,27–30] Headache usually starts at the beginning of the symptomatic phase[1,9,16,18,20,27,31] and is the first symptom presented in around a quarter of those with headache.[1,9,18,20,27,31,32] Some symptoms such as fever, sore throat, anosmia, ageusia, myalgia, and fatigue occur more frequently associated with headache and often occur grouped together.[1]

The most common pattern of headache presents an insidious onset, is bilateral, has tight/pressure quality, and is moderate to severe in intensity.[1,17–19,26,27,30,31,33] There may also be nausea, vomiting, photophobia, and phonophobia associated to the

Table 1		
Diagnostic criteria for headaches associated with COVID-19		
Acute Headache Attributed to Systemic Viral Infection (Headache Has Been Present for <3 mo)	**Chronic Headache Attributed to Systemic Viral Infection (Headache Has Been Present for >3 mo)**	**New Daily Persistent Headache**
Systemic viral infection has been diagnosed; No evidence of meningitic or encephalitic involvement	Systemic viral infection has been diagnosed; No evidence of meningitic or encephalitic involvement	Persistent headache present for more than 3 mo
Evidence of causation demonstrated by at least two of the following:	Evidence of causation demonstrated by at least two of the following:	Distinct and clearly remembered onset, with pain becoming continuous and unremitting within 24 h
1. Headache has developed in temporal relation to onset of the systemic viral infection	1. Headache has developed in temporal relation to onset of the systemic viral infection	Not better accounted for by another ICHD-3 diagnosis
2. Headache has significantly worsened in parallel with worsening of the systemic viral infection	2. Headache has significantly worsened in parallel with worsening of the systemic viral infection	
3. Headache has significantly improved or resolved in parallel with improvement in or resolution of the systemic viral infection	3. Headache has significantly improved or resolved in parallel with improvement in or resolution of the systemic viral infection	
4. Headache has either or both of the following characteristics	4. Headache has either or both of the following characteristics	
A. Diffuse pain	A. Diffuse pain	
B. Moderate or severe intensity	B. Moderate or severe intensity	
Not better accounted for by another ICHD-3 diagnosis	Not better accounted for by another ICHD-3 diagnosis	

Abbreviation: ICHD-3, International Classification of Headache Disorders, 3rd edition.

headache.[1,16,18,19,26,27,33] There is no consensus in the literature as to whether the most frequent pattern of headache in acute COVID-19 resembles a pattern similar to tension-type headache[1,20,26,33,34] or migraine.[7,16,28]

Acute phase headache is often aggravated by coughing.[18,26] However, the pattern triggered by the Valsalva maneuver (cough headache), despite being frequent, has rarely been studied. It is estimated that this pattern occurs in 2% to 16% of patients.[7,16,18] Some patients present a transient increase in intracranial pressure during the acute phase of the headache.[35] It is possible that this contributes to the occurrence of cough headache. However, none of the studies that reported this headache pattern measured patient intracranial pressure.

Cases of trigeminal neuralgia have also been described in the acute phase of COVID-19.[36,37]

There are no clinical trials assessing treatments for headache in the acute phase of COVID-19. Patients should be kept hydrated and measures should be taken to avoid hypoxia in cases with greater pulmonary involvement.

The most commonly used drugs for acute headache are acetaminophen, metamizole, triptans, and nonsteroidal anti-inflammatory drugs.[18,27,38] A series of cases with refractory headaches demonstrated an improvement with indomethacin (50 mg orally, twice per day for 5 days).[39] As the kidneys may be affected during COVID-19, renal function must be monitored if nonsteroidal anti-inflammatory drugs are used.

A Turkish study reported a good response to headache with greater occipital nerve block using lidocaine.[38] A case series also reported an improvement with sphenopalatine ganglion block.[40] Two retrospective cohort studies reported divergent results regarding an improvement in headache after using corticosteroids.[20,31]

SECONDARY HEADACHES

Complications of COVID-19 may cause acute and persistent headaches. **Box 1** presents the main complications.

Cerebrovascular diseases are particularly outstanding among the potentially serious complications that may cause headaches. Ischemic and hemorrhagic strokes and cerebral venous thrombosis are among the most reported complications.[3,6,7,41] The incidence of cerebral venous thrombosis is estimated at 0.8 per 1000 hospitalized patients. In 2% of the cases of cerebral venous thrombosis, headache is the patient's only symptom.[41]

There are reports of reversible cerebral vasoconstriction syndrome associated with COVID-19. Most cases occurred within 30 days of the acute phase of the disease. Endothelial invasion and endotheliitis caused by the virus as well as the downregulation of angiotensin two receptors caused by severe acute respiratory syndrome coronavirus 2 (SARS-Cov-2) with consequent sympathetic and/or renin-angiotensin hyperactivity could justify vasoconstriction.[42,43]

Infectious and postinfectious inflammatory complications of COVID-19, such as acute disseminated encephalomyelitis, syndrome of transient headache, and neurologic deficits with cerebrospinal fluid (CSF) lymphocytosis (HaNDL syndrome), meningitis, and meningoencephalitis may also cause headaches.[44–48] Cases of HaNDL have occurred a few weeks after acute COVID-19.[47,48]

Box 1
Main complications of COVID-19 that can cause headaches

Cerebrovascular Diseases
  Ischemic stroke
  Hemorrhagic stroke
  Cerebral venous thrombosis
  Reversible cerebral vasoconstriction syndrome

Inflammatory and Infectious Causes
  Acute rhinosinusitis
  Meningoencephalitis
  Meningitis
  Acute disseminated encephalomyelitis
  Syndrome of transient headache and neurologic deficits with cerebrospinal fluid lymphocytosis

Other Causes
  Intracranial hypertension

Patients with acute rhinosinusitis are three times more likely to experience headache in the acute phase of COVID-19. In patients with headache and rhinosinusitis, the pain is often exacerbated when pressing on the paranasal sinuses during physical examination. The absence of fever does not rule out this diagnosis.[33]

There may be an increase in intracranial pressure during the acute phase of COVID-19, even in individuals without meningitis, parenchymal lesions, or hydrocephalus, and this may contribute to the persistence of headache.[35] There are rare reports of intracranial hypertension associated with visual loss ("idiopathic intracranial hypertension").[49,50]

Therefore, the neurologic complications of COVID-19 that may place the patient's life at risk must be carefully ruled out through anamnesis, clinical and neurologic examination and, if necessary, complementary examinations such as brain MRI, magnetic resonance angiography, or tomography angiography of the brain and CSF.

PERSISTENT POST-COVID-19 HEADACHE
Pathophysiology

The neurologic symptoms of COVID-19 may persist after the acute phase of the disease, thereby forming part of the long COVID syndrome. These symptoms include cognitive changes, headache, anosmia, ageusia, fatigue, myalgia, and sleep disorders.[2] The presence of headache in the acute phase of COVID-19[21] and a previous history of migraines[51,52] are associated with a greater number of post-COVID-19 symptoms.

Several hypotheses have been raised to explain these persistent symptoms, such as SARS-CoV2 viral persistence and neuroinvasion, abnormal immunologic response, autoimmunity, coagulopathies, and endotheliopathy.[53]

This session discusses the studies that have specifically aimed to study persistent post-COVID-19 headache.

A case-control study compared patients who had COVID-19 with and without persistent headache in terms of cardiorespiratory function. An echocardiogram, spirometry pulmonary function test, and cardiopulmonary exercise tests were performed. There was no difference between the two groups.[54]

A case-control study compared the levels of the neurofilament light chain (NfL) (marker of neuronal injury) and glial fibrillary acidic protein (marker of reactive astrogliosis and neuroinflammation) in the blood of patients with persistent post-COVID-19 headache ($n = 6$) and seronegative patients for COVID-19. There was no difference between the groups.[55]

The same research group compared patients with persistent, daily headache for at least 3 weeks after mild COVID-19 ($n = 7$) versus patients with mild COVID-19, and neuroCOVID (peripheral facial nerve palsy, impaired gait, seizures, or encephalopathy) versus negative COVID-19 patients with other diseases (primary headaches, facial paralysis, multiple sclerosis/optic neuritis, Parkinson's disease, epileptic seizure, psychiatric disease). NfL, ubiquitin carboxyl-terminal hydrolase L1, Tau, and glial fibrillary astrocytic protein were measured in the CSF. The levels of these substances were not higher in patients with persistent headache when compared with those with NeuroCOVID and those with negative COVID-19.[56] The findings of these two studies speak out against the participation of neuronal injury and neuroinflammation in the physiopathology of persistent headache. It should be noted, however, that these studies included few patients with persistent headache.

Another unpublished study, which is on a preprint server, compared patients with long COVID with headache, with those with long COVID without headache and healthy controls using multi-omics analyzes of blood and plasma. Patients with long COVID presented a state of hyperinflammation before the chronic headache, which remained after the headache developed.[57]

Altunisik and colleagues compared the diameter of the optic nerve sheath and the transverse diameter of the eyeball (indirect measurements of intracranial pressure) of 32 people presenting with persistent post-COVID-19 headache and 74 people with normal resonance. MRI scans were performed 2 to 12 weeks after a diagnosis of COVID-19. There was no difference between the groups. This suggests no involvement of intracranial hypertension in the pathophysiology of persistent headache.[58]

Two studies carried out with MRI reported anatomic differences in patients with persistent post-COVID-19 headache.

Planchuelo-Gómez and colleagues compared patients with a new headache that persisted for more than 3 months after COVID-19 ($n = 40$) with healthy controls ($n = 41$), patients with episodic migraine ($n = 43$) and chronic migraine ($n = 43$). MRI of the brain was used and gray matter morphometry and diffusion tensor imaging-based measurements of white matter were studied. Patients with persistent post-COVID-19 headache presented several changes in both the gray and white matter. Those with persistent post-COVID-19 headache presented a significantly lower volume of the gray matter and cortical thickness in the inferior frontal lobe and the fusiform cortex than in healthy controls. They also presented a greater volume and thickness of the cortical gray matter in the cingulate and frontal gyri, paracentral lobule and superior temporal sulcus, and a smaller volume in the subcortical regions and a lower curvature in the precuneus and cuneus than those with migraine. The changes in the white matter were more diffuse. Those with persistent post-COVID-19 headache presented lower fractional anisotropy and higher radial diffusivity than healthy controls in 15 regions of the white matter, involving the white matter tracts, with a predominance in the left hemisphere. The investigators concluded that changes in the white matter are different from those found in chronic and episodic migraine, but that those in the gray matter, although milder, are similar to those in migraine.[59]

Kim and colleagues compared the MRI scans of 23 children and adolescents with persistent post-COVID-19 headache that lasted more than 3 months ($n = 23$), with 23 children and adolescents with primary headaches (tension-type headache, migraine, and new daily persistent headache [NDPH]). Machine learning was used to assess what differentiated the two groups. It was possible to classify correctly those who had COVID-19 with an area under the curve of 0.73 (accuracy = 63.4%). Changes in the gray matter of the orbitofrontal and medial regions of the temporal lobes were suggestive of post-COVID headache, whereas altered thalamic connectivity was suggestive of primary headaches.[60]

EPIDEMIOLOGY

A systematic review that included 36 articles, either published or on preprint servers until May 2021, estimated the prevalence of persistent headache after 30, 60, 90, and more than 180 days of the acute phase of COVID-19 at 10.2% (95% CI: 5.4%–18.5%); 16.5% (95% CI: 5.3%–39.7%); 10.6% (95% CI: 4.7%–22.3%); and 8.4% (95% CI: 4.6%–14.8%), respectively.[15]

A post hoc analysis of six Spanish cohort studies that followed 905 patients with headache in the acute phase of COVID-19 for 9 months reported a prevalence of persistent headache in the first, second, third, sixth, and ninth months of 31% (95% CI: 28.1%–34.3%); 21.5% (95% CI: 18.9%–24.4%); 19% (95% CI: 16.5%–21.8%); 16.8 (95% CI: 14.4%–19.5%); and 16% (95% CI: 13.7%–18.7%), respectively. Hence, the prevalence of headache fell in the first 3 months and then remained stable in the subsequent 6 months.[61]

A prospective cohort study carried out in Turkey followed 85 patients for 3 months and reported that for 20% of the patients the headache persisted for more than 3 months.[29]

Sex,[29,61] age,[29,61] having been hospitalized due to COVID-19,[15,61,62] the severity of COVID-19,[62] and having a headache before COVID-19[29,61] are not risk factors for persistent headache.

Two cohort studies assessed whether migraine was a risk factor. In one study, there was no difference between those with and without migraine in terms of persistent headache.[51] In the other study, those with migraine had a higher prevalence of persistent headache.[52]

Thus, to date, no relevant risk factor for this headache has been reported.

Most studies that assessed the persistence of headache were conducted only with patients infected by the original variant of SARS-CoV2. However, subsequent variants seem to have a greater potential for causing persistent headache.

A study conducted in Spain assessed the medical records of unvaccinated patients hospitalized in Madrid for COVID-19 in the first (Wuhan variant), third (alpha variant), and fifth (delta variant) waves of the disease. Patients were interviewed by telephone 6 months after hospital discharge. The prevalence of post-COVID-19 headache was significantly higher among those with the delta variant (12.9%) than those with the Wuhan (5.5%) or alpha (3.8%) variant. The occurrence of headache at the beginning of the acute phase of COVID-19 was a risk factor for the development of persistent headache only in those who presented the Wuhan and delta variants. No other risk factors were observed. The most common post-COVID-19 headache pattern was similar to tension-type headache (90%), with no difference between the variants.[34]

A study carried out in a clinic that treated post-COVID-19 symptoms in Japan divided patients into three periods according to the predominant variant in the region: "the preceding period," the delta-dominant period, and the omicron-dominant period. Those who had COVID-19 in the omicron-dominant phase (61%) presented with more headaches that persisted for 4 weeks after the acute phase than those in the delta-dominant (24%) or the preceding (15%) phases.[14]

Diagnostic Criteria and Clinical Characteristics

Systemic viral infections may cause persistent headaches. In the third edition of the International Classification of Headaches Disorders, the diagnostic possibilities described for these headaches are chronic headache attributed to systemic viral infection and NDPH. The diagnostic criteria for these headaches are presented in **Box 1**. For the diagnosis of chronic headache attributed to systemic viral infection, this headache should persist for more than 3 months after the acute phase of this infection, regardless of its monthly frequency.[25]

In NDPH, the patient is able to remember clearly the moment that the pain started, which becomes continuous and without remission within a period of 24 hours. In order for a definitive diagnosis to be made, the headache should persist for a period equal to or longer than 3 months. The presence of another previous primary headache does not rule out a diagnosis of NDPH, as long as a progressive increase in headache has not been identified.[25]

Forty percent of patients with NDPH are able to identify a precipitating event. The most frequently cited triggers are systemic infections (often viral respiratory conditions), stressful events, and extracranial surgeries that require intubation.[63,64]

Its physiopathology may involve an immunologic/inflammatory disorder, especially in postinfectious cases. The elevation of tumor necrosis factor alpha in the CSF of patients with NDPH reinforces this hypothesis.[63–66]

Cases of NDPH associated with COVID-19 have been described.[52,67–71]

Both a migraine-like pattern and tension-type headache may occur in post-COVID-19 persistent headache. It has not been well established which pattern is most common.[7,34,52,71,72]

MANAGEMENT

COVID-19 may aggravate preexisting primary headaches.[21,28] Therefore, headaches that existed before COVID-19 and their behavior after the disease should be characterized through careful anamnesis.

Pain-perpetuating factors should be investigated and treated. Patients with this headache often have associated myofascial pain syndrome. This is particularly important in those who needed hospitalization, who were bedridden for a long period of time, and who needed mechanical ventilation. However, those who had mild cases may have prolonged myalgia, with the recruitment of latent myofascial trigger points. Therefore, the presence of craniocervical myofascial trigger points ought to be assessed on physical examination and these should be treated.

Patients who have had COVID-19 may have associated psychiatric illnesses such as depressive and anxiety disorders and post-traumatic stress disorder. Those with persistent headaches have more depressive symptoms than those without headaches.[14] Although the importance of this for the perpetuation of headache has not yet been specifically studied, the importance of these for the impact and prognosis of other primary and secondary headaches has been demonstrated.[73–77] Therefore, investigating these conditions in the anamnesis and their treatments is recommended.

Around 30% of patients who have had COVID-19 present sleep disorders.[2] Those with persistent headaches have more insomnia than those without headaches.[14,72] Insomnia is associated with a greater impact of primary headaches.[78] Although this has not yet been demonstrated for post-COVID headache, it would be reasonable to investigate and treat sleep disorders in these patients, because these may also have an impact on their lives.[14]

There are no clinical trials that have assessed the treatment of persistent post-COVID-19 headache. As a general rule, the treatments for most secondary headaches are much the same as for primary headaches. The pattern of the secondary headache is identified (eg, tension-type headache-like pattern, migraine-like pattern) and thereafter treated in a similar manner to the corresponding primary headache.

A retrospective cohort study assessed the use of amitriptyline for the treatment of headaches that persisted for more than 3 months after COVID-19. When compared with the period before using the drug, there was a significant decrease in the number of days with headache, the number of days with severe headache, and the number of days in which acute pain medication was used. Those with a previous history of tension-type headache and those with nausea presented a greater chance of responding to amitriptyline.[79]

There is one report of a case that improved after sphenopalatine ganglion block with lidocaine. The patient had suffered with headaches for 5 months and remained headache-free during the month of follow-up.[80]

In cases of NDPH that were triggered by COVID-19, there are reports of a good response with the use of amitriptyline, onabotulinumtoxinA, pulse therapy with methylprednisolone, and venlafaxine.[23,67,68]

CLINICS CARE POINTS

- The headache that occurs in the acute phase of COVID-19 affects around half of patients with this disease and is more common in younger people and those with primary headaches, particularly those with migraines.

- The headache that occurs in the acute phase of COVID-19 generally occurs at the beginning of the symptomatic phase, with insidious onset, is bilateral, of moderate to severe intensity and may be associated with nausea, vomiting, photophobia, and phonophobia. It may be treated with common analgesics and nonhormonal anti-inflammatory drugs. Most patients experience partial or complete pain relief with these drugs.

- Complications brought on by COVID-19 may cause headaches. These include cerebrovascular diseases, rhinosinusitis, meningitis, and meningoencephalitis and intracranial hypertension.

- In 10% to 20% of patients with COVID-19, headache may persist beyond the acute phase. These patients present subtle changes in both white matter and gray matter. It is speculated that they have persistent immunologic activation. In general, the headache improves over time.

- Although there are no clinical trials that have assessed the treatment of post-COVID-19 headache, in general, the treatment is much the same as treatments for primary headaches. The pattern of post-COVID-19 headache is identified and treated in a similar way to the corresponding primary headache. Amitriptyline has provided the best evidence for the treatment of this headache.

DISCLOSURE

The author has nothing to disclose.

REFERENCES

1. Sampaio Rocha-Filho PA, Albuquerque PM, Carvalho LCLS, et al. Headache, anosmia, ageusia and other neurological symptoms in COVID-19: a cross-sectional study. J Headache Pain 2022;23(1):2.
2. Premraj L, Kannapadi NV, Briggs J, et al. Mid and long-term neurological and neuropsychiatric manifestations of post-COVID-19 syndrome: A meta-analysis. J Neurol Sci 2022;434:120162.
3. Karadaş Ö, Öztürk B, Sonkaya AR. A prospective clinical study of detailed neurological manifestations in patients with COVID-19. Neurol Sci 2020;41(8):1991–5.
4. Lechien JR, Chiesa-Estomba CM, Place S, et al. Clinical and epidemiological characteristics of 1420 European patients with mild-to-moderate coronavirus disease 2019. J Intern Med 2020;288(3):335–44.
5. Lapostolle F, Schneider E, Vianu I, et al. Clinical features of 1487 COVID-19 patients with outpatient management in the Greater Paris: the COVID-call study. Intern Emerg Med 2020;15(5):813–7.
6. Sampaio Rocha-Filho PA, Magalhães JE, Fernandes Silva D, et al. Neurological manifestations as prognostic factors in COVID-19: a retrospective cohort study. Acta Neurol Belg 2022;122(3):725–33.
7. Amanat M, Rezaei N, Roozbeh M, et al. Neurological manifestations as the predictors of severity and mortality in hospitalized individuals with COVID-19: a multicenter prospective clinical study. BMC Neurol 2021;21(1):116.
8. Romero-Sánchez CM, Díaz-Maroto I, Fernández-Díaz E, et al. Neurologic manifestations in hospitalized patients with COVID-19: The ALBACOVID registry. Neurology 2020;95(8):e1060–70.

9. Trigo J, García-Azorín D, Planchuelo-Gómez Á, et al. Factors associated with the presence of headache in hospitalized COVID-19 patients and impact on prognosis: A retrospective cohort study. J Headache Pain 2020;21(1):94.

10. Gonzalez-Martinez A, Fanjul V, Ramos C, et al. Headache during SARS-CoV-2 infection as an early symptom associated with a more benign course of disease: a case–control study. Eur J Neurol 2021;28(10):3426–36.

11. Saniasiaya J, Islam MA, Abdullah B. Prevalence of Olfactory Dysfunction in Coronavirus Disease 2019 (COVID-19): A Meta-analysis of 27,492 Patients. Laryngoscope 2021;131(4):865–78.

12. Gallardo VJ, Shapiro RE, Caronna E, et al. The relationship of headache as a symptom to COVID-19 survival: A systematic review and meta-analysis of survival of 43,169 inpatients with COVID-19. Headache 2022;62(8):1019–28.

13. Rodríguez-Pérez MP, Sánchez-Herrera-Baeza P, Rodríguez-Ledo P, et al. Headaches and Dizziness as Disabling, Persistent Symptoms in Patients with Long COVID–A National Multicentre Study. J Clin Med 2022;11(19):5904.

14. Fujita K, Otsuka Y, Sunada N, et al. Manifestation of Headache Affecting Quality of Life in Long COVID Patients. J Clin Med 2023;12(10):3533.

15. Fernández-de-las-Peñas C, Navarro-Santana M, Gómez-Mayordomo V, et al. Headache as an acute and post-COVID-19 symptom in COVID-19 survivors: A meta-analysis of the current literature. Eur J Neurol 2021;28(11):3820–5.

16. Rocha-Filho PAS, Magalhães JE. Headache associated with COVID-19: Frequency, characteristics and association with anosmia and ageusia. Cephalalgia 2020;40(13):1443–51.

17. Caronna E, Ballvé A, Llauradó A, et al. Headache: A striking prodromal and persistent symptom, predictive of COVID-19 clinical evolution. Cephalalgia 2020;40(13):1410–21.

18. Membrilla JA, de Lorenzo Í, Sastre M, et al. Headache as a Cardinal Symptom of Coronavirus Disease 2019: A Cross-Sectional Study. Headache 2020;60(10):2176–91.

19. Souza DD, Shivde S, Awatare P, et al. Headaches associated with acute SARS-CoV-2 infection: A prospective cross-sectional study. SAGE open Med 2021;9. 205031212110502.

20. Hussein M, Fathy W, Eid RA, et al. Relative frequency and risk factors of COVID-19 related headache in a sample of Egyptian population: A hospital-based study. Pain Med 2021;22(2):2092–9.

21. Fernández-de-las-Peñas C, Gómez-Mayordomo V, Cuadrado ML, et al. The presence of headache at onset in SARS-CoV-2 infection is associated with long-term post-COVID headache and fatigue: A case-control study. Cephalalgia 2021;41(13):1332–41.

22. Magalhães JE, Sampaio Rocha-Filho PA. Neurological manifestations of COVID-19 in pregnancy: a cross-sectional study. J Neurovirol 2023;29(4):472–8.

23. Sampaio Rocha-Filho PA. Headache associated with COVID-19: Epidemiology, characteristics, pathophysiology, and management. Headache 2022;62(6):650–6.

24. Gárate G, Toriello M, González-Quintanilla V, et al. Serum alpha-CGRP levels are increased in COVID-19 patients with headache indicating an activation of the trigeminal system. BMC Neurol 2023;23(1):109.

25. Headache Classification Committee of the International Headache Society. The International Classification of Headache Disorders, 3rd edition. Cephalalgia. 2018;38(1):1-211. doi:10.1177/0333102417738202.

26. López JT, García-Azorín D, Planchuelo-Gómez Á, et al. Phenotypic characterization of acute headache attributed to SARS-CoV-2: An ICHD-3 validation study on 106 hospitalized patients. Cephalalgia 2020;40(13):1432–42.

27. García-Azorín D, Sierra Á, Trigo J, et al. Frequency and phenotype of headache in covid-19: a study of 2194 patients. Sci Rep 2021;11(1):14674.

28. Al-Hashel JY, Abokalawa F, Alenzi M, et al. Coronavirus disease-19 and headache; impact on pre-existing and characteristics of de novo: a cross-sectional study. J Headache Pain 2021;22(1):97.

29. Akıncı T. Post-discharge persistent headache and smell or taste dysfunction after hospitalisation for COVID-19: a single-centre study. Ir J Med Sci 2023;192(1): 369–75.

30. Sahin BE, Celikbilek A, Kocak Y, et al. Patterns of COVID-19-related headache: A cross-sectional study. Clin Neurol Neurosurg 2022;219:107339.

31. Magdy R, Hussein M, Ragaie C, et al. Characteristics of headache attributed to COVID-19 infection and predictors of its frequency and intensity: A cross sectional study. Cephalalgia 2020;40(13):1422–31.

32. García-Azorín D, Trigo J, Talavera B, et al. Frequency and Type of Red Flags in Patients With Covid-19 and Headache: A Series of 104 Hospitalized Patients. Headache 2020;60(8):1664–72.

33. Straburzyński M, Nowaczewska M, Budrewicz S, et al. COVID-19-related headache and sinonasal inflammation: A longitudinal study analysing the role of acute rhinosinusitis and ICHD-3 classification difficulties in SARS-CoV-2 infection. Cephalalgia 2022;42(3):218–28.

34. Fernández-de-las-Peñas C, Cuadrado ML, Gómez-Mayordomo V, et al. Headache as a COVID-19 onset symptom and post-COVID-19 symptom in hospitalized COVID-19 survivors infected with the Wuhan, Alpha, or Delta SARS-CoV-2 variants. Headache 2022;62(9):1148–52.

35. Silva MTT, Lima MA, Torezani G, et al. Isolated intracranial hypertension associated with COVID-19. Cephalalgia 2020;40(13):1452–8.

36. Molina-Gil J, González-Fernández L, García-Cabo C. Trigeminal neuralgia as the sole neurological manifestation of COVID-19: A case report. Headache 2021; 61(3):560–2.

37. Daripa B, Lucchese S. Unusual Presentation of COVID-19 Headache and Its Possible Pathomechanism. Cureus 2022;14(9):e29358.

38. Karadaş Ö, Öztürk B, Sonkaya AR, et al. Latent class cluster analysis identified hidden headache phenotypes in COVID-19: impact of pulmonary infiltration and IL-6. Neurol Sci 2021;42(5):1665–73.

39. Krymchantowski AV, Silva-Néto RP, Jevoux C, et al. Indomethacin for refractory COVID or post-COVID headache: a retrospective study. Acta Neurol Belg 2022;122(2):465–9.

40. Machado FC, Carone Neto G, Carone RSD. Sphenopalatine ganglion block for refractory COVID-19 headache: a descriptive case series. Brazilian J Anesthesiol 2021;71(6):667–9.

41. Baldini T, Asioli GM, Romoli M, et al. Cerebral venous thrombosis and severe acute respiratory syndrome coronavirus-2 infection: A systematic review and meta-analysis. Eur J Neurol 2021;28(10):3478–90.

42. Arandela K, Samudrala S, Abdalkader M, et al. Reversible Cerebral Vasoconstriction Syndrome in Patients with Coronavirus Disease: A Multicenter Case Series. J Stroke Cerebrovasc Dis 2021;30(12):106118.

43. Ray S, Kamath VV, Raju PA, et al. Fulminant Reversible Cerebral Vasoconstriction Syndrome in Breakthrough COVID 19 Infection. J Stroke Cerebrovasc Dis 2022; 31(2):106238.

44. de Oliveira FAA, Palmeira DCC, Rocha-Filho PAS. Headache and pleocytosis in CSF associated with COVID-19: case report. Neurol Sci 2020;41(11):3021–2.

45. François G, Cleuziou P, Vannod-Michel Q, et al. Acute Corticosteroid Responsive Meningoencephalitis with Cerebral Vasculitis after COVID-19 Infection in a Thirteen-Year-Old. Neuropediatrics 2023;54(1):68–72.

46. de Miranda Henriques-Souza AM, de Melo ACMG, de Aguiar Coelho Silva Madeiro B, et al. Acute disseminated encephalomyelitis in a COVID-19 pediatric patient. Neuroradiology 2021;63(1):141–5.

47. García JCN, Isasi MTA, Parada C M, et al. HaNDL syndrome after COVID-19. Neurol Perspect 2022;2(4):253–5.

48. Marzoughi S, Plecash A, Chen T. Transient Headache and Neurological Deficits with Cerebrospinal Fluid Lymphocytosis following COVID-19. Can J Neurol Sci 2023. https://doi.org/10.1017/CJN.2023.51.

49. Thakur S, Mahajan M, Azad RK, et al. Covid 19 Associated Idiopathic Intracranial Hypertension and Acute Vision loss. Indian J Otolaryngol Head Neck Surg 2023; 75(2):1031–4.

50. Ilhan B, Cokal B, Mungan Y. Intracranial hypertension and visual loss following COVID-19: A case report. Indian J Ophthalmol 2021;69(6):1625–7.

51. Fernández-de-las-Peñas C, Gómez-Mayordomo V, García-Azorín D, et al. Previous History of Migraine Is Associated With Fatigue, but Not Headache, as Long-Term Post-COVID Symptom After Severe Acute Respiratory SARS-CoV-2 Infection: A Case-Control Study. Front Hum Neurosci 2021;15:678472.

52. Magdy R, Elmazny A, Soliman SH, et al. Post-COVID-19 neuropsychiatric manifestations among COVID-19 survivors suffering from migraine: a case-control study. J Headache Pain 2022;23(1):101.

53. Leng A, Shah M, Ahmad SA, et al. Pathogenesis Underlying Neurological Manifestations of Long COVID Syndrome and Potential Therapeutics. Cells 2023; 12(5):816.

54. Á Aparisi, Ybarra-Falcón C, Iglesias-Echeverría C, et al. Cardio-Pulmonary Dysfunction Evaluation in Patients with Persistent Post-COVID-19 Headache. Int J Environ Res Publ Health 2022;19(7):3961.

55. de Boni L, Odainic A, Gancarczyk N, et al. No serological evidence for neuronal damage or reactive gliosis in neuro-COVID-19 patients with long-term persistent headache. Neurol Res Pract 2022;4(1):53.

56. de Boni L, Odainic A, Gancarczyk N, et al. No evidence for neuronal damage or astrocytic activation in cerebrospinal fluid of Neuro-COVID-19 patients with long-term persistent headache. Neurol Res Pract 2023;5(1):49.

57. Foo S-S, Chen W, Jung KL, et al. Immunometabolic rewiring in long COVID patients with chronic headache. bioRxiv Prepr Serv Biol 2023. https://doi.org/10.1101/2023.03.06.531302.

58. Altunisik E, Sut SK, Sahin S, et al. Is Increased Intracranial Pressure a Factor in Persistent Headache After Coronavirus Disease 2019? J Nerv Ment Dis 2021; 209(9):640–4.

59. Planchuelo-Gómez Á, García-Azorín D, Guerrero ÁL, et al. Structural brain changes in patients with persistent headache after COVID-19 resolution. J Neurol 2023;270(1):13–31.

60. Kim M, Sim S, Yang J, et al. Multivariate prediction of long COVID headache in adolescents using gray matter structural MRI features. Front Hum Neurosci 2023;17:1202103.
61. Garcia-Azorin D, Layos-Romero A, Porta-Etessam J, et al. Post-COVID-19 persistent headache: A multicentric 9-months follow-up study of 905 patients. Cephalalgia 2022;42(8):804–9.
62. Ali M. Severe acute respiratory syndrome coronavirus 2 infection altered the factors associated with headache: evidence from a multicenter community-based case-control study. Pain reports 2022;7(6):E1051.
63. Cheema S, Mehta D, Ray JC, et al. New daily persistent headache: A systematic review and meta-analysis. Cephalalgia 2023;43(5). 3331024231168089.
64. Peng KP, Rozen TD. Update in the understanding of new daily persistent headache. Cephalalgia 2023;43(2). 3331024221146314.
65. Riddle EJ, Smith JH. New Daily Persistent Headache: a Diagnostic and Therapeutic Odyssey. Curr Neurol Neurosci Rep 2019;19(5):21.
66. Robbins MS, Smith JH. Other Primary Headache Disorders. Continuum 2021; 27(3):652–64.
67. Caronna E, Alpuente A, Torres-Ferrus M, et al. Toward a better understanding of persistent headache after mild COVID-19: Three migraine-like yet distinct scenarios. Headache 2021;61(8):1277–80.
68. Dono F, Consoli S, Evangelista G, et al. New daily persistent headache after SARS-CoV-2 infection: a report of two cases. Neurol Sci 2021;42(10):3965–8.
69. Simmons AC, Bonner A, Giel A, et al. Probable New Daily Persistent Headache After COVID-19 in Children and Adolescents. Pediatr Neurol 2022;132:1–3.
70. Sampaio Rocha-Filho PA, Voss L. Persistent headache and persistent anosmia associated with COVID-19. Headache 2020;60:1797–9.
71. Torrente A, Alonge P, Di Stefano V, et al. New-onset headache following COVID-19: An Italian multicentre case series. J Neurol Sci 2023;446:120591.
72. Rodrigues AN, Dias ARN, Paranhos ACM, et al. Headache in long COVID as disabling condition: A clinical approach. Front Neurol 2023;14:1149294.
73. Rocha-Filho PAS, Gherpelli JLD, De Siqueira JTT, et al. Post-craniotomy headache: Characteristics, behaviour and effect on quality of life in patients operated for treatment of supratentorial intracranial aneurysms. Cephalalgia 2008; 28(1):41–8.
74. Magalhães JE, Azevedo-Filho HRC, Rocha-Filho PAS. The risk of headache attributed to surgical treatment of intracranial aneurysms: A cohort study. Headache 2013;53(10):1613–23.
75. Sousa Melo E, Pedrosa RP, Carrilho Aguiar F, et al. Dialysis headache: characteristics, impact and cerebrovascular evaluation. Arq Neuropsiquiatr 2022;80(2):129–36.
76. de Mélo Silva Júnior ML, Melo TS, de Sousa Menezes NC, et al. Headache in Medical Residents: A Cross-Sectional Web-Based Survey. Headache 2020; 60(10):2320–9.
77. Zwart JA, Dyb G, Hagen K, et al. Depression and anxiety disorders associated with headache frequency. The Nord-Trøndelag Health Study. Eur J Neurol 2003;10(2):147–52.
78. Corrêa Rangel T, Falcão Raposo MC, Sampaio Rocha-Filho PA. The prevalence and severity of insomnia in university students and their associations with migraine, tension-type headache, anxiety and depression disorders: a cross-sectional study. Sleep Med 2021;88:241–6.

79. Gonzalez-Martinez A, Guerrero-Peral ÁL, Arias-Rivas S, et al. Amitriptyline for post-COVID headache: effectiveness, tolerability, and response predictors. J Neurol 2022;269(11).

80. Levin D, Acquadro M, Cerasuolo J, et al. Persistent Coronavirus Disease 2019 Headache Relieved with Sphenopalatine Ganglion Block. Turkish J Anaesthesiol Reanim 2022;50(Supp1):S68–70.

Headaches Attributed to Disorders of Homeostasis

Ana Marissa Lagman-Bartolome, MD, FRCPC, FAHS[a,b,*],
James Im, MD[c], Jonathan Gladstone, MD, FRCPC[a,d]

KEYWORDS

- Hypoxia • High altitude • Sleep apnea • Dialysis • Hypertension • Hypothyroidism
- Fasting • Cardiac cephalalgia

KEY POINTS

- Headaches attributed to disorders of homeostasis are secondary headache disorders associated with different metabolic, endocrine, and systemic diseases.
- Detailed history and examination is crucial in the assessment and diagnosis of patients with these headache disorders.
- Investigations are always considered and necessary to confirm diagnosis.
- Recognition and careful identification of the causes of these headache disorders is important to implement appropriate treatment and management of these patients.

HEADACHES ATTRIBUTED TO DISORDERS OF HOMEOSTASIS

Headaches attributed to disorders of homeostasis were referred to as "headaches associated with metabolic or systemic diseases" in the first edition of the International Classification of Headache Disorders (ICHD).[1] In the ICHD-3, if a headache occurs for the first time in close temporal relation to a disorder of homoeostasis, it is coded as a secondary headache attributed to that disorder specifically (even when the new headache has the characteristics of any of the primary headache disorders).[2] The headaches attributed to disorders of homeostasis include headaches attributed to (i) hypoxia and/or hypercapnia (high altitude, diving, sleep apnoea); (ii) dialysis; (iii) arterial hypertension (pheochromocytoma, hypertensive crisis without hypertensive encephalopathy, hypertensive encephalopathy, pre-eclampsia or eclampsia, autonomic dysreflexia); (iv)

[a] Department of Pediatrics, Division of Neurology, The Hospital for Sick Children, University of Toronto; [b] Department of Pediatrics, Division of Neurology, Children's Hospital, London Health Sciences Center, Schulich School of Medicine & Dentistry, University of Western Ontario, 800 Commissioner's Road East, London, Ontario N6A5W9, Canada; [c] Department of Medicine, Division of Adult Neurology, St. Michael's Hospital, University of Toronto, 30 Bond Street, Toronto, Ontario M5B1W8, Canada; [d] Gladstone Headache Clinic, 1333 Sheppard Avenue E, Suite 122, North York, Ontario M2J1V1, Canada
* Corresponding author.
E-mail address: marissa.lagman@lhsc.on.ca

Neurol Clin 42 (2024) 521–542
https://doi.org/10.1016/j.ncl.2023.12.007
0733-8619/24/© 2023 Elsevier Inc. All rights reserved.

neurologic.theclinics.com

hypothyroidism; (v) fasting; (vi) cardiac cephalalgia; and (vii) other disorder of homoeostasis. Although there are varied mechanisms behind causation of these different subtypes of headache attributed to disorder of homoeostasis (10.0), there are general diagnostic criteria applicable in most cases (**Box 1**).[2,3]

Headache Attributed to Hypoxia or Hypercapnia

This is a group of headache disorders caused by hypoxia and/or hypercapnia and occurring in conditions of exposure to one or both. It is difficult to separate the effects of hypoxia and hypercapnia (**Box 2**). The ICHD-2 criteria for headache secondary to hypoxia stated that headache begins within 24 hours after acute onset of hypoxia with a partial pressure of oxygen (PaO_2) less than 70 mm Hg or in chronically hypoxic patients with a PaO_2 persistently at or below these levels; the ICHD-3 does not specify the parameters for the hypoxia/hypercapnia. Diseases that are related to acute or chronic hypoxia/hypercapnia may be associated with headache. Any disease that induces a hypoxic state, such as pulmonary diseases (asthma, chronic obstructive pulmonary disease), cardiac disease (congestive heart failure), or hematological disorders (with significant anemia), may be associated with headache.

A proposed pathophysiologic mechanism is the activation of spinal trigeminal neurons with meningeal afferent input as demonstrated in rat models.[4] Another study suggests that an increase in fraction of inspired carbon dioxide ($FiCO_2$) can induce cerebral vasodilatation and increased cerebral pulsatility, which can lead to multiple symptoms including dyspnea, fatigue, sweating, dizziness, nausea, cognitive impairment, but also headaches.[5] There is also research in hypoxia-inducing migraine in patients with pre-existing episodic migraine utilizing normobaric hypoxia to induce migraine in 63.3% of their participants.[6]

There are 4 unique situations associated with headaches attributed to hypoxia that are cited in the ICHD-3: headaches attributed to high altitude, airplane travel, diving, and sleep apnea, and each will be discussed in detail in this section.

With the coronavirus disease 2019 (COVID-19) pandemic, personal protective equipment (PPE) has been proposed to adversely influence pulmonary gas exchange, resulting in systemic hypercapnic hypoxemia and subsequently cerebral hyperperfusion-induced cephalalgia.[5] In a study of healthy individuals who wore N95 masks greater than 6 hours per day, MRI-blood oxygenation level-dependent imaging revealed a significant drop in brain oxygenation as compared with the control group.[7] One study described an increase in $FiCO_2$ to almost 8%, a 260-fold increase

---

Box 1
Headache attributed to a disorder of homoeostasis

A. Headache fulfilling criterion C.

B. A disorder of homoeostasis known to be able to cause headache has been diagnosed.

C. Evidence of causation demonstrated by at least 2 of the following:
  1. Headache has developed in temporal relation to the onset of the disorder of homoeostasis
  2. Either or both of the following:
    a. Headache has significantly worsened in parallel with worsening of the disorder of homoeostasis
    b. Headache has significantly improved after resolution of the disorder of homoeostasis
  3. Headache has characteristics typical for the disorder of homoeostasis.

D. Not better accounted for by another International Classification of Headache Disorders (ICHD)-3 diagnosis.

Box 2
Headache attributed to hypoxia or hypercapnia

A. Any headache fulfilling criterion C.

B. Exposure to conditions of hypoxia and/or hypercapnia.

C. Evidence of causation demonstrated by either or both of the following:
   1. Headache has developed in temporal relation to the exposure
   2. Either or both of the following:
      a. Headache has significantly worsened in parallel with increasing exposure to hypoxia and/or hypercapnia
      b. Headache has significantly improved in parallel with improvement in hypoxia and/or hypercapnia.

D. Not better accounted for by another ICHD-3 diagnosis.

---

in atmospheric carbon dioxide (0.03%). This however remains under debate as another study revealed no marked changes in global cerebral blood flow with prolonged use of type 3 PPE. They did find however that this was associated with increased headache scores alongside impaired executive motor function.[8]

High Altitude Headache

ICHD-3 defines high-altitude headache (HAH) as typically a bilateral headache, aggravated by exertion, and caused by ascent above 2500 m, which resolves spontaneously within 24 hours after descent (**Box 3**). Although the criteria suggest that the headaches are more often bilateral, unilateral headaches can occur, and this is seen more often in migraineurs.[9]

Headache is the most frequent symptom of acute exposure to high altitude, with an incidence as high as 73.3% to 86.7%.[10–12] HAH is often associated with nausea, photophobia, vertigo, and poor concentration. In severe cases, impaired judgment and symptoms or signs suggestive of brain edema can occur. Risk factors for HAH include a history of migraine, low arterial oxygen saturation, high perceived degree of exertion, fluid intake less than 2 L within 24 hours, insomnia, high heart rate, and high Self-Rating Anxiety Scale score.[9,10]

The pathophysiological process that causes HAH remains unknown. Hypoxia elicits neurohumoral and hemodynamic responses that result in over-perfusion of

---

Box 3
Headache attributed to high altitude

A. Headache fulfilling criterion C.

B. Ascent to altitude above 2500 m has occurred.

C. Evidence of causation demonstrated by at least 2 of the following:
   1. Headache has developed in temporal relation to the ascent
   2. Either or both of the following:
      a. Headache has significantly worsened in parallel with continuing ascent
      b. Headache has resolved within 24 hours after descent to below 2500 m
   3. Headache has at least 2 of the following 3 characteristics:
      a. Bilateral location
      b. Mild or moderate intensity
      c. Aggravated by exertion, movement, straining, coughing, and/or bending.

D. Not better accounted for by another ICHD-3 diagnosis.

---

microvascular beds, increased hydrostatic capillary pressure, capillary leakage, and consequent edema.[13] Neuroimaging studies have demonstrated a mild increase in brain volume associated with an increased T2 relaxation time and apparent diffusion coefficient that were associated with the severity of neurologic symptoms. The authors suggested that the brain edema is predominantly vasogenic rather than a cytotoxic edema. Mild extracellular vasogenic edema contributes to the generalized brain swelling observed at high altitude and may be of significance in headache attributed to altitude.[14,15] This was supported by findings that elderly people have fewer headaches after exposure to high altitude, proposed because of varying degrees of brain atrophy.[16] An observational study described with high-altitude exposures, increased retinal nerve fiber layer thickness, potentially reflecting increased intracranial pressure affecting the lamina cribosa.[17] HAH has been associated with a history of migraine in 2 large prospective studies, though the implication of this is unknown.[18,19]

Efforts to demonstrate a specific genotype associated with HAH led to the suggestion that low mRNA expression of the ATP1A1 subunit of the ATPase gene may be of importance.[20] Another study noted a 72.6% prevalence of HAH in a young healthy Han Chinese male population with polymorphisms in EPAS1 and PPARA after high-altitude exposure.[21]

Medical treatment of HAH varies and involves simple analgesics such as paracetamol (acetaminophen) or ibuprofen, antiemetic agents, as well as acetazolamide, at 125 to 375 mg twice daily ± dexamethasone.[22–24]

Randomized, placebo-controlled trials and systematic reviews demonstrated efficacy with the use of acetylsalicylic acid at a dose of 320 mg taken 3 times at 4-h intervals, starting 1 hour before ascent,[25] or ibuprofen at a dose of 600 mg 3 times daily,[26,27] starting a few hours before ascent. Evidence for the addition of 10 mg of metoclopramide also exists, affecting both headache and nausea symptoms.[28]

Nonpharmacological strategies include at least 2 days of acclimatization prior to engaging in strenuous exercise at high altitudes, slow ascent, liberal fluid intake, and avoidance of alcohol.[23]

A related condition is acute mountain sickness (AMS). As defined by the Lake Louise Consensus Group, AMS is the presence of a headache in an unacclimatized person reaching an altitude of 2500 m that is moderate to severe in severity combined with 1 or more of nausea, anorexia, fatigue, photophobia, dizziness, and sleep disturbances.[29] This can also develop into chronic mountain sickness where some patients may develop cerebral edema and encephalopathy.[30]

The proposed pathophysiology of AMS primarily surrounds hypoxemia and its effects on autonomic imbalance causing increased parasympathetic tone, vascular permeability, and potentially cytotoxic edema.[31] The hypoxia-induced cerebral vasodilation or its effectors, such as nitrc oxide (NO), most likely produce the headache, perhaps through the activation of the trigeminovascular system.[29]

Treatment typically involves modulation of the altitude where ascent should be discontinued until symptoms have resolved. Medications including acetazolamide, dexamethasone and ibuprofen have been reported to improve symptoms.[29]

Headache Attributed to Airplane Travel

Headache attributed to airplane travel (**Box 4**), also called "airplane headache(AH)," was first introduced in the ICHD-3 (see also Chapter 56[2]). It is described to be often severe, usually unilateral and periocular, and without autonomic symptoms, occurring during and caused by airplane travel, remitting after landing.[2]

A large case series of AH reported stereotyped attacks, which include the short duration of pain (lasting <30 minutes in up to 95% of cases), a clear relationship

---

Box 4
Headache attributed to airplane travel

A. At least 2 episodes of headache fulfilling criterion C.

B. The patient is traveling by airplane.

C. Evidence of causation demonstrated by at least 2 of the following:
  1. Headache has developed during the aeroplane flight
  2. Either or both of the following:
    a. Headache has worsened in temporal relation to ascent following take-off and/or descent prior to landing of the aeroplane
    b. Headache has spontaneously improved within 30 minutes after the ascent or descent of the aeroplane is completed
  3. Headache is severe, with at least 2 of the following 3 characteristics:
    a. Unilateral location
    b. Orbitofrontal location
    c. Jabbing or stabbing quality.

D. Not better accounted for by another ICHD-3 diagnosis.

---

with the landing phase, a male preponderance, and the absence of accompanying signs and/or symptoms.[32] According to a Scandinavian survey, AH occurred in up to 8.3% of Scandinavian air travellers.[33] A larger cross-sectional study of 50,000 travellers showed a prevalence of 101 (0.2%) that fit the ICHD-3 criterion for AH.[34]

Although the pathophysiology of AH remains unclear, speculation exists that inflammation produces a squeezing effect on the frontal sinus wall, when air trapped inside it contracts, producing a negative pressure leading to mucosal edema, transudation, and intense pain.[35] A proportion of subjects experiencing headache attributed to aeroplane travel report similar headache during free snorkelling and/or rapid descent from mountains, suggesting these headaches may be due to imbalance between intra-sinus and external air pressures. A sinus disorder should be excluded before this diagnosis is considered.[34]

Another proposed theory is that this type of headache generally results from local inflammation caused by hypoxia or dryness in the sinus mucosa or sinus barotraumas.[35,36] A systematic review on AH showed that the most common theoretic mechanism in the development of AH includes changes in cabin pressure during take-off and landing, leading to sinus barotrauma and local inflammation (prostaglandin E2 or PGE-2) with vasodilation in the cerebral arteries.[37,38]

There are no specific guidelines for the treatment of AH since it is considered short-lasting and aborted after the flight travel is over. Prophylactic therapy for AH may include trials of simple analgesics, non-steroidal anti-inflammatory drugs(NSAIDs), antihistamines, triptans, and nasal decongestants administered 30 minutes up to 1 hour prior to travel.[33,34,37,38] Among these medications, ibuprofen, naproxen, and triptans (sumatriptan, naratriptan, zolmitriptan, and eletriptan) have been found the most effective[37]; however, there is a need for randomized controlled trials. Performing specific maneuvers (ie, pressure on the pain area, valsalva maneuvers, relaxation methods, chewing, and extension of the earlobe) has been shown to decrease pain intensity.[33,39]

The most common symptoms of AH include severe, short lasting (<30 minutes in most cases) unilateral, throbbing, or stabbing headache over the fronto-orbital area with parietal spread, which can side-shift between different flights in 10% of cases, with autonomic features like restlessness and unilateral tearing, and migraine features like nausea, photophobia, and phonophobia.[32,37,38]

Diving Headache

Diving headache (**Box 5**) is a headache caused by diving below 10 m, occurring during the dive and often intensified on resurfacing, in the absence of decompression illness. It is usually accompanied by symptoms of carbon dioxide (CO_2) intoxication. It remits quickly with oxygen or spontaneously within 3 days after the dive has ended.[2] There is some evidence that hypercapnia (arterial partial pressure of CO_2 (Pco_2) > 50 mm Hg) causes relaxation of cerebrovascular smooth muscle, leading to intracranial vasodilatation and increased intracranial pressure potentially leading to headache.[39,40]

The diving reflex may contribute as cerebral blood flow is significantly increased at this time. Cerebral hypotension precedes migraine headaches and inducing the diving reflex in migraine patients during aura could alter and potentially prevent the migraine itself.[41]

CO_2 may accumulate in divers who intermittently hold their breath in a mistaken attempt to conserve air or take shallow breaths to minimize buoyancy variations in narrow passages. Divers may also hypoventilate unintentionally when a tight wetsuit or buoyancy compensator jacket restricts chest wall expansion, or when ventilation is inadequate in response to physical exertion. Notably, strenuous exercise increases the rate of CO_2 production more than 10- fold, resulting in a transient elevation of PCO_2 to greater than 60 mm Hg. Inadequate ventilation of compressed gases can lead to CO_2 accumulation, cerebral vasodilation, and headache.[39,40] Diving headache usually intensifies during the decompression phase of the dive or on resurfacing.

Notably, a study by Di Fabio and colleagues[42] suggested that the prevalence of headache among male divers and matched controls was not significant (16% vs 22%).

Headache in divers can occasionally signify serious consequences of hyperbaric exposure, such as arterial gas embolism, decompression sickness, and otic or paranasal sinus barotrauma and should be considered.[39,43–45] Focal neurologic symptoms should be treated with 100% oxygen acutely, and the patient should be referred without delay to a facility with a hyperbaric chamber.[3]

Interestingly, a relationship between patent foramen ovale and migraine with aura was first observed in scuba divers.[46] Interestingly, a relationship between patent

---

Box 5
Diving headache

A. Any headache fulfilling criterion C.

B. Both of the following:
1. The patient is diving at a depth greater than 10 m
2. No evidence of decompression illness.

C. Evidence of causation demonstrated by at least 1 of the following:
1. Headache has developed during the dive
2. Either or both of the following:
   a. Headache has worsened as the dive is continued
   b. Either of the following:
      i. Headache has spontaneously resolved within 3 days of completion of the dive
      ii. Headache has remitted within 1 hour after treatment with 100% oxygen
3. At least 1 of the following symptoms of CO_2 intoxication:
   a. Mental confusion
   b. Light-headedness
   c. Motor incoordination
   d. Dyspnea
   e. Facial flushing.

D. Not better accounted for by another ICHD-3 diagnosis.

foramen ovale (PFO) using a bubble contrast transthoracic echocardiography with provocative maneuvers in divers with high risk factors, including a history of migraine with aura, cerebral, spinal, inner ear or cutaneous decompression illness, a family history of PFO or atrial septal defect, or those with other forms of congenital heart disease.[40,47]

Sleep Apnea Headache

Sleep apnea headache (**Box 6**) is a recurrent morning headache, usually bilateral and typically with a duration of less than 4 hours, caused by sleep apnea diagnosed using polysomnography with an apnoea– hypopnoea index (AHI)$\geq$5.[2] Importantly, this headache disorder resolves with successful treatment of the sleep apnea.[48,49]

The relationship between headache and sleep disorders is complex and incompletely understood (see also Chapter 57). Firstly, sleep disturbances may trigger migraine.[50] Secondly, snoring and other sleep disorders are risk factors for migraine progression.[51] Thirdly, sleep apnea is a risk factor for cluster headache and morning headaches.[52,53] Although morning headache is more frequent in patients with obstructive sleep apnea (OSA) (11.8% vs 4.6%) than those without OSA, headache present on awakening is a non-specific symptom that occurs in a variety of headache disorders, in other sleep-related respiratory (eg, Pickwickian syndrome, chronic obstructive pulmonary disease), and in other primary sleep disorders such as periodic leg movements of sleep.[54]

Studies have demonstrated higher prevalence (27.2%–74%) of morning headaches in patients with OSA,[49,55–57] habitual snoring (23.5%),[55] and insomnia (48%). Other predictors for sleep apnea headache include female sex, history of migraine, psychological distress, and obesity.[55,57]

The current proposed pathophysiology is due to recurrent apneic-hypopneic episodes resulting in transient depressions in cerebral oxygenation and even micro ischemic events.[58] Studies have found that a higher apnea-hypopnea index (AHI) and lower oxygen saturation specifically in the rapid eye movement (REM) sleep period were associated with morning headache in patients with OSA.[59] However, a Norwegian epidemiologic survey did not reveal significant differences between OSA patients with and without headache in total sleep time, average oxygen saturation, minutes below 90% oxygen

---

Box 6
Headache attributed to sleep apnea

A. Headache present on awakening after sleep and fulfilling criterion C.

B. Sleep apnea with apnea– hypopnea index $\geq$ 5 has been diagnosed.

C. Evidence of causation demonstrated by at least 2 of the following:
   1. Headache has developed in temporal relation to the onset of sleep apnea
   2. Either or both of the following:
      a. Headache has worsened in parallel with worsening of sleep apnea
      b. Headache has significantly improved or remitted in parallel with improvement in or resolution of sleep apnea
   3. Headache has at least 1 of the following 3 characteristics:
      a. Recurring on $\geq$ 15 days/month
      b. All of the following:
         i. Bilateral location
         ii. Pressing quality
         iii. Not accompanied by nausea, photophobia, or phonophobia.
      c. Resolving within 4 hours.

D. Not better accounted for by another ICHD-3 diagnosis

saturation (23.1 minutes vs 22.4 minutes), higher level of average oxygen desaturation (5.9% vs 5.8%) or lower average of the lowest oxygen saturation (80.9% vs 81.8%).[60] Thus, oxygen desaturation alone may not explain the pathophysiology of sleep apnea headache. Other contributors may include hypercapnia, obesity or disturbance in sleep architecture (ie, shorter rapid eye movement sleep), and increases in intracranial pressure.[49,55–58,61]

Treatment for OSA is multimodal and case-specific but can include lifestyle education and modification including diet and weight loss, continuous positive airway pressure, oral appliances, or surgical options.[61] Weight loss especially has been noted with a study showing patients with mild OSA who gain 10% of their body weight are at a 6-fold increased risk of progression in the severity of OSA, and an equivalent weight loss can result in a more than 20% improvement.[62]

An association exists between positive airway pressure (PAP) therapy and decreased chronic headache outcomes in patients with OSA. Additionally, research shows that PAP therapy may increase pain tolerance and threshold.[63]

Dialysis Headache

Dialysis headache (**Box 7**) is a type of secondary headache disorder with no specific characteristics occurring during or after (most often after the second hour) hemodialysis.[3,64,65] It resolves spontaneously within 72 hours of a hemodialysis session completing or headache episodes may also stop altogether after a successful kidney transplant and termination of hemodialysis in as high as 27.3% in a study.[2,66]

Dialysis headache occurs in 27% to 73% of patients receiving hemodialysis.[65,67–69] However, in a prospective study, one-third of patients with typical dialysis headache also had similar headache in between their dialysis sessions.[67] This has led to studies using the term "headache after hemodialysis" which has a causal relationship but does not fulfill the ICHD-3 criterion.[70]

This type of headache is described as a mild to moderate (73%), bilateral frontotemporal (50%) ache, which can escalate to severe throbbing (87%) pain lasting for less than 4 hours (63%), that worsens in the reclined position and is accompanied by nausea and vomiting.[65] One study found that women, younger individuals, individuals with higher schooling levels, and individuals who had been on hemodialysis programs for longer times presented with dialysis headache significantly more frequently.[71]

Box 7
Dialysis headache

A. At least 3 episodes of acute headache fulfilling criterion C.

B. The patient is on hemodialysis.

C. Evidence of causation demonstrated by at least 2 of the following:
   1. Each headache has developed during a session of hemodialysis
   2. Either or both of the following:
      a. Each headache has worsened during the dialysis session
      b. Each headache has resolved within 72 hours after the end of the dialysis session
   3. Headache episodes cease altogether after successful kidney transplantation and termination of hemodialysis.

D. Not better accounted for by another ICHD-3 diagnosis.

Additionally, since caffeine is rapidly removed by dialysis, caffeine-withdrawal headache should be considered in patients who consume large quantities of caffeine as a confounder of this headache (ICHD-3).

The pathophysiology of dialysis headache is thought to occur in association with hypotension and dialysis disequilibrium syndrome. Dialysis disequilibrium syndrome may begin as a headache and then progress to obtundation and coma, with or without seizures. The concentration gradient between the brain and the blood that occurs during dialysis, with consequent passage of free water through the blood–brain barrier may lead to cerebral edema, thus causing symptoms including headache.[71]

The most consistent triggers for dialysis headache include arterial hypertension (38%), arterial hypotension (12%), and changes in weight during the hemodialysis sessions.[69,72] Reduced serum osmolality, low magnesium, and high sodium levels may also be risk factors for developing dialysis headache.[68] Variations in NO, Calcitonin gene-related peptide (CGRP) and subtance P levels related to dialysis pose another potential contributor to dialysis headache.[65]

Dialysis headache may be prevented by changing dialysis parameters. There is no specific treatment for dialysis headache. Acute treatment is mainly symptomatic and complicated by the chronic renal insufficiency status. Analgesics and NSAIDs are often used during dialysis sessions. The use of preventative medication may be necessary to improve headache burden; however, evidence for this is limited. Angiotensin-converting enzyme inhibitors were given in a case, with a good response reported.[73] According to ICHD-3 criteria, dialysis headache should resolve after a successful kidney transplantation and suspension of hemodialysis. However in the same study where 27.3% of the patients had a complete resolution of their headaches after transplant, 7.2% instead reported worsening.[66]

Headache Attributed to Hypertension

Headache attributed to hypertension (**Box 8**) is caused by arterial hypertension, usually during an acute rise in systolic (to $\geq$180 mm Hg) and/or diastolic (to $\geq$120 mm Hg) blood pressure. The headache is often bilateral and pulsating. The headache remits after normalization of blood pressure.

Some studies have suggested that ambulatory blood pressure monitoring in patients with mild (140–159/90–99 mm Hg) and moderate (160–179/100–109 mm Hg) hypertension demonstrated no convincing relationship between blood pressure fluctuations over a 24-h period and the presence or absence of headache.[74,75] Others report a significant correlation between blood pressure levels and headache, as well as reduced headache frequency with treatment of hypertension.[76–78] Whether moderate hypertension predisposes to headache at all remains unclear. In a national survey in the United States based on the National Hospital Medical Care Survey data from

---

Box 8
Headache attributed to hypertension

1. Any headache fulfilling criterion C

2. Hypertension, with systolic pressure $\geq$180 mm Hg and/or diastolic pressure $\geq$120 mm Hg, has been demonstrated

3. Evidence of causation demonstrated by either or both of the following:

1. Headache has developed in temporal relation to the onset of hypertension

2. Either or both of the following:
   a. Headache has significantly worsened in parallel with worsening hypertension
   b. Headache has significantly improved in parallel with improvement in hypertension

3. Not better accounted for by another ICHD-3 diagnosis.

2016 to 2019, with severely elevated BP defined as $\geq$180 mm Hg systolic and/or $\geq$120 mm Hg diastolic, 36.39% of patients reported headache as a symptom.[79]

Several studies have documented association of headache with pheochromocytoma,[80–82] hypertensive encephalopathy,[83,84] pre-eclampsia and eclampsia,[85,86] as well as autonomic dysreflexia.[87] The proposed mechanism for this type of headache is failure of the normal baroreceptor reflex in which pathologic changes occur at the limit of compensatory cerebrovascular vasoconstriction, which acts to prevent hyperperfusion as blood pressure rises.[77,88]

Headache Attributed to Pheochromocytoma

A pheochromocytoma is a rare neuroendocrine tumor characterized by intermittent surges of catecholamines.[89]

Headaches attributed to pheochromocytoma (**Box 9**) are usually severe and of short duration (<1 hour) with attacks accompanied by sweating, palpitations, pallor, and/or anxiety.[2] This type of headache occurs as a paroxysmal headache in 51% to 80% of patients with pheochromocytoma.[80,81] The headache is often severe, frontal or occipital, and usually described as either pulsating or constant in quality. A notable feature of the headache is its short duration: less than 15 minutes in 50% and less than 1 hour in 70% of patients.[80] The variable duration and intensity of the headache appear to correlate with the pressor and cranial vasoconstrictor effects of the secreted amines.[82]

Associated features include apprehension and/or anxiety, a sense of impending death, tremor, visual disturbances, abdominal or chest pain, nausea, vomiting, facial flushing, andparaesthesias[80,82] and in severe cases with multi-organ failure and cardiopulmonary collapse known as pheochromocytoma crisis.[89]

The diagnosis of pheochromocytoma is established by the demonstration of increased excretion of catecholamines or catecholamine metabolites usually with analysis of a 24-h urine sample collected when the patient is hypertensive or symptomatic.[84,86,87] A computed tomography (CT) scan is the imaging test of choice to locate the tumor. Iodine meta-iodobenzylguanidine scintigraphy further confirms the diagnosis and is particularly important for the detection of metastatic lesions.[90]

Box 9
Headache attributed to pheochromocytoma

A. Recurrent discrete short-lasting headache episodes fulfilling criterion C.

B. Pheochromocytoma has been demonstrated.

C. Evidence of causation demonstrated by at least 2 of the following:
1. Headache episodes have commenced in temporal relation to development of the phaeochromocytoma, or led to its discovery
2. Either or both of the following:
   a. Individual headache episodes develop in temporal relation to abrupt rises in blood pressure
   b. Individual headache episodes remit in temporal relation to normalization of blood pressure
3. Headache is accompanied by at least 1 of the following:
   a. Sweating
   b. Palpitations
   c. Anxiety
   d. Pallor
4. Headache episodes remit entirely after removal of the pheochromocytoma.

D. Not better accounted for by another ICHD-3 diagnosis.

Treatment involves blood pressure management and the eventual removal of the tumor with special considerations taken in the pre, peri, and postoperative periods by expert surgeons, endocrinologists, and anesthesiologists.[91]

Headache Attributed to Hypertensive Crisis Without Hypertensive Encephalopathy

Headache attributed to hypertensive crisis (**Box 10**) without hypertensive encephalopathy is usually a bilateral and pulsating headache, caused by a paroxysmal rise of arterial hypertension (systolic $\geq$180 mm Hg and/or diastolic $\geq$120 mm Hg). It remits after normalization of blood pressure.[2] Paroxysmal hypertension may occur in association with failure of baroreceptor reflexes (after carotid endarterectomy or irradiation of the neck) or in patients with enterochromaffin cell tumors.

Headache Attributed to Hypertensive Encephalopathy

Headache attributed to hypertensive encephalopathy (**Box 11**) consists of a headache (usually bilateral and pulsating), during this condition which is defined by persistent blood pressure elevation to 180/120 mm Hg or above and accompanied by at least 2 of confusion, reduced level of consciousness, visual disturbances including blindness, and seizures[83,84] It improves after normalization of blood pressure.[2] Headache is one of the most frequent signs (22%–36%) at presentation in hypertensive urgencies.[84] It is thought to occur when compensatory cerebrovascular vasoconstriction can no longer prevent cerebral hyperperfusion as blood pressure rises.[92] As normal cerebral autoregulation of blood flow is overwhelmed, endothelial permeability increases, and cerebral edema occurs.[83] On MRI, this is often most prominent in the parieto-occipital white matter.[93]

Although hypertensive encephalopathy in patients with chronic arterial hypertension is usually accompanied by a diastolic blood pressure of greater than 120 mm Hg, and by grade III or IV hypertensive retinopathy (Keith–Wagener–Barker classification), previously normotensive individuals can, occasionally, develop signs of encephalopathy with blood pressures as low as 160/100 mm Hg.[94]

Headache Attributed to Pre-eclampsia or Eclampsia

The diagnosis of pre-eclampsia and eclampsia require hypertension (>140/90 mm Hg) documented on 2 blood pressure readings at least 4 hours apart, or a rise in diastolic

---

Box 10
Headache attributed to hypertensive crisis without hypertensive encephalopathy

A. Headache fulfilling criterion C.

B. Both of the following:
   1. A hypertensive crisis is occurring
   2. No clinical features or other evidence of hypertensive encephalopathy.

C. Evidence of causation demonstrated by at least 2 of the following:
   1. Headache has developed during the hypertensive crisis
   2. Either or both of the following:
      a. Headache has significantly worsened in parallel with increasing hypertension
      b. Headache has significantly improved or resolved in parallel with improvement in or resolution of the hypertensive crisis
   3. Headache has at least 1 of the following 3 characteristics:
      a. Bilateral location
      b. Pulsating quality
      c. Precipitated by physical activity.

D. Not better accounted for by another ICHD-3 diagnosis.

Box 11
Headache attributed to hypertensive encephalopathy

A. Headache fulfilling criterion C.

B. Hypertensive encephalopathy has been diagnosed.

C. Evidence of causation demonstrated by at least 2 of the following:
   1. Headache has developed in temporal relation to the onset of the hypertensive encephalopathy
   2. Either or both of the following:
      a. Headache has significantly worsened in parallel with worsening of the hypertensive encephalopathy
      b. Headache has significantly improved or resolved in parallel with improvement in or resolution of the hypertensive encephalopathy.
   3. Headache has at least 2 of the following 3 characteristics:
      a. Diffuse pain
      b. Pulsating quality
      c. Aggravated by physical activity.

D. Not better accounted for by another ICHD-3 diagnosis.

As noted in the ICHD-3 criterion, any cause of hypertension can lead to hypertensive encephalopathy and should be coded as 10.3.3 Headache attributed to hypertensive encephalopathy regardless of the underlying cause.

---

pressure of $\geq$15 mm Hg or in systolic pressure of $\geq$30 mm Hg, coupled with urinary protein excretion greater than 0.3 g/24 h.[85]

Headache attributed to pre-eclampsia or eclampsia (**Box 12**) is usually a bilateral and pulsating headache, occurring in women with pre-eclampsia or eclampsia during pregnancy or the immediate puerperium.[95] It remits after resolution of the pre-eclampsia or eclampsia.[2]

They are considered as multisystemic disorders that may present with tissue edema, thrombocytopenia, and abnormalities in liver function,[85] as well as seizures in patients with eclampsia. A case–control study found that headache was significantly more frequent in patients with pre-eclampsia (63%) than in controls (25%).[96]

Box 12
Headache attributed to pre-eclampsia or eclampsia

A. Headache, in a woman who is pregnant or in the puerperium (up to 4 weeks postpartum), fulfilling criterion C.

B. Pre-eclampsia or eclampsia has been diagnosed.

C. Evidence of causation demonstrated by at least 2 of the following:
   1. Headache has developed in temporal relation to the onset of the pre-eclampsia or eclampsia
   2. Either or both of the following:
      a. Headache has significantly worsened in parallel with worsening of the pre-eclampsia or eclampsia
      b. Headache has significantly improved or resolved in parallel with improvement in or resolution of the pre-eclampsia or eclampsia
   3. Headache has at least 2 of the following 3 characteristics:
      a. Bilateral location
      b. Pulsating quality
      c. Aggravated by physical activity.

Treatment of the headache will generally involve antihypertensive therapies considering the health of the carrier, placenta, and fetus in conjunction with expert consultation. Intravenous labetalol is often used for reduction of blood pressure though a large case-series study on nicardipine showed high efficacy with an acceptable safety profile in pregnancy as a potential alternative.[97] Delivery of the infant and placental tissues are the definitive treatments and may be instituted.[98–101]

Headache Attributed to Autonomic Dysreflexia

Headache attributed to autonomic dysreflexia (**Box 13**) is a throbbing, severe headache, in patients with spinal cord injury (SCI) and autonomic dysreflexia.[2] It is a sudden-onset severe headache associated with sudden increase in blood pressure, altered heart rate, and diaphoresis cranial to the level of SCI.[87] This is typically described to be at or above T6, though it has been described in case reports with injuries as low as T12.[102,103]

Severe headaches occur in 56% to 85% of the patients with autonomic dysreflexia.[104,105] Triggers include noxious or non-noxious stimuli, usually of visceral origin (bladder distension, urinary tract infection, bowel distension, gastric ulcers), but also of somatic origin (pressure ulcers, burns, trauma, or invasive diagnostic procedures).[105] The time to onset of autonomic dysreflexia after SCI is variable and has been reported to be from 4 days to 15 years.[104] The most important predictors of autonomic dysreflexia are the level and severity of SCI. Patients with complete SCI are at greater risk of development of autonomic dysreflexia and, consequently, more susceptible to develop headaches.[87]

It has been postulated that this type of headache has a vasomotor nature and may result from passive dilation of cerebral vessels or increased circulating PGE-2.[87] Autonomic dysreflexia can be life-threatening, thus prompt recognition and management are critical. The primary treatment of autonomic headache involves management of the autonomic dysreflexia, which includes close monitoring of blood pressure and heart rate with the following measures: (i) patient is placed in a sitting position; (ii) removal/loosening of clothing or constrictive devices; (iii) scrutinize for potential triggers (ie, bladder distension and bowel impaction); (iv) pharmacologic treatment with a rapid-onset and short-duration antihypertensive agent (ie, nifedipine or nitrates) for elevated systolic blood pressure ($\geq$150 mm Hg).[87]

Box 13
Headache attributed to autonomic dysreflexia

A. Headache of sudden onset, fulfilling criterion C.

B. Presence of spinal cord injury and autonomic dysreflexia documented by a paroxysmal rise above baseline in systolic pressure of $\geq$30 mm Hg and/or diastolic pressure of $\geq$ 20 mm Hg.

C. Evidence of causation demonstrated by at least 2 of the following:
  1. Headache has developed in temporal relation to the rise in blood pressure
  2. Either or both of the following:
     a. Headache has significantly worsened in parallel with increase in blood pressure
     b. Headache has significantly improved in parallel with decrease in blood pressure
  3. Headache has at least 2 of the following 4 characteristics:
     a. Severe intensity
     b. Pounding or throbbing (pulsating) quality
     c. Accompanied by diaphoresis cranial to the level of the spinal cord injury
     d. Triggered by bladder or bowel reflexes.

D. Not better accounted for by another ICHD-3 diagnosis

Headache Attributed to Hypothyroidism

Headache attributed to hypothyroidism (**Box 14**) is usually bilateral and non-pulsatile, occurring in patients with hypothyroidism and remitting after normalization of thyroid hormone levels[2,106] occurring in approximately 30% of patients with hypothyroidism with female preponderance.[106,107] In migraineurs with subclinical hypothyroidism, treatment of borderline hypothyroidism is sometimes followed by dramatic improvement in headache.[108] This type of headache is described as intermittent, unilateral, throbbing pain associated with nausea and/or vomiting, which begins within 2 months of the onset of hypothyroidism and lasts less than 3 months after its effective treatment.[109]

The mechanism of headache attributed to thyroid disease is unclear. There is a female preponderance and often a history of migraine in childhood.[108] There is evidence examining genetic relationships between thyroid traits and headache where some significant genetic correlations were found between headache and hypothyroidism and free T4 levels.[110]

Hypothyroidism has also been identified as a potential risk factor for new daily persistent headache in a clinic-based case–control study, when the control group was migraine.[108] In the presence of hypothyroidism, it is important to remember that headache can also be a manifestation of pituitary adenoma.[111]

Treatment with levothyroxine produces relief or complete remission of headache in the majority of patients. Headache has shown to decrease in intensity and duration within the first 2 weeks of treatment. The degree of hypothyroidism does not seem to affect potential for improvement with levothyroxine treatment.[88]

Headache Attributed to Fasting

Headache attributed to fasting (**Box 15**) is typically a diffuse non-pulsating headache, usually mild to moderate, occurring during and caused by fasting for at least 8 hours that is relieved after eating (see also Chapter 7).[2] Even though the typical headache attributed to fasting is diffuse, non-pulsating, and mild to moderate in intensity, in those with a prior history of migraine, the headache may resemble migraine without aura.[112]

The etiology of fasting-induced headaches is uncertain.[113] Headache attributed to fasting is significantly more common in people who have a prior history of headache,

---

Box 14
Headache attributed to hypothyroidism

A. Headache fulfilling criterion C.

B. Hypothyroidism has been demonstrated.

C. Evidence of causation demonstrated by at least 2 of the following:
   1. Headache has developed in temporal relation to the onset of the hypothyroidism, or led to its discovery
   2. Either or both of the following:
      a. Headache has significantly worsened in parallel with worsening of the hypothyroidism
      b. Headache has significantly improved or resolved in parallel with improvement in or resolution of the hypothyroidism
   3. Headache has either or both of the following characteristics:
      a. Bilateral location
      b. Constant over time.

D. Not better accounted for by another ICHD-3 diagnosis.

Box 15
Headache attributed to fasting

A. Diffuse headache not fulfilling the criteria for "1. migraine" or any of its types but fulfilling criterion C below.

B. The patient has fasted for $\geq$ 8 hours.

C. Evidence of causation demonstrated by both of the following:
   1. Headache has developed during fasting
   2. Headache has significantly improved after eating.

D. Not better accounted for by another ICHD-3 diagnosis.

---

particularly migraine. However, in individuals without a well-defined history of headache, prolonged fasting may also be associated with the development of headaches. This is often seen in religious fasting and has been documented as "Yom Kippur headache"[114] and "'first of Ramadan headache."[115] The likelihood of headache developing due to fasting increases with the duration of the fast. Fasting headache can occur in the absence of hypoglycemia, suggesting that other factors play an important role (eg, caffeine withdrawal, duration of sleep, and circadian factors).

In terms of treatment, a study suggested that pre-emptive cyclooxygenase 2 inhibitor treatment (rofecoxib, 50 mg just before the onset of fasting) is effective in reducing these forms of headache.[112] Pre-emptive treatment with NSAIDs or long-acting triptans may be a reasonable alternative.[114]

There is a potentially related phenomenon known as post prandial headaches or post-iftar headaches. In a study of 16,037 respondents in Saudi Arabia during the month of Ramadan, 3144 reported fasting-related postprandial headaches following Iftar time or when breaking their fast (19.5%) occurring within 2 hours following the meal.[116] Descriptions of this headache were variable but generally described to be episodic, with a tension type quality and relieved with lying down or sleep.[116] As of yet, the ICHD has not described or incorporated this headache description.

Cardiac Cephalalgia

Cardiac cephalalgia (**Box 16**) is a headache with migraine features, usually but not always aggravated by exercise, occurring during an episode of myocardial ischemia that is relieved by nitroglycerin (see also Chapter 28).[2] Lipton and colleagues[117] proposed that this type of headache during a stess test correlated with electrocardiography changes indicative of myocardial ischemia. In both patients, coronary angiography revealed 3-vessel disease, and myocardial revascularization procedures were followed by complete resolution of headaches.

ICHD-3 states that the diagnosis must include a detailed headache history and simultaneous cardiac ischemia during treadmill or nuclear cardiac stress testing. However, cardiac cephalalgia occurring at rest has been described.[118] Several authors reported that this type of headache may be the sole manifestation of myocardial ischemia.[118–121] A previous literature review of cardiac cephalalgia showed that in more than half of the 35 reviewed cases, the headache was triggered by high myocardial oxygen consumption (ie, exertion, sexual activity, and emotional fluctuation); however, in 6 cases, the headache occurred during rest.

Cardiac cephalalgia, like migraine, can present with severe headaches associated with photophobia, phonophobia, osmophobia, nausea, or vomiting, and triggered by exertion.[121,122] It is therefore crucial to distinguish this disorder from migraine

---

Box 16
Cardiac cephalalgia

A. Any headache fulfilling criterion C.

B. Acute myocardial ischemia has been demonstrated.

C. Evidence of causation demonstrated by at least 2 of the following:
  1. Headache has developed in temporal relation to the onset of acute myocardial ischemia
  2. Either or both of the following:
     a. Headache has significantly worsened in parallel with worsening of the myocardial ischemia
     b. Headache has significantly improved or resolved in parallel with improvement in or resolution of the myocardial ischemia.
  3. Headache has at least 2 of the following 4 characteristics:
     a. Moderate to severe intensity
     b. Accompanied by nausea
     c. Not accompanied by photophobia or phonophobia
     d. Aggravated by exertion
  4. Headache is relieved by nitroglycerin or its derivatives.

D. Not better accounted for by another ICHD-3 diagnosis.

---

without aura, particularly as vasoconstrictor medications (eg, triptans, ergots) are indicated in the treatment of migraine but contraindicated in patients with ischemic heart disease.

The mechanisms involved in cardiac cephalalgia remain unclear; however, possible mechanisms reported are related to neural convergence, including somatic and sympathetic impulses converging in the posterior horn of the spinal cord, mixing neural supply to cervical area and cranial vessels; transient increases of intracardiac pressure that cause intracranial pressure elevation secondary to cerebral venous congestion[123,124] and severe headache; a functioning ventricular pacemaker producing the headache; and release of inflammatory mediators during cardiac ischemia such as substance P, bradykinin, and histamine causing vasodilation in intracranial arteries.[3,119,123,124] A case report by Wang and colleagues described cardiac cephalalgia with evidence of cerebral hypoperfusion, including reversible cerebral vasoconstriction and possible sympathetic hyperfunction through activation of cardiac sympathetic afferents during myocardial ischemia, which can increase the sympathetic outflow through cardiac sympathetic nerve reflexes, as well as abnormal hypothalamic functional connectivity.[122] It has also been proposed that these processes could cause cortical cerebral hypoperfusion and subsequent cortical spreading depression which are potential mechanisms implicated in cardiac cephalalgia.[123,124]

DISCLOSURE

Dr Ana Marissa Lagman-Bartolome received royalties as an author from Canadian Pharmacists Association, participated in advisory boards for TEVA, Miravo/Searchlight, Lundbeck and Pfizer as well as received research and unrestricted educational grants from Amgen, Lundbeck, TEVA and Abbvie which were submitted to the Center for Headache at Women's College Hospital and Hospital for Sick Children Research Institute. Dr James Im has nothing to disclose. Dr Jonathan Gladstone participated in advisory boards for, and designed, chaired or participated in continuing medical education programs via unrestricted educational grants for Abbvie, Eli Lily, Lundbeck, Novartis, Miravo/Searchlight and TEVA Canada.

REFERENCES

1. Headache Classification Subcommittee of the International Headache Society. Classification and diagnostic criteria for headache disorders, cranial neuralgia, and facial pain. Cephalalgia 1988;8(Suppl. 7):1–96.
2. Headache Classification Subcommittee of the International Headache Society. The International Classification of Headache Disorders. Cephalalgia 2018;38: 1–211.
3. Bigal M, Gladstone J. The metabolic headaches. Curr Pain Headache Rep 2008;12:292–5.
4. Waldmann D, Messlinger K. Transient activation of spinal trigeminal neurons in a rat model of hypoxia-induced headache. Pain 2021 Apr 1;162(4):1153–62.
5. James OP, Stacey B, Hopkins L, et al, Welsh Surgical Research Initiative and Neurovascular Research Laboratory collaborators. Personal protective equipment impairs pulmonary gas exchange causing systemic hypercapnia-hypoxaemia and cerebral hyperperfusion-induced cephalalgia. Br J Surg 2021;108(5):e205–6.
6. Frank F, Faulhaber M, Messlinger K, et al. Migraine and aura triggered by normobaric hypoxia. Cephalalgia 2020;40(14):1561–73.
7. Vakharia RJ, Jani I, Yadav S, et al. To Study Acute Changes in Brain Oxygenation on MRI in Healthcare Workers Using N95 Mask and PPE Kits for Six Hours a Day. Indian J Radiol Imaging 2022;31(4):893–900.
8. Luton OW, Stacey BS, Mellor K, et al. Personal protective equipment-induced systemic hypercapnic hypoxaemia: translational implications for impaired cognitive-clinical functional performance. Br J Surg 2023;110(5):606–13.
9. Queiroz LP, Rapoport AM. High-altitude headache. Curr Pain Headache Rep 2007;11:293–6.
10. Bian SZ, Zhang JH, Gao XB, et al. Risk factors for high-altitude headache upon acute high-altitude exposure at 3700 m in young Chinese men: a cohort study. J Headache Pain 2013;14:35.
11. Alizadeh R, Ziaee V, Aghsaeifard Z, et al. Characteristics of headache at altitude among trekkers; a comparison between acute mountain sickness and non-acute mountain sickness headache. Asian J Sports Med 2012;3:126–30.
12. Marmura MJ, Hernandez PB. High-altitude headache. Curr Pain Headache Rep 2015;19:483.
13. Hackett PH, Roach RC. High-altitude illness. N Engl J Med 2001;345:107–44.
14. Kallenberg K, Bailey DM, Christ S, et al. Magnetic resonance imaging evidence of cytotoxic cerebral edema in acute mountain sickness. J Cereb Blood Flow Metab 2006;27:1064–71.
15. Lawley J, Oliver S, Mullins P, et al. Investigation of whole-brain white matter identifies altered water mobility in the pathogenesis of high-altitude headache. J Cereb Blood Flow Metab 2013;33:1286–94.
16. Silber E, Sonnenberg P, Collier DJ, et al. Clinical features of headache at altitude: a prospective study. Neurology 2003;60:1167–71.
17. Yin X, Li Y, et al. Thickened Retinal Nerve Fiber Layers Associated With High-Altitude Headache. Front Physiol 2022;13:864222.
18. Burtscher M, Mairer K, Wille M, et al. Risk factors for high-altitude headache in mountaineers. Cephalalgia 2011;31:706–11.
19. Canoui-Poitrine F, Veerabudun K, Larmignat P, et al. Risk prediction score for severe high altitude illness: A cohort study. PLoS One 2014;9:e100642.

20. Appenzeller O, Minko T, Qualls C, et al. Migraine in the Andes and headache at sea level. Cephalalgia 2005;25:1117–21.
21. Shen Y, Zhang J, Yang J, et al. Association of EPAS1 and PPARA Gene Polymorphisms with High-Altitude Headache in Chinese Han Population. BioMed Res Int 2020;2020, 1593068.
22. Carlsten C, Swenson ER, Ruoss S. A dose-response study of acetazolamide for acute mountain sickness prophylaxis in vacationing tourists at 12,000 feet (3630 m). High Alt Med Biol 2004;5:33–9.
23. Bärtsch P, Swenson ER. Clinical practice: acute high-altitude illnesses. N Engl J Med 2013;368:2294–302.
24. Dumont L, Mardirosoff C, Tramèr MR. Efficacy and harm of pharmacological prevention of acute mountain sickness: quantitative systematic review. BMJ 2000;321(7256):267–72.
25. Burtscher M, Likar R, Nachbauer W, et al. Effects of aspirin during exercise on the incidence of high-altitude headache: a randomized, double-blind, placebo-controlled trial. Headache 2001;41(6):542–5.
26. Xiong J, Lu H, Wang R, et al. Efficacy of ibuprofen on prevention of high altitude headache: a systematic review and meta-analysis. PLoS One 2017;12: e0179788.
27. Gertsch JH, Lipman GS, Holck PS, et al. Prospective, double-blind, randomized, placebo-controlled comparison of acetazolamide versus ibuprofen for prophylaxis against high altitude headache: the Headache Evaluation at Altitude Trial (HEAT). Wilderness Environ Med 2010;21(3):236–43.
28. Irons HR, Salas RN, et al. Prospective Double-Blinded Randomized Field-Based Clinical Trial of Metoclopramide and Ibuprofen for the Treatment of High Altitude Headache and Acute Mountain Sickness. Wilderness Environ Med 2020;31(1): 38–43.
29. Hackett PH, Roach RC. High-altitude illness. N Engl J Med 2001;345(2):107–14.
30. Bao H, He X, Wang F, et al. Study of Brain Structure and Function in Chronic Mountain Sickness Based on fMRI. Front Neurol 2022;12:763835.
31. Acute mountain sickness: Do different time courses point to different pathophysiological mechanisms? Berger MM, Sareban M, Bärtsch P. J Appl Physiol (1985) 2020;128(4):952–9.
32. Bui SBD, Petersen T, Poulsen JN, et al. Headache attributed to airplane travel: a Danish survey. J Headache Pain 2016;17:33.
33. Mainardi F, Maggioni F, Lisotto C, et al. Diagnosis and management of headache attributed to airplane travel. Curr Neurol Neurosci Rep 2013;13:335.
34. Konrad F, Moritz A, Moritz M, et al. The epidemiology of airplane headache: A cross-sectional study on point prevalence and characteristics in 50,000 travelers. Cephalalgia 2022;42(10):1050–7.
35. Cherian A, Mathew M, Iype T, et al. Headache associated with airplane travel: a rare entity. Neurol India 2013;61:164.
36. Berilgen MS, Müngen B. A new type of headache, headache associated with airplane travel: preliminary diagnostic criteria and possible mechanisms of aetiopathogenesis. Cephalalgia 2011;31:1266–73.
37. Bui SBD, Gazerani P. Headache attributed to airplane travel: diagnosis, pathophysiology, and treatment—a systematic review. J Headache Pain 2017;18:84.
38. Niereburg H, Jackfert K. Headache attributed to airplane travel: a review of literature. Curr Pain Headache Rep 2018;22:48.
39. Chesire WP. Headache and facial pain in scuba divers. Curr Pain Headache Rep 2004;8:315–20.

40. Burkett JG, Nahas-Geiger SJ. Diving headache. Diving Hyperb Med 2015;45: 129–31.

41. Panneton WM, Gan Q. The Mammalian Diving Response: Inroads to Its Neural Control. Front Neurosci 2020;14:524.

42. Di Fabio R, Vanacore N, Davassi C, et al. Scuba diving is not associated with high prevalence of headache: a cross-sectional study in men. Headache 2012;52:385–92.

43. Cheshire WP Jr, Ott MC. Headache in divers. Headache 2001;41:235–47.

44. Englund M, Risberg J. Self-reported headache during saturation diving. Aviat Space Environ Med 2003;74:236241.

45. Arieli R, Shochat T, Adir Y. CNS toxicity in closed-circuit oxygen diving: symptoms reported from 2527 dives. Aviat Space Environ Med 2006;77:526–32.

46. Wilmshurst P, Nightingale S. Relationship between migraine and cardiac and pulmonary right-to-left shunts. Clin Sci 2001;100:215–20.

47. Smart D, Mitchell S, Wilmurst P, et al. Joint position statement on persistent foramen ovale (PFO) and diving. South Pacifc Underwater Medicine Society (SPUMS) and the United Kingdom Sports Diving Medical Committee (UKSDMC). Diving Hyper Med 2015;45:129–31.

48. Rains JC, Poceta JS. Headache and sleep disorders: review and clinical implications for headache management. Headache 2006;46:1344–63.

49. Loh NK, Dinner DS, Foldvary N, et al. Do patients with obstructive sleep apnea wake up with headaches? Arch Intern Med 1999;159:1765–8.

50. Poceta JS. Sleep-related headache. Curr Treat Options Neurol 2002;4:121–8.

51. Scher AI, Stewart WF, Lipton RB. Factors associated with the onset and remission of chronic daily headache in a population-based study. Pain 2003; 106:81–9.

52. Graf-Radford SB, Newman A. Obstructive sleep apnea and cluster headache. Headache 2004;44:607–10.

53. Chen PK, Fuh JL, Lanue HY, et al. Morning headache in habitual snorers: frequency, characteristics, predictors and impacts. Cephalalgia 2011;31:829–36.

54. Kristiansen HA, Kvaerner KJ, Akre H, et al. Sleep apnoea headache in the general population. Cephalalgia 2011;32:451–8.

55. Chen PK, Fuh JL, Lane HY, et al. Morning headache in habitual snorers: Frequency, characteristics, predictors and impacts. Cephalalgia 2011;31:829–36.

56. Goksan B, Gunduz A, Karadeniz D, et al. Morning head- ache in sleep apnoea: clinical and polysomnographic evaluation and response to nasal continuous positive airway pressure. Cephalalgia 2009;29:635–41.

57. Alberti A, Mazzotta G, Gallinela E, et al. Headache characteristics in obstructive sleep apnea syndrome and insomnia. Acta Neurol Scand 2005;111:309–16.

58. Russell MB, Kristiansen HA, Kværner KJ. Headache in sleep apnea syndrome: Epidemiology and pathophysiology. Cephalalgia 2014;34:752–5.

59. KoÇ G, Metİn KM, AkÇay BD, et al. Relationship between Apnea-Hypopnea Index and Oxygen Desaturation in REM-Sleep Period and Morning Headache in Patients with Obstructive Sleep Apnea Syndrome. Noro Psikiyatr Ars 2019; 57(4):294–8.

60. Kristiansen HA, Kværner KJ, Akre H, et al. Sleep apnoea headache in the general population. Cephalalgia 2012;32(6):451–8.

61. Headache Secondary. Current Update. Zhu K, Born DW, Dilli E. Headache 2020;60(10):2654–64.

62. Peppard PE, Young T, Palta M, et al. Longitudinal study of moderate weight change and sleep-disordered breathing. JAMA 2000;284:3015–21.

63. McCarthy K, Saripella A, Selvanathan J, et al. Positive airway pressure therapy for chronic pain in patients with obstructive sleep apnea-a systematic review. Sleep Breath 2022;26(1):47–55.

64. Sav MY, Sav T, Senocak E, et al. Hemodialysis-related headache. Hemodial Int 2014;18:725–9.

65. Sousa Melo E, Carrilho Aguiar F, Sampaio Rocha-Filho PA. Dialysis headache: a narrative review. Headache 2017;57:161–4.

66. Viticchi G, Falsetti L, Salvemini S, et al. Headache changes after kidney transplant. Acta Neurol Belg 2022;122(1):83–90.

67. Antoniazzi AL, Bigal ME, Bordini CA, et al. Headache associated with dialysis: the International Headache Society criteria revisited. Cephalalgia 2003;23:146–9.

68. Goksel BK, Torun D, Karaca S, et al. Is low magnesium level associated with hemodialysis headache? Headache 2006;46:40–5.

69. Goksan B, Karaali-Savrun F, Ertan S, et al. Hemodialysis related headache. Cephalalgia 2004;24:284–7.

70. Yang Y, Meng F, Zhu H, et al. The applicability research of the diagnostic criteria for 10.2 Heamodialysis-related headache in the international classification of headache disorders. J Headache Pain 2023;24(1):19.

71. Sousa Melo E, Pedrosa RP, Carrilho Aguiar F, et al. Dialysis headache: characteristics, impact and cerebrovascular evaluation. Arq Neuropsiquiatr 2022;80(2):129–36.

72. Antoniazzi AL, Corrado AP. Dialysis headache. Curr Pain Headache Rep 2007;11:297–303.

73. Leinisch-Dahlke E, Schmidt-Wilcke T, Krämer BK, et al. Improvement of dialysis headache afer treatment with ACEinhibitors but not angiotensin II receptor blocker: a case report with pathophysiological considerations. Cephalalgia 2004;25:71–4.

74. Kruszewski P, Bieniaszewski L, Neubauer J, et al. Headache in patients with mild to moderate hypertension is generally not associated with simultaneous blood pressure elevation. J Hypertens 2000;18:437–44.

75. Gus M, Fuchs FD, Pimentel M, et al. Behavior of ambulatory blood pressure surrounding episodes of headache in mildly hypertensive patients. Arch Intern Med 2001;161:252–5.

76. Cooper WD, Glover DR, Hormbrey JM, et al. Headache and blood pressure: evidence of a close relationship. J Hum Hypertens 1989;3:41–4.

77. Dodick DW. Recurrent short-lasting headache associated with paroxysmal hypertension: a clonidine-responsive syndrome. Cephalalgia 2000;20:509–14.

78. Gipponi S, Venturelli E, Rao R, et al. Hypertension is a factor associated with chronic daily headache. Neurol Sci 2010;31(Suppl. 1):171–3.

79. Liberman AL, Kamel H, Lappin R, et al. Prevalence of neurological complaints among emergency department patients with severe hypertension. Am J Emerg Med 2023;64:90–5.

80. Tomas JE, Rooke ED, Kvale WF. The neurologists experience with pheochromocytoma. JAMA 1966;197:754–8.

81. Mannelli M, Ianni L, Cilotti A, et al. Pheochromocytoma in Italy: a multicentric retrospective study. Eur J Endocrinol 1999;141:619–24.

82. Lance JW, Hinterberger H. Symptom of pheochromocytoma with particular reference to headache, correlated with catecholamine production. Arch Neurol 1976;33:281–8.

83. Vaughan CJ, Delanty N. Hypertensive emergencies. Lancet 2000;356:411–7.

84. Zampaglione B, Pascale C, Marchisio M, et al. Hypertensive urgencies and emergencies. Prevalence and clinical presentation. Hypertension 1996;27: 144–7.

85. Walker JJ. Pre-eclampsia. Lancet 2000;56:1260–5.

86. Land SH, Donovan T. Pre-eclampsia and eclampsia headache: classifcation recommendation. Cephalalgia 1999;19:67–9.

87. Furlan JC. Headache attributed to autonomic dysrefexia. Neurology 2011;77: 792–8.

88. Cocores AN, Monteith TS. Headache as a Neurologic Manifestation of Systemic Disease. Curr Treat Options Neurol 2022;24(1):17–40.

89. Bartikoski SR, Reschke DJ. Pheochromocytoma Crisis in the Emergency Department. Cureus 2021;13(3):e13683.

90. Anyfanti P, Mastrogiannis K, Lazaridis A, et al. Clinical presentation and diagnostic evaluation of pheochromocytoma: case series and literature review. Clin Exp Hypertens 2023;45(1):2132012.

91. Patel D, Phay JE, Yen TWF, et al. Update on Pheochromocytoma and Paraganglioma from the SSO Endocrine and Head and Neck Disease Site Working Group, Part 2 of 2: Perioperative Management and Outcomes of Pheochromocytoma and Paraganglioma. Ann Surg Oncol 2020;27(5):1338–47.

92. Immink R, van den Born BJ, van Montfrans GA, et al. Impaired cerebral autoregulation in patients with malignant hypertension. Circulation 2004;110:2241–5.

93. Schwartz R, Jones K, Kalina P, et al. Hypertensive encephalopathy: fndings on CT, MR imaging and SPECT imaging in 14 cases. AJR Am J Roentgenol 1992; 159:379–83.

94. Amraoui F, van Montfrans GA, van den Born BJ. Value of retinal examination in hypertensive encephalopathy. J Hum Hypertens 2010;24:274–9.

95. Macgregor EA. Headache in pregnancy. Continuum 2014;20:128–47.

96. Facchinetti F, Allais G, D'Amico R, et al. Te relationship between headache and preeclampsia: a case–control study. Eur J Obstet Gynaecol Reprod Biol 2005; 121:143–8.

97. Nij Bijvank SW, Hengst M, Cornette JC, et al. Nicardipine for treating severe antepartum hypertension during pregnancy: Nine years of experience in more than 800 women. Acta Obstet Gynecol Scand 2022;101(9):1017–25.

98. Gestational Hypertension and Preeclampsia: ACOG Practice Bulletin, Number 222. Obstet Gynecol 2020;135(6):e237–60.

99. Chao AS, Chen YL, Chang YL, et al. Severe pre-eclamptic women with headache: is posterior reversible encephalopathy syndrome an associated concurrent finding? BMC Pregnancy Childbirth 2020;20(1):336.

100. Umar T, Gilani A, Tasnim A, et al. MRI Changes Among Patients Of Eclampsia And Preeclampsia With Associated Neurological Symptom Analysis. J Ayub Med Coll Abbottabad 2022;34(2):269–72.

101. Zhang N, Yang L, Han A, et al. Advances in imaging findings of preeclampsia-related reversible posterior leukoencephalopathy syndrome. Front Neurosci 2023;17:1144867.

102. Iser C, Arca K. Headache and Autonomic Dysfunction: a Review. Curr Neurol Neurosci Rep 2022;22(10):625–34.

103. Hubbard ME, Phillips AA, Charbonneau R, et al. PRES secondary to autonomic dysreflexia: A case series and review of the literature. J Spinal Cord Med 2021; 44(4):606–12.

104. Kewalramani LS. Autonomic dysrefexia in traumatic myelopathy. Am J Phys Med 1980;59:1–21.

105. Lindan R, Joiner E, Freehafer AA, et al. Incidence and clinical features of autonomic dysrefexia in patients with spinal cord injury. Paraplegia 1980;18:285–92.

106. Moreau T, Manceau E, Giraud L. Headache in hypothyroidism. Prevalence and outcome under thyroid hormone therapy. Cephalalgia 1998;18:687–9.

107. Lima Carvalho MF, de Medeiros JS, Valença MM. Headache in recent onset hypothyroidism: prevalence, characteristics and outcome after treatment with levothyroxine. Cephalalgia 2017;37:938–46.

108. Bigal ME, Shefell FD, Tepper S. Chronic daily headache: identifcation of factors associated with induction and transformation. Headache 2002;42:575–8.

109. Tepper DE, Tepper SJ, Shefell FD, et al. Headache attributed to hypothyroidism. Curr Pain Headache Rep 2007;11:304–9.

110. Tasnim S, Wilson SG, Walsh JP, et al. Cross-Trait Genetic Analyses Indicate Pleiotropy and Complex Causal Relationships between Headache and Thyroid Function Traits. Genes 2022;14(1):16.

111. Arafah B, Prunty D, Ybarra J, et al. Te dominant role of increased intrasellar pressure in the pathogenesis hypopituitarism, hyperprolactinemia, and headache in patients with pituitary adenomas. J Clin Endocrinol Metab 2000;85:1789–93.

112. Drescher MJ, Elstein Y. Prophylactic COX-2 inhibitor: an end to the Yom Kippur headache. Headache 2006;46:1487–91.

113. Dalkara T, Kilic K. How does fasting trigger migraine? A hypothesis. Curr Pain Headache Rep 2013;17:368.

114. Kundin JE. Yom Kippur headache. Neurology 1996;47:854, 87.

115. Awada A, al Jumah M. The first-of-Ramadan headache. Headache 1999;39: 490–3.

116. AlAmri A, AlMuaigel M, AlSheikh M, et al. Postprandial fasting related headache during Ramadan in Saudi Arabia: A cross-sectional study 2021;41(11–12): 1201–7.

117. Lipton RB, Lowenkopf T, Bajwa ZH, et al. Cardiac cephalgia: a treatable form of exertional headache. Neurology 1997;49:813–6.

118. Chen SP, Fuh JL, Yu WC, et al. Cardiac cephalalgia: Case series and review of the literature with new ICDH-II criteria revisited. Eur Neurol 2004;24:231–4.

119. Wei JH, Wang HF. Cardiac cephalalgia: case reports and review. Cephalalgia 2008;28:892–6.

120. Seow VK, Chong CF, Wang TF, et al. Severe explosive headache: a sole presentation of acute myocardial infarction in a young man. Am J Emerg Med 2007;25: 250–1.

121. Bini A, Evangelista A, Castellini P, et al. Cardiac cephalalgia. J Headache Pain 2009;10:3–9.

122. Wang M, Wang L, Liuc Bain X, et al. Cardiac cephalalgia: one case with cortical hypoperfusion in headaches and literature review. J Headache Pain 2017;18:24.

123. Navarro-Pérez MP, Bellosta-Diago E, Olesen J, et al. Cardiac cephalalgia: a narrative review and ICHD-3 criteria evaluation. J Headache Pain 2022; 23(1):136.

124. Kobata H. Cardiac cephalalgia: a case series of four patients and updated literature review. Int J Emerg Med 2022;15(1):33.

Cervicogenic Headaches

A Literature Review and Proposed Multifaceted Approach to Diagnosis and Management

Aishwarya V. Pareek, MD[a], Everton Edmondson, MD[b],
Doris Kung, DO[b],*

KEYWORDS

- Cervicogenic headaches • Secondary headaches • Neck pain

KEY POINTS

- A standardized approach to diagnosing cervicogenic headaches can not only provide sustained relief for patients but also clarity for future research.
- Cervicogenic headaches can manifest in variable symptoms and overlap with other primary headaches, with or without neck pain.
- A confirmatory diagnosis of cervicogenic headaches requires certain clinical features, establishing a cervical origin, and identifyin.

INTRODUCTION

The relationship between headache and the cervical spine has been well described. However, the concept of cervicogenic headaches, or headaches that originate from disease or injury affecting the cervical spine, has only been accepted in the last 4 decades. Since then, there has been considerable controversy surrounding the diagnosis of cervicogenic headaches and around whether it is in fact a unique entity at all. This is largely due to its variable and wide range of clinical presentations and that the clinical symptoms tend to overlap with several primary and secondary headaches, as well as nonheadache neurologic diagnoses.

There are 3 general approaches to the diagnosis of cervicogenic headaches. The first aims to make the diagnosis based on clinical features, as is common practice with most primary headaches. The second is focused on establishing a cervical source for head pain. Finally, there is increasing support for the use of various treatment modalities

[a] Department of Pediatrics, Section of Neurology and Developmental Neuroscience, Baylor College of Medicine at Texas Children's Hospital, 7200 Cambridge Street, 9th Floor, Houston, TX 77030, USA; [b] Department of Neurology, Baylor College of Medicine, 7200 Cambridge Street, 9th Floor, Houston, TX 77030, USA
* Corresponding author.
E-mail address: Kung@bcm.edu

Neurol Clin 42 (2024) 543–557
https://doi.org/10.1016/j.ncl.2023.12.008

aimed at the cervical spine resulting in headache alleviation as a confirmation of diagnosis. Here, we aim to provide a review of the current available literature on cervicogenic headaches including its epidemiology and pathophysiology and provide a holistic framework for its diagnosis and management.

BACKGROUND AND DEFINITION

In its broadest sense, cervicogenic headache is a condition that presents with head pain with or without accompanying neck pain secondary to dysfunction in the cervical spine, specifically with its component bony, disc and/or soft tissue elements. In its earliest form, it was described by French neurologist Barre in 1926 with the term "syndrome cervical sympathetique posterieur," which linked headache with a supposed posterior sympathetic deficiency.[1] The term cervicogenic headaches was finally coined in 1983 by Sjaastad after he presented a case series of 22 patients with a uniform clinical presentation of headache in the setting of evidence suggesting a cervical etiology.[2] In 1988, the International Headache Society amended its diagnostic classification system to include a category for headaches associated with disorders of the neck. Finally, after various iterations, clinical diagnostic criteria were published in 1998 by the Cervicogenic Headache International Study Group (CHISG) and remain the most current clinical criteria for the entity.[3]

EPIDEMIOLOGY

There is considerable variability in the reporting of the prevalence of cervicogenic headaches. The reason for this is that prevalence studies have been undertaken on heterogenous patient populations, the study methodologies have been varied, and several different diagnostic criteria have been used. In the general population, cervicogenic headache has an estimated prevalence of between 0.4% and 2.5%.[4] Cervicogenic headaches seem more common among women. The average age of presentation is 42.9 years with an average duration of symptoms lasting 6.8 years.[5,6]

PATHOPHYSIOLOGY

The most common source implicated in cervicogenic headache is upper cervical joint dysfunction. It is thought that pain in cervicogenic headache results from the interaction of nociceptive afferents of the descending trigeminal nerve (trigeminal nucleus caudalis) and the C1 to C3 segments of the cervical spine. Accordingly, pain signals can travel bidirectionally between the neck and regions of the face and head that receive innervation from the trigeminal nerve (**Fig. 1**).[7] The best studied and most implicated joint in cervicogenic headache is the C2–3 zygapophyseal joint. Stimulation of C2–C3 intervertebral disc or cervical facet joints produced characteristic and distinguishable pain in normal subjects.[8] The second commonly implicated joint is the C1–2 atlanto-axial joint, which innervates the posterior fossa and portions of the dens.[7] In one study, head pain was demonstrated in human subjects following electrical stimulation of C1 or noxious stimulation of the greater occipital nerve.[9] The C2 nerve root is the main contributor to the greater occipital nerve and due to the unique anatomy of C1 and C2 relative to other vertebrae, the greater occipital nerve is not protected by a cervical facet leaving it prone to injury. This is supported by a study in which direct compression of the greater occipital nerve was achieved in cadavers between the atlas and axis in extension and by adjacent muscles and connective tissue traveling to the occipital scalp in flexion.[10] Less commonly, cervicogenic headache may result from involvement of the C3–C4 zygapophyseal joint,

MECHANISM OF PAIN REFERRAL FROM CERVICAL SPINE TO THE HEAD

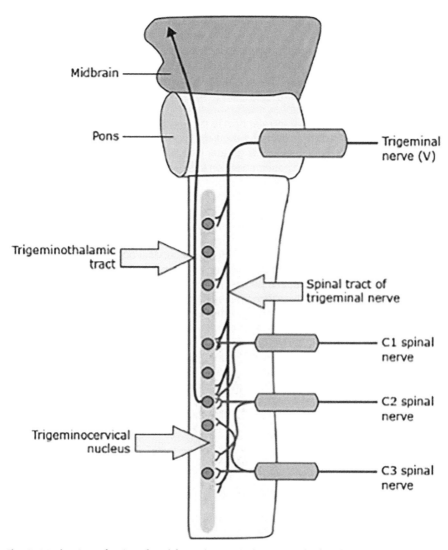

Fig. 1. Mechanism of pain referral from the cervical spine to the head showing nociceptive afferents of the trigeminal and upper 3 cervical spinal nerves converge onto second-order neurons in the trigeminocervical nucleus in the upper cervical spinal cord. This convergence mediates the referral of pain signals from the neck to regions of the head innervated by cervical nerves or the trigeminal nerve. (*Reprinted with permission from* Elsevier. The Lancet Neurology, 2009, 8 (10), October 2009, 959-968.)

upper cervical intervertebral discs, or intraspinal processes affecting the upper cervical roots.[10]

CLINICAL PRESENTATION

Cervicogenic headaches have a varied clinical presentation, particularly because the cervical cause of these headaches is heterogeneous. The most salient and specific features of cervicogenic headaches are concerning the involvement of the neck. Neck pain is typically described as constant, dull, nonthrobbing. It is typically localized to the occiput and is ipsilateral to the side of the headache. The headache is similarly unilateral at the onset, although it may progress to bilateral. It is typically occipital but there have been reports of periorbital, temporal, frontal, and parietal distributions. Myofascial trigger point tenderness may be present in the ipsilateral suboccipital, cervical, or shoulder regions and may refer pain to the head with stimulation.[11] There have been rare reports of radicular symptoms on the side of the headache and sensory dysfunction of the occipital scalp if the greater occipital nerve is involved.

The first diagnostic criterion based solely on clinical features was formalized by the CHISG in 1990 and further amended in 1998 to improve specificity (**Box 1**).[3] The revised criteria were evaluated for interrater reliability and showed fair-to-good agreement with higher scores obtained by expert neurologists and anesthesiologists with more experience diagnosing cervicogenic headache.[11] The criteria prioritize clinical features pertaining to neck involvement, such as precipitation of pain with awkward head positioning of external pressure over the upper cervical/occipital region. Patients may describe protective behaviors to limit neck motion or avoid certain precipitating neck positions.[11] These protective behaviors may also be visible in the examination room before attempting provocative maneuvers. They may present as abnormal posture at baseline or awkward head movements. Restriction of neck range of motion is a critically important clinical feature of cervicogenic headache. Patients with cervicogenic headache typically show at least 10° of restriction on the affected side, and this restriction correlates to headache frequency and associated disability.[12,13]

The characteristics of the head pain itself as well as the additional, although less important, clinical characteristics such as nausea, photophobia, phonophobia, and neck pain are not specific to cervicogenic headaches. Thus, when relying solely on clinical criteria, there exists a substantial possibility of overdiagnosis of cervicogenic headaches.

Box 1
Diagnostic criteria for cervicogenic headache per CHISG

Diagnostic Criteria
  I. Symptoms and signs of neck involvement
      A. Precipitation of head pain, similar to the usually occurring one
          1. By neck movement and/or sustained awkward head positioning, and/or
          2. By external pressure over the upper cervical or occipital region on the symptomatic side
      B. Restriction of the range of motion in the neck
      C. Ipsilateral neck, shoulder, or arm pain of a rather vague nonradicular nature or, occasionally, arm pain of a radicular nature
  II. Confirmatory evidence by diagnostic anesthetic blockades
  III. Unilaterally of the head pain, without side shift

Important notations added to the diagnostic criteria are as follows: points 1A suffices as the sole criterion for the diagnosis whereas points 1B and 1C do not; provisionally, the combination of 1B and 1C is satisfactory; and "unilaterality on two sides" may be acceptable

INTERNATIONAL CLASSIFICATION OF HEADACHE DISORDERS-3 CRITERIA AND CAUSATION

The third edition of the International Classification of Headache Disorders (ICHD-3) is a hierarchical classification system and is widely accepted as the current gold standard diagnostic classification for headache disorders. Cervicogenic headaches are coded under Part II of the ICHD-3 classification, secondary headaches, which, by definition, are headaches that develop as a secondary symptom due to another disorder that is known to cause headaches. The diagnosis is specifically listed under subsection 11.2, headaches attributed to disorders of the neck. It is 1 of 3 headache diagnoses in this subsection, along with headache attributed to retropharyngeal tendonitis and headache attributed to craniocervical dystonia (HACCD).

Per the ICHD-3, cervicogenic headaches are headaches caused by a disorder of the cervical spine and its component bony, disc, and/or soft tissue elements, usually but not invariably accompanied by neck pain and have the following diagnostic criteria (**Box 2**).[14] The diagnosis requires the presence of a headache with or without neck pain (criterion A), the presence of a cervical source for the headache (criterion B), and evidence of causation (criterion C). Causation in cervicogenic headaches is, however, a hotly debated concept because neck involvement in the form of pain or restricted mobility can be a component of primary headache versus a nidus for secondary headache. The ICHD-3 lists causes that certainly and possibly fulfill the criteria of causation, although this list is not exhaustive, and care must be taken to investigate causes outside this list (**Box 3**).[14]

INTERVENTIONAL PROCEDURES: A ROUTE TO DIAGNOSIS, PROBABLE CAUSATION, AND TREATMENT

Interventional procedures can be useful in the treatment and diagnosis of cervicogenic headaches. Here we present 2 clinical vignettes as an avenue to narrow the differential diagnoses and decipher the most reasonable treatment plan.

Vignette #1

A 55-year-old woman presents with a 6-month history of left occipital-temporal headaches, which are dull and aching in quality. She sought care with her primary care doctor who initially treated her for presumed tension headache with a nonsteroidal anti-

---

Box 2

Diagnostic criteria for cervicogenic headache per ICHD-3

Diagnostic Criteria

A. Any headache fulfilling criterion C

B. Clinical, laboratory, and/or imaging evidence of a disorder or lesion within the cervical spine or soft tissues of the neck, known to be able to cause headache

C. Evidence of causation demonstrated by at least 2 of the following:
1. Headache has developed in temporal relation to the onset of the cervical disorder or appearance of the lesion
2. Headache has significantly improved or resolved in parallel with improvement in or resolution of the cervical disorder or lesion
3. Cervical range of motion is reduced, and headache is made significantly worse by provocative maneuvers
4. Headache is abolished following diagnostic blockade of a cervical structure or its nerve supply

D. Not better accounted for by another ICHD-3 beta diagnosis

Box 3
Etiologies of causation in cervicogenic headaches per ICHD-3

Certainly fulfill
1. Tumor
2. Fracture
3. Infection
4. Rheumatoid arthritis of the upper cervical spine

May fulfill
1. Cervical spondylosis
2. Osteochondritis

---

inflammatory drug and a muscle relaxant. She did not improve. On returning, she also complains of bilateral neck pain, although worse on the left side. Radiograph of the cervical spine is obtained, and she is noted to have multiple levels of spondylosis from C2 to C6. She then receives 6 weeks of physical therapy during which she worsens with persistent headaches ranging from moderate to sometimes severe intensity. MRI of the cervical spine confirms similar findings from C2 to C6—spondylosis with mild-to-moderate lateral recess narrowing and facet hypertrophy but no root impingement. MRI of the brain is obtained, and it is normal.

Given the presentation of occipital and temporal headache with ipsilateral neck pain, a provocative maneuver is attempted and produces accentuation of pain without radicular spread. A reasonable next step is a diagnostic and therapeutic block. The highest likely target is the C2–3 facet joint or the third occipital nerve. This assertion is based on the distribution of pain and noted prevalence of cervicogenic headache being most common in the C2–3 area followed by C1–2, then C3–4.[10] A zygapophyseal joint injection at the left C2–3 facet can be achieved via C-arm guided localization and injection with either bupivacaine or a combination of bupivacaine and a nonparticulate steroid such as preservative-free dexamethasone. If the facet injection provides 2 weeks of 70% to 80% relief, then the next therapeutic goal is to achieve more enduring relief with a medial branch block at the superior articular pillar of C3 subjacent to the C2–3 facet. There, the third occipital nerve courses onward along a medial and cephalad course to the occipital scalp (**Figs. 2 and 3**). If at least 90% relief from local anesthetic injection at the medial branch is achieved, then a medial branch radiofrequency ablation can be performed. Relief is apt to last 6 to 12 months with repeat radiofrequency ablation providing similar relief.[15–17] Some clinicians rely on greater than 50% relief but false-positive results increase with a lower bar.

If there is no relief from a facet or medial branch block an atlanto-occipital (C0–1) or atlanto-axis (C1–2) joint injection are potential targets. Lee and colleagues provided data from a study of 29 patients, 20 of whom had at least 50% relief from C0–1 joint injection.[18] This relieved pain in the posterior neck and occipital area but in some patients, there was referred pain extending to the lower neck and scapula that disappeared after the injection. Atlanto-axial involvement causes pain in the upper neck radiating to the suboccipital zone and laterally. However, similar to all the upper cervical joints, referred pain patterns can vary and spread to the ear or scapula. Bogduk and Govind sites referral patterns for the C0–1-related and C1–2-related cervicogenic pain patterns. Volunteers were given injections to expand the joint to induce pain, which mapped the distribution of pain referral.[8,19] Given the varied presentation, a tailored approach to injections for patients' refractory to facet or medial branch blocks is warranted.

UPPER CERVICAL SPINE NERVES

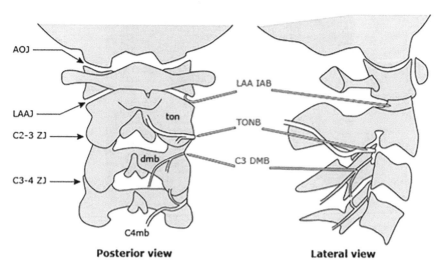

Posterior view   **Lateral view**

Fig. 2. Posterior and lateral views of the upper cervical spine nerves, showing the leading articular sources of cervicogenic headache, the related nerves, and where needles are placed for diagnostic blocks of these structures.[7] Red labels and needles point to target sites for diagnostic blocks. AOJ, atlanto-occipital joint; C3 DMB, C3 deep medial branch block; C4mb, medical branch of the C4 dorsal ramus; DMB, deep medial branch of the C3 dorsal ramus; LAA IAB, intra-articular block of the lateral atlanto-axial join; LAAJ, lateral atlanto-axial joint; ton, third occipital nerve; TONB, third occipital nerve block; ZJ, zygapophysial joint. (*Reprinted with permission from* Elsevier. The Lancet Neurology, 2009, 8 (10), October 2009, 959-968.)

Vignette #2

A 44-year-old man presents with a history of acute onset severe neck pain associated with lancinating pain along the anterior frontotemporal region extending down the preauricular region, posterior jaw on the left side, and shoulders bilaterally but significantly worse on the left side. There is no numbness or weakness in the upper limbs and cervical spasm is noted. His pain is refractory to treatment with 1 week of scheduled naproxen and methocarbamol. Given the presence of lancinating facial pain and severe neck pain, MRI of the internal auditory canal with and without contrast is obtained and does not reveal vascular compression in the trigeminal region of the pons or ambient cistern. However, MRI of the cervical spine reveals a C4–5 broad disc protrusion with more leftward extension compressing the cord at this level. Neurosurgical consultation is obtained, and although there is no myelopathic physical finding, anterior cervical decompression and fixation is entertained given the trigeminal neuralgic pain and concurrent neck pain. A course of oral steroids helps partially but the severe pain returns as the steroid dosing is tapered and discontinued.

In this patient, possible interventions include epidural steroid injection versus neurosurgical intervention. Given his presentation with spinal stenosis created by a broad disc protrusion with left-sided deviation, it may be appropriate to proceed directly to neurosurgical intervention. However, some interventionalists would first try a less-invasive approach with either interlaminar or transforaminal epidural steroid injection.

POSTERIOR AND LATERAL VIEWS OF THE UPPER CERVICAL SPINE

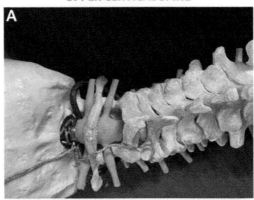

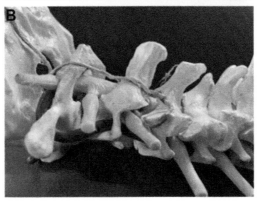

Fig. 3. Posterior and lateral anatomic views of the occipital nerve. (*A*) Posterior view of the upper cervical spine with the third occipital nerve coursing around the superior facet endplate at C3 then cephalad to the occipital skull. The facet joint is purposely separated from the inferior endplate of C2 facet to emphasize the course of the third occipital nerve from its inception as the superficial branch of the dorsal ramus of C3 root-a medical branch path. (*B*) Lateral view of the upper cervical spine demonstrating the location of the vertebral artery and the lack of a true foramen transversarium cephalad to the C2 vertebra. The root and the vertebral artery are relatively nakedly exposed.

Some risks do still exist, including nerve injury particularly with injectate volumes greater than 1 to 2 mL or quick injection causing a pressure surge. Interlaminar injection has less of a risk compared with transforaminal epidural injection with the latter being closer to the vertebral artery increasing the risk of arterial insult. In this case, pursuing surgery will be necessary if conservative measures fail to mitigate this patient's pain. Unrelenting severity of pain would typically prompt surgical intervention sooner rather than later.

COMPLICATIONS FROM CERVICAL INTERVENTIONAL PROCEDURES

Machikanti and colleagues conducted a prospective, nonrandomized study examining the records looking for adverse events for 7500 episodes related to 43,000 facet injections. About 11.4% of the adverse events were due to intravascular penetration, with 20% cervical, 4% lumbar, and 6% thoracic injections.[20] A meta-analysis study performed by Ekhator and colleagues revealed superior reduction in pain and duration of relief in radiofrequency ablation procedures versus epidural steroid injections with a complication rate of 12%.[21] Only a few anecdotal reports have noted serious side effects such as intravascular injection into the vertebral artery due to error in localization of its trajectory causing vertebral dissection or stroke. Injection of an anesthetic intra-arterially could cause vertigo, ataxia, seizure, stroke, or death. If the needle penetrates the facet joint and the tip advances beyond the facet joint anterior margin, inadvertent epidural injection will occur. Local anesthetic spread could cause respiratory depression. Proximity of the dorsal root and thecal envelope of the nerve root at that level could be violated at the distal lateral recess or the foramen resulting in root injury or intrathecal spread of the injectate. In **Fig. 3**, the lateral view of the spine shows the proximity of the vertebral artery to the facet region. The occipital-axial joint and C1–2 are especially notable for vulnerable vessels and exposed nerve roots. Given this anatomy, the risk factor for interventional measures increases at these upper cervical spine levels. This region requires caution and exceptional skills to avoid adverse events. There is also a risk of inadvertent intrathecal entry at the nerve root level. The C7/T1 space is the most capacious epidural space, and it is the most favored level to do an interlaminar epidural injection. A more proximate site near the area of interest can be considered if there is concern for impedance from a stenotic region, fibrosis, or other obstructions. Transforaminal epidural injection in the cervical region accounts for only 2.4% of epidural injections performed, and it has a higher complication rate.[22] Scanlon and colleagues performed a survey study of US physician members of the American Pain Society with 287 respondents.[23] Complications were noted in 78 patients out of 287 who received transforaminal epidural steroids. There were 12 cervical spine infarcts; 13 fatalities from posterior circulation infarcts, combined brain, and cervical infarcts with seizure; and 5 unspecified adverse events. Inamasu and Guiot reviewed the incidence of vertebral artery injury from diagnostic and therapeutic cervical procedures including embolic events, arterial dissection, or inadvertent intra-arterial injection of anesthetic causing seizures, respiratory depression, or other serious events.[24] Recognition of the presentation of arterial dissection requires vigilance especially since some patients' symptoms may evolve subacutely. Neck pain and occipital pain is commonly seen and if unrecognized, occlusion of the vertebral artery could be devastating. Serious complications are reported as notably rare, nonetheless, it should be stressed that appropriate measures should be implemented to minimize risk. There is a likelihood that adverse events are underreported. Further studies and mandatory reporting mechanisms should be instituted to truly reflect the procedural risk and adverse events.

A MULTIFACETED APPROACH TO DIAGNOSIS

The successful diagnosis of cervicogenic headache relies on a careful history including thorough review of systems, as well as a physical examination. We recommend a combined approach to diagnosis that includes careful consideration of clinical criteria, assessment of causation, and evaluation of response to treatment to most accurately diagnose cervicogenic headaches. Here, we propose a diagnostic algorithm that combines the most pertinent and specific clinical features per the CHISG, the causative recommendations of the ICHD-3 criteria, and the response to validated treatment options (**Fig. 4**).

Per the CHISG, the presence of characteristic head pain precipitated by neck movement and/or sustained awkward head positioning and/or external pressure over the

CERVICOGENIC HEADACHES DIAGNOSTIC ALGORITHM

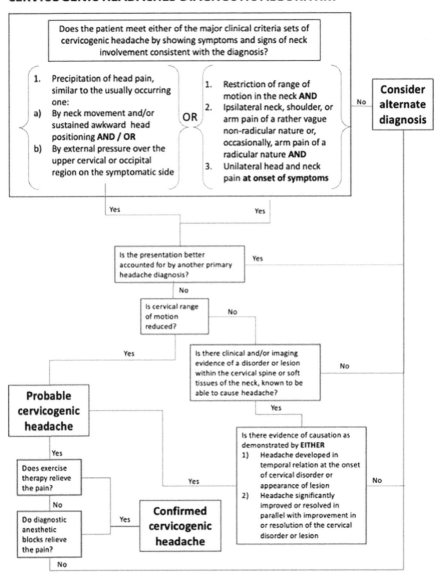

Fig. 4. A proposed diagnostic algorithm for cervicogenic headaches incorporating clinical features (*blue boxes*), causation criteria (*green boxes*), and intervention-based confirmation (*red boxes*). Endpoints are either confirmed cervicogenic headache, probable cervicogenic headache, or alternate diagnosis. A confirmed diagnosis of cervicogenic headache will, at a minimum, meet ICHD-3 criteria.

upper cervical or occipital region on the symptomatic side secures a diagnosis of cervicogenic headache. It is also proposed that a combination of (1) restriction of the range of motion in the neck, (2) characteristic ipsilateral neck, shoulder, or arm pain and (3) unilaterality of the headache at onset of symptoms secures the diagnosis. For research purposes, CHISG recommends that the combination of these clinical features must be supported by confirmatory evidence with diagnostic anesthetic blockades. For our clinical diagnostic purposes that aim to be practical and prioritize noninvasive measures, diagnostic anesthetic blockades are not required to fulfill the initial clinical diagnostic criteria and are only introduced later.

Although the CHISG suggests that the clinical points outlined are sufficient to provide a diagnosis, the ICHD-3 criteria require additional proof of causation, as well as a concerted effort to rule out common mimicking entities. Thus, if clinical criteria are fulfilled per the CHISG criteria and the presentation is not better accounted for by an alternate ICHD-3 diagnosis, the algorithm moves on to establish causation, specifically by introducing criterion B, followed by criterion C1 and C2 which are 2 clinical features that both help establish causation and are not accounted for by the CHISG. At this stage in the algorithm, workup will likely be expanded to include laboratory testing to rule out alternate systemic sources of pain, and imaging of the head and neck with either MRI or computed tomography (CT). Cervical spine MRI or CT do adequately demonstrate cervical facet hypertrophy when examined in the sagittal or axial plane and so may be useful in establishing a cervical source of pain.[11] Imaging also aids in ruling out sources of pain that may warrant alternate intervention such as vertebral artery dissection, aneurysm, or myelopathy.

Fulfillment of the most salient clinical features per the CHISG as well as establishment of causation per the ICHD-3 result in a diagnosis of probable cervicogenic headache, which warrants intervention in a stepwise manner with priority given to the most noninvasive treatment options. To further solidify and confirm the diagnosis of cervicogenic headache, the algorithm offers therapeutic diagnostic modalities. We recommend intervention with physical therapy followed by or concurrently with diagnostic anesthetic blocks at the discretion of the provider based on degree of pain and disability. Substantial improvement in pain or full resolution results in a diagnosis of confirmed cervicogenic headache.

This diagnostic algorithm is novel in that it provides a more practical and stepwise manner for the diagnosis of cervicogenic headaches, an entity often clouded by alternate contributing sources of pain such as primary headaches, alternate secondary headaches, or nonheadache neurologic diagnoses. It first establishes clear clinical criteria per the most validated criteria available, and priority is given to features that have a higher degree of specificity for cervicogenic headaches. This is followed by a rigorous evaluation of causation per ICHD-3 consensus criteria. This step often requires laboratory testing and imaging to rule out alternate causes and possibly establish a cervical source of pain. Only after both these criteria are met are therapeutic diagnostic modalities offered. This approach is important because simultaneous treatment of the various etiologies on the differential for cervicogenic headaches is usually underway. It becomes difficult to tease out the true cause of headache when multiple interventions are performed simultaneously. A high clinical and causative degree of suspicion is required before the initiation of therapeutic intervention targeted to treat cervicogenic headaches, especially when considering invasive options.

This approach may also reduce the burden of health-care costs associated with jumping straight to anesthetic blocks. There are multiple checkpoints in the algorithm that lead the practitioner to consider alternate diagnoses and halt their progress down the cervicogenic headache diagnostic and therapeutic path. In addition, invasive therapeutic interventions are often not immediately covered by insurance companies. Insurance companies often rely on evidence-based metrics or a preponderance of expert consensus to finance treatment, both of which are lacking in the research and literature surrounding cervicogenic headache. Adherence to this stepwise path may also reduce unnecessary invasive measures and subsequently reduce the financial burden on the patient.

DIFFERENTIATING FROM PRIMARY OR OTHER SECONDARY HEADACHES

The definitive diagnosis of cervicogenic headaches is complicated by the fact that patients may not present purely with one type of headache. Thus, treating a patient without considering wider differential diagnoses and management options can be detrimental and ineffective for the patient. Often it is useful to treat the headache phenotype depending on the presentation.[25] It is helpful to categorize headaches based on whether it is a primary headache disorder or a secondary headache disorder. Primary headaches that may be confused with or coexist with cervicogenic headaches include migraine and tension-type headaches.

Migraines are characterized by paroxysmal moderate-to-severe headaches associated with nausea and/or vomiting or photophobia and phonophobia. Neck pain may be present in up to 76% of patients with migraines.[26] The pathophysiology of cervicogenic headaches through the activation of the trigeminal nerve may also consequently activate nociceptive afferents involved in migraines resulting in a mixed clinical picture such that it is difficult to differentiate between the 2 headache types.

Similarly, patients with primary tension-type headaches often have neck pain and may be present in up to 88% of these patients.[26] Tension-type headaches are characterized by mild-to-moderate headaches often bilateral and nonpulsating and are not associated with nausea or vomiting, although phonophobia or photophobia may exist.[14] Cervical myofascial pain is common in patients with tension-type headaches and cervicogenic headaches. Thus, similar pathophysiology is noted with peripheral sensitization through the trigeminal nucleus caudalis causing increased pain in both headache types. Fortunately, management options for the primary headache types often overlap but do not aid in differentiating the type of headache.

DIFFERENTIATING FROM OTHER NEUROLOGIC DIAGNOSES

Disorders such as cervical or vertebral artery dissection, posterior fossa tumor, multiple sclerosis, or retropharyngeal abscess may present with similar symptoms as cervicogenic headache but the associated symptoms including focal neurologic signs, fever, meningismus, and acuity would effectively lower the suspicion for cervicogenic headaches. Other neurologic conditions to consider when diagnosing cervicogenic headaches include occipital neuralgia and cervical dystonia.

Cervicocerebral artery dissection is an important differential diagnosis to consider for cervicogenic headaches. Extracranial or intracranial dissections can present with acute severe unilateral head and neck pain typically ipsilateral to the side of the dissection accompanied by focal neurologic symptoms. Dissections involving the anterior circulation often present with temporal or frontal pain, whereas vertebrobasilar dissections involve occipital and nuchal pain thus mimicking cervicogenic headaches.[27] Persistent headache and neck pain after cervicocerebral artery dissection can also occur and in many studies reveal that this affects about 20% of patients 6 months to 3 years after the dissection.[28] Posterior circulation dissections and a history of primary headaches could predispose to persistent headache and neck pain after a cervicocerebral artery dissection.

Occipital neuralgia is characterized by unilateral or bilateral severe paroxysmal shooting, stabbing, or sharp pain around the greater, lesser, or third occipital nerves.[14] The pain is associated with allodynia and tenderness on applying pressure to the area. The greater occipital nerve is most often affected, 90% of the time, compared with

10% of patients with lesser occipital nerve involvement, and rare involvement of the third occipital nerve.[29] Occipital nerve blocks can provide sustained relief for occipital neuralgia but have also been shown to alleviate both migraine and cervicogenic headaches.

Cervical dystonia is an idiopathic condition causing involuntary muscle contractions of isolated muscle groups in the cervical region resulting in twisting movements and abnormal postures. HACCD is characterized by neck pain that is in the location of the dystonic muscle, has either worsened or developed around the time of the cervical dystonia, and/or has improved as the cervical dystonia improved. In one study, pain and disability were significantly worse in patients with HACCD compared with patients with cervical dystonia without headaches and can be seen in up to 29% of patients with cervical dystonia.[30]

SUMMARY

Cervicogenic headache is a unique clinical entity, which presents with head and neck pain due to a cervical source and affects a significant proportion of the population. Since its recognition as a secondary headache disorder, there has been debate regarding the most sensitive and specific diagnostic measures, and this has posed a dilemma for diagnosing practitioners and researchers. This is further clouded by the many neurologic and nonneurologic mimickers of cervicogenic headache pain.

We provide a systematic algorithm for diagnosis that serves as a practical approach that prioritizes ruling in patients based on a critical assessment of their clinical presentation and physical examination, followed by the establishment of causation, and finally confirmation of suspicion with interventions that are simultaneously therapeutic. Further research is required to better define treatment options for this patient population. This, and other studies of cervicogenic headache, will be facilitated by this consistent and standardized approach to diagnosis.

CLINICS CARE POINTS

- Given the varied presentations of cervicogenic headaches, it is important to utilize a standardized algorithm for diagnosis and treatment.
- Interventional procedures are useful for the treatment and diagnosis of cervicogenic headaches and require a careful targeted approach.
- Treatment and confirmation of cervicogenic headaches includes diagnostic anesthetic blockade and exercise therapy to relieve pain.
- The differential diagnosis of cervicogenic headaches, although extensive, can often involve similar management strategies such as with migraine, tension-headache, and occipital neuralgia.

DISCLOSURE

The authors have no conflicts of interest or relevant financial disclosures.

REFERENCES

1. Barré M. Sur un syndrome sympathique cervical postérieur et sa cause fréquente: l'arthrite cervicale. Rev Neurol (Paris) 1926;33:1246–8.
2. Sjaastad O, Saunte C, Hovdahl H, et al. Cervicogenic headache. A hypothesis. Cephalalgia 1983;3(4):249–56.

3. Sjaastad O, Fredriksen TA, Pfaffenrath V. Cervicogenic headache: diagnostic criteria. The Cervicogenic Headache International Study Group. Headache 1998;38(6):442–5.

4. U Nilsson N. The prevalence of cervicogenic headache in a random population sample of 20-59 year olds. Spine 1995;20(17):1884–8.

5. Haldeman Scott, Dagenais Simon. Cervicogenic Headaches: a Critical Review. Spine J 2001;1(1):31–46.

6. Sjaastad O, Fredriksen TA. Cervicogenic headache: criteria, classification and epidemiology. Clin Exp Rheumatol 2000;18(2 Suppl 19):S3–6.

7. Bogduk N, Govind J. Cervicogenic headache: an assessment of the evidence on clinical diagnosis, invasive tests, and treatment. Lancet Neurol 2009;8:959.

8. Dwyer A, Aprill C, Bogduk N. Cervical zygapophysial joint pain patterns I: a study in normal volunteers. Spine 1990;15:453–7.

9. Piovesan EJ, Kowacs PA, Tatsui CE, et al. Referred pain after painful stimulation of the greater occipital nerve in humans: evidence of convergence of cervical afferences on trigeminal nuclei. Cephalalgia 2001;21:107–9.

10. Cooper G, Bailey B, Bogduk N. Cervical zygapophysial joint pain maps. Pain Med 2007;8(4):344–53.

11. Cooper WM, Masih Amit K. "Chapter 16 - Cervicogenic Headache." Headache and Migraine Biology and Management. Elsevier 2015;203–12.

12. Vavrek D, Haas M, Peterson D. Physical examination and self reported pain outcomes from a randomized trial on chronic cervicogenic headache. J Manip Physiol Ther 2010;33:338 348.

13. Hall TM, Briffa K, Hopper D, et al. Comparative analysis and diagnostic accuracy of the cervical flexion rotation test. J Headache Pain 2010;11:391–7.

14. Headache Classification Committee of the International Headache Society (IHS). The international classification of headache disorders, 3rd edition. Cephalalgia, vol. 38, no. 1, 2018, pp. 1–211.

15. Bogduk N. The Neck and Headaches. Neurol Clin 2014;32:471–87.

16. Centeno CJ, Thacker J, Elkins W. Radiofrequency Lesioning of the Cervical Medial Branches. Tech Reg Anesth Pain Manag 2004;8(1):10–6.

17. Dermont A, Simon L, Benaissa L, et al. Cervicogenic Headache, an easy diagnosis A systematic review and meta-analysis of diagnostic studies. Musculoskeletal Science and Practice 2022;62:1026–40.

18. Lee DG, Cho YW, Jang SH, et al. Effectiveness of Intra-articular steroid injection for atlanto-occipital joint pain. Pain Med 2015;16:1077–82.

19. Dreyfuss P, Michaelsen M, Fletcher D. Atlanto-occipital and lateral atlanto-axial joint pain patterns. Spine 1994;19:1125–31.

20. Machikanti L, Malla Y, Waro BW, et al. Complications of Fluoroscopically Directed Facet Joint Nerve Blocks: A Prospective Evaluation of 7, 500 Episodes with 43, 000 Nerve Blocks. Pain Physician 2012;15:E143–50.

21. Ekhator C, Urbi A, Nduma BN, et al. Safety and efficacy of radiofrequency ablation and epidural steroid injection for management of cervicogenic headaches and neck pain: meta-analysis and literature review. Curēus (Palo Alto, CA) 2023;15(2):e34932.

22. Machikanti L, Hirsch J. Neurological complications associated with epidural steroid injections. Curr Pain Headache Rep 2015;19(5):482–92.

23. Scanlon GC, Moeller-Bertram T, Romanowsky SM, et al. Cervical transforaminal epidural steroid injections—more dangerous than we think? Spine 2007;32(11): 1249–56.

24. Inamasu J, Guiot BH. Iatrogenic vertebral artery injury. Acta Neurol Scand 2005; 112:349–57.
25. Blumenfeld A, Siavoshi S. The challenges of cervicogenic headache. Curr Pain Headache Rep 2018;22(7):47.
26. Ashina S, Bendtsen L, Lyngberg AC, et al. Prevalence of Neck Pain in Migraine and Tension-Type Headache: A Population Study. Cephalalgia 2015;35(3):211–9.
27. Vidale S. Headache in cervicocerebral artery dissection. Neurol Sci 2020; 41(Suppl 2):395–9.
28. Martins BP, Mesquita I, Sousa JM, et al. Persistent headache attributed to past cervicocephalic artery dissection: clinical characteristics and contributors to headache persistence. Cephalalgia 2023;43(2).
29. Dougherty C. Occipital Neuralgia. Curr Pain Headache Rep 2014;18(5):411.
30. Eugenio Ramalho Bezerra M, Pedro A. Sampaio Rocha-Filho. Headache Attributed to Craniocervical Dystonia: A Prospective Cohort Study. Eur J Pain 2020; 24(8):1484–94.

Painful Eyes in Neurology Clinic: A Guide for Neurologists

Saif Aldeen Alryalat, MD[a,b], Osama Al Deyabat, MD[a],
Andrew G. Lee, MD[a,b,c,d,e,f,g,h,*]

KEYWORDS

• Eye pain • Ophthalmoplegia • Orbital • Dry eye • Headache

KEY POINTS

• Patients with eye pain can present to neurology clinics, either as first-time patients or as a comorbidity in patients with pre-existing neurological conditions.
• Eye pain can be due to intraocular, intraorbital, or intracranial lesions and can also be referred pain to the eye from the neck.
• Neurologists should consider consultation with an ophthalmologist to perform a complete eye and orbital exam including ocular surface, pupil, lid, motility, intraocular pressure, and optic nerve evaluation.
• Knowledge about ocular conditions in addition to signs and symptoms of these conditions enable neurologists to appropriately triage such patients, avoiding unnecessary imaging and invasive testing.

BACKGROUND

One of the most common ocular complaints is eye pain.[1] Overall, more than 60% of all eye pain cases are related to localized ocular and orbital etiologies (eg, conjunctivitis, episcleritis, scleritis, uveitis, dry eye, and keratitis).[2] However, eye pain in the neurology clinic (with a normal eye examination) is most commonly associated with a primary headache syndrome, particularly migraine.[2] One study reviewed eye pain

Funding Statement: The authors report no funding received for this work.
[a] Department of Ophthalmology, Blanton Eye Institute, Houston Methodist Hospital, Houston, TX, USA; [b] Department of Ophthalmology, The University of Jordan, Amman, Jordan; [c] Sam Houston State, Conroe, TX, USA; [d] Department of Ophthalmology, Cullen Eye Institute, Baylor College of Medicine, Houston, TX, USA; [e] Departments of Ophthalmology, Neurology, and Neurosurgery, Weill Cornell Medicine, New York, NY, USA; [f] Department of Ophthalmology, University of Texas MD Anderson Cancer Center, Houston, TX, USA; [g] Texas A&M College of Medicine, Bryan, TX, USA; [h] Department of Ophthalmology, The University of Iowa Hospitals and Clinics, Iowa City, IA, USA
* Corresponding author. Department of Ophthalmology, Blanton Eye Institute, Houston Methodist Hospital, 6560 Fannin Street 450, Houston, TX 77030.
E-mail address: aglee@houstonmethodist.org

Neurol Clin 42 (2024) 559–571
https://doi.org/10.1016/j.ncl.2023.12.009
0733-8619/24/© 2023 Elsevier Inc. All rights reserved.
neurologic.theclinics.com

from two referral centers and more than 90% were seen in the eye clinic, whereas only 6%–8% were seen in neurology clinic.[2]

In this review, the authors describe an approach to eye pain for the neurologist. A complete eye examination is necessary for these cases to exclude intraocular and intraorbital etiologies. The authors describe the main clinical scenarios: (1) eye pain in a non-inflamed eye (ie, the "white" eye); (2) eye pain with a "red eye" of interest to neurologists; and (3) eye pain in a proptotic eye. The authors describe the specific entities for each scenario including the specific primary headache syndromes with eye manifestations. Although eye pain for the neurologist has been the subject of prior issues in 2004 and 2014,[3,4] the authors update the literature and recommendations in this monograph.

APPROACH TO EYE PAIN
Signs and Symptoms Suggestive of Eye Disease

The comprehensive management of eye pain requires evaluation for specific signs and symptoms that might indicate an underlying intraocular, intraorbital, or intracranial disease. **Table 1** summarizes the critical "red flags" in eye pain that should prompt timely and complete evaluation. The loss of visual acuity, anisocoria, relative afferent pupillary defect, ptosis, proptosis, ophthalmoplegia, anterior or posterior uveitis, glaucoma, and optic disc edema are all findings suggesting potentially dangerous etiologies for they eye pain. Although all eye pain patients should be considered for a complete ophthalmic examination, a recent history of intraocular surgery or acute trauma should prompt more urgent evaluation.

Eye Pain in White Eye

In patients presenting with a white, yet painful, eye, the characteristics of the eye pain may suggest the underlying pathology. A burning "foreign body" sensation often typifies

Table 1 "Red flags" in eye pain	
Red Flags Prompting Ophthalmic Referral	**Associated Concerns or Potential Conditions**
New visual disturbances	Visual acuity, color vision defects, visual field loss
Relative afferent pupillary defect	Retinal or optic nerve pathology
Extraocular muscle abnormalities	Ocular motor nerve or extraocular muscle pathologies causing ocular misalignment or diplopia
Proptosis	Orbital tumors, inflammation, or other mass effect
Lid retraction or ptosis	Neurogenic, myogenic, or mechanical causes
Conjunctival changes	Chemosis, injection, inflammation, or infection
Corneal opacity	Infections, dystrophies, or other corneal diseases
Hyphema or hypopyon	Blood (hyphema) can suggest ocular trauma, whereas pus (hypopyon) in the anterior chamber suggest active infection or inflammation (uveitis)
Iris irregularity or nonreactive pupil	Trauma, iris damage, posterior synechiae, elevated intraocular pressure, or uveitis
Fundus abnormalities	Retinal hemorrhages, optic disc edema, optic atrophy
Recent intraocular surgery (<3 mo)	Potential complications or issues related to the surgery (eg, endophthalmitis)
Recent ocular trauma	Wide range of potential injuries or conditions related to the trauma

Table 2
Pain characteristics and differentiating findings that help to define eye pain syndromes

Pain Characteristics	Associated Entities	Differentiating Signs and Symptoms
Burning, foreign body sensation	Ocular surface disease, dry eyes	Pain improve with blinking, worst in the evening, stinging sensation, improve with lubrication
Stabbing	Primary headache syndromes (eg, migraine, tension)	Associated photophobia or phonophobia, dysautonomia, nausea, or vomiting in migraine
Straining	Accommodative effort	Young patients who have accommodative effort and existing uncorrected refractive error
Sharp pain worse with eye movement	Optic neuritis	Optic nerve dysfunction tests (RAPD, automated perimetry, optical coherence tomography (OCT)

ocular surface diseases (eg, dry eye, recurrent erosions, corneal epithelial defect). Patients commonly describe improvement with blinking, a stinging sensation that worsens as the day progresses, and relief with the application of artificial tears and lubricants.[5]

The characteristics (timing, duration, severity, frequency, quality [eg, stabbing or throbbing pain], associated features, palliating, and precipitating factors) of the eye pain and any associated headache should be documented (**Table 2**).

Specific diagnostic criteria may be helpful in defining the primary headache syndromes.[6,7] The pain may present with accompanying photophobia or phonophobia and may even involve sympathetic signs and symptoms. Young patients who describe an eye-straining type of pain with reading, particularly those with uncorrected refractive errors, frequently have accommodative insufficiency or spasm. The pain is related to a physiologic attempt of the eye to maintain clear vision at near but some cases are nonorganic.[8]

Alternatively, a sharp pain exacerbated by eye movement, particularly when paired with findings from optic nerve dysfunction tests (eg, relative afferant pupillary defect [RAPD]) is suggestive of optic neuropathy (eg, optic neuritis).[9] Recognizing these pain patterns and their associated signs can significantly enhance a neurologist's ability to pinpoint and address the underlying causes of ocular discomfort.

Eye Pain with Red Eye: Patterns of Eye Redness and Their Associated Etiologies

For neurologists encountering patients with eye pain, understanding the various patterns of eye redness can be invaluable in differentiating between etiologies and can allow multidisciplinary care and communication if systemic or neurologic disorders could be causing the red eye.

The ocular surface's vascular response to various insults or diseases often presents in characteristic patterns; however, none of these patterns are specific. For instance, a diffuse redness might indicate a broad inflammatory or irritative process such as conjunctivitis or dry eyes. In contrast, ciliary injection, with its telltale ring of redness encircling the cornea, often signifies deeper intraocular inflammation (ie, uveitis) or acutely elevated intraocular pressure.[10] Localized or sectoral redness can be indicative of conditions affecting specific regions of the eye, including episcleritis or scleritis.[11] Distinctive presentations, such as arterialization of conjunctival vessels, may hint at intracranial vascular anomalies like carotid-cavernous fistulas,[12] whereas redness specifically at the origins

Table 3	
Pattern of eye redness and potential association with systemic or neurologic disease	
Pattern of Eye Redness	**Associated Etiology**
Diffuse redness	• Conjunctivitis (viral, bacterial, chemical, allergic)
Ciliary injection (around the cornea)	• Iritis or anterior uveitis • Acute angle closure glaucoma • Keratitis
Sectoral redness (localized)	• Episcleritis • Scleritis • Localized inflammation or trauma
Conjunctival hemorrhage (bright red spot)	• Trauma (even minor) • Hypertension • Blood thinners or clotting disorders • Spontaneous
Palpebral (eyelid) redness	• Blepharitis • Hordeolum (stye) • Dacryocystitis (lacrimal sac inflammation)
Arterialization of conjunctival vessels	• Carotid-cavernous fistula (CCF)
Redness at rectus muscle origin	• Thyroid eye disease (often seen in the early inflammatory phase, especially with increased blood flow to the inflamed extraocular muscles)

of the rectus muscles might point toward thyroid eye disease.[13] Thus, the meticulous observation of redness patterns, coupled with other clinical signs and symptoms, can guide neurologists in their diagnostic process and subsequent referrals (**Table 3**).

Eye Pain and Proptosis

In the domain of neurology, the convergence of eye pain with proptosis warrants a multi-dimensional evaluation, as these signs can be harbingers of diverse and occasionally grave intraorbital or intracranial etiologies. Traumatic events can precipitate this presentation, with underlying factors such as orbital fractures or hemorrhages instigating both pain and the forward displacement of the eye. Infectious processes, such as orbital cellulitis or the more serious septic cavernous sinus thrombosis, must also be judiciously considered. Localized inflammatory conditions (eg, orbital inflammatory pseudotumor, IgG4 disease, Tolosa–Hunt syndrome) and systemic inflammation can affect the orbit (eg, granulomatosis with polyangiitis (previously termed Wegener granulomatosis), sarcoidosis, lymphoid, and atypical lymphoid hyperplasia).[14]

In addition, vascular anomalies such as orbital arteriovenous or cavernous malformations or carotid-cavernous fistulas can induce pain and proptosis.[12] Neoplasms include primary orbital tumors, metastatic lesions, lymphoma, and tumors extending from the sinus or brain that can produce eye pain. Thyroid ophthalmopathy (Graves orbitopathy) is a common cause of eye pain, lid retraction, proptosis, lid, conjunctival and caruncular discomfort, redness, and edema.[15] **Table 4** outlines some orbital etiologies and findings.

Specific Ocular Diseases for Neurologists

Neurologists may encounter patients presenting with eye pain as the initial or major manifestation of underlying neurologic or systemic disease. Dry eye can occur in primary or secondary Sjogren syndrome. Optic neuritis may occur due to demyelinating disease (eg, multiple sclerosis) or antibody-mediated optic neuropathies (eg, neuromyelitis optica, myelin oligodendrocytic glycoprotein). Large- (eg, giant cell arteritis,

Table 4
Orbital findings in eye pain

Category	Causes of Pain and Proptosis
Trauma	• Orbital fracture • Orbital hemorrhage • Subperiosteal hematoma
Infectious	• Orbital cellulitis • Septic cavernous sinus thrombosis
Inflammation	• Tolosa-Hunt syndrome • Orbital inflammatory pseudotumor • Sarcoidosis, granulomatosis with polyangiitis (ie, Wegener granulomatosis), systemic lupus erythematosus
Vascular	• Orbital arteriovenous malformation • Carotid-cavernous fistula
Neoplastic	• Orbital tumors (eg, rhabdomyosarcoma, dermoid, hemangioma) • Metastatic • Lymphoma • Contiguous or perineural spread of sinus neoplasm
Thyroid ophthalmopathy	• Typically associated with Grave's disease but can occur in any systemic thyroid state; characterized by inflammation of the extraocular muscles, leading to proptosis, pain, and potential vision loss

Takayasu arteritis), medium-, and small-vessel vasculitis can present with eye pain or uveitis. Vascular intracranial aneurysms, carotid cavernous fistula, or carotid artery dissection can present with eye pain. **Table 5** summarizes several neurologic conditions that can present with eye pain.

Primary Headache Syndromes with Eye Manifestations

Primary headache syndromes can present with eye pain. According to the International Headache Society (IHS),[19] there are four main types of primary headaches: (1) migraine, (2) tension type, (3) trigeminal autonomic cephalalgia (TAC), and (4) others. Each of these primary level diagnoses has second- and third-degree diagnoses (eg, retinal migraine is 1.2.4). The main two types that may present to ophthalmic clinic are.

- Migraine and its subtypes due to visual phenomena
- TAC due to periorbital pain and autonomic stimulation.

Migraine

Migraine with aura or aura without migraine: The visual aura patients may experience can include monocular tunnel vision to total vision loss (lasting hours rather than few seconds in amaurosis fugax), geometric or bolt like colors or scotomas (geometric jagging and scintillating scotoma), and polyopia (multiple images in one eye). The duration of the attack is key in differentiating the migraine (5–60 minutes) from transient ischemic attack (TIA) (seconds), especially if aura without headache. The migraine visual aura can have different patterns, with a prior review described around 25 distinctive patterns of visual aura that previously reported in the literature.[20] Here is the specific aura description from the IHS: a zigzag figure near the point of fixation that may gradually spread right or left and assume a laterally convex shape with an angulated scintillating edge, leaving absolute or variable degrees of relative scotoma in its wake. In other cases, scotoma without positive phenomena may occur; this is often perceived as being of acute onset but, on scrutiny, usually enlarges gradually.

Table 5
Eye pain in neurologic and systemic disease

Etiology	Distinctive Symptoms and Signs	Management
Dry eye	The prevalence of dry eye syndrome per definition can reach up to 50% based on signs; however, only up to 20% are symptomatic.[16] Higher prevalence in patients with degenerative brain diseases.[17] Symptoms include burning, blurred vision, photophobia, and monocular diplopia.	Over-the-counter lubricating eye drops. More severe cases need referral to specialized eye clinic. Evaluation for Sjogren syndrome if moderate to severe dry eye and dry mouth.
Corneal inflammation (ie,. keratitis), infection (microbial keratitis), or exposure keratopathy	Foreign body sensation. Epithelial defect may be visible with fluorescein dye and cobalt blue light on the cornea (detailed below). Such examination is pertinent in cases of herpetic infections or autoimmune disease, which can lead to neurotrophic keratitis.[18]	Ophthalmic referral is generally recommended. Patients with epithelial keratitis or ulceration may have underlying trigeminal neuropathy (corneal anesthesia). Stromal keratitis can be seen in infectious and inflammatory (eg, syphilis, Cogan syndrome) disorders.
Acute angle closure glaucoma	Severe pain, blurred vision, markedly elevated intraocular pressure, or cloudy cornea. May have acute nausea or vomiting mimicking an acute abdomen or migraine attack.	Requires referral to emergency ophthalmic care. Medications such as topiramate can precipitate angle closure.
Uveitis	Pain, halos around lights, blurred vision, and a "red eye" may be present. Layered white cells may be present in the anterior chamber in severe cases (ie, hypopyon).	Urgent ophthalmic referral. Some patients with uveitis have concomitant neurologic syndromes (ie, Uveo-meningeal syndromes) and the type, location, and laterality of the uveitis may be helpful in the neurologic differential diagnosis for these conditions.
Hyphema	Layered red blood cells seen in the anterior chamber. Typically follows trauma but may occur in patients on anticoagulation. Pain and blurred vision common.	Urgent ophthalmic referral recommended.
Conjunctivitis	Conjunctival injection and irritation. Typically not severely painful. May have purulent or nonpurulent discharge. Severe pain with conjunctivitis is a red flag for more severe	Ophthalmic referral recommended.

Episcleritis and scleritis	Often more injected and more painful than simple allergic or viral infectious conjunctivitis. Deeper involvement of vessels may be apparent and may have violaceous hue to sclera (ie, scleromalacia).	Urgent ophthalmic referral recommended.
Optic neuritis and perineuritis	Visual loss is the predominant complaint, with pain with eye movement as a secondary symptom.	Ophthalmologic consultation recommended. Neuroimaging (eg, MRI) might show contrast enhancement of optic nerve (optic neuritis) or the optic nerve sheath (optic perineuritis).
Trochlear pain (trochleitis)	Localized superomedial pain and tenderness in orbit is characteristic and the pain may be exacerbated with eye movement.	Treatment with local injection of lidocaine or local or systemic corticosteroids is often helpful.
Myositis, orbital inflammatory pseudotumor	Conjunctival redness or chemosis, pain with eye movement, proptosis, or diplopia.	Orbital imaging might show extraocular muscle enlargement or enlargement or enhancement of orbital structures. Urgent ophthalmologic consultation recommended.
Giant cell arteritis	Isolated eye pain is an unusual presenting symptom. Visual loss typically predominates. Headache, scalp tenderness, and jaw claudication are additional classic symptoms.	Serum stat erythrocyte sedimentation rate, platelet count, and C-reactive protein are often elevated. Temporal artery biopsy may be diagnostic. Start empirical corticosteroids immediately. Urgent ophthalmologic consultation recommended.
Orbital masses and vascular malformation	Rapid painful expanding orbital mass, proptosis, lid or conjunctival edema, vision loss, ophthalmoplegia, and elevated intraocular pressure are red flags for diagnosis.	Ophthalmic consultation is recommended.
Abscess and cellulitis	Orbital cellulitis typically produces eyelid edema, erythema, exophthalmos, partial or total ophthalmoplegia, pain with eye movement, chemosis, decreased visual function, and relative afferent pupillary defect.	Urgent ophthalmic referral is recommended.

(continued on next page)

Table 5
(continued)

Etiology	Distinctive Symptoms and Signs	Management
Thyroid eye disease (TED) or Graves orbitopathy	The characteristic signs are eyelid retraction and lid lag, proptosis, chemosis, periorbital edema, corneal exposure, diplopia, and sometimes a compressive optic neuropathy.	Orbital imaging (eg, CT, MRI) looking for enlargement of the extraocular muscle enlargement with sparing of the tendons is the distinctive radiographic sign. Typically, the inferior and medial recti are affected first. Ophthalmic referral is recommended.
Microvascular ocular motor cranial mononeuropathies	Ocular motor nerve palsies produce diplopia. Third nerve palsy may have ptosis and pupil involvement.	Ophthalmic consultation is generally recommended.
Carotid artery dissection	Ipsilateral head, neck, face, or jaw. Pain may be located in the forehead or periocular region. Conjunctival injection may occur due to conjunctival vessel dilation from sympathetic block.	Neuroimaging is generally recommended for the head and neck to exclude carotid dissection. Ophthalmic consultation is recommended.

Table 6 Distinctive features of for retinal migraine (1.2.4) versus migraine aura without headache (1.2.2)		
Criteria	Retinal Migraine	Migraine Aura Without Headache
Affected eyes	One eye only	Both eyes
Associated headache	Typically follows visual symptoms; may also occur before or during	No headache (also called "acephalgic" or "silent" migraine)
Duration of visual symptoms	Usually less than an hour	Typically, 20–30 min
Type of visual phenomena	Partial or complete temporary blindness	Flashing lights, zigzag lines, blind spots (scotomas), and so forth.
Risk of transient ischemic attack	Higher risk for misdiagnosis and confusion with TIA (considered more serious as it can signify underlying vascular issues)	Generally less concerning if typical migraine aura medically, but still distressing for the patient and may require vascular evaluation if new onset without prior migraine history or in vasculopathic patients.
Other aura symptoms	Usually not present	Can include tingling, auditory, olfactory hallucinations, or difficulty speaking.
Diagnosis	Requires eye examination and possibly imaging to rule out other causes	Often based on patient history if other causes can be excluded

Of note, IHS gave separate description for retinal migraine (1.2.4) versus migraine aura without headache (1.2.2).

- Retinal migraine affects one eye and is usually followed by a headache on the same side. It is considered more serious and requires thorough evaluation to rule out other causes of monocular blindness.
- Migraine aura without headache affects both eyes, does not progress to a headache, and the visual symptoms can be more varied. It is typically less concerning from a medical standpoint but can still be distressing for the patient.

Table 6 summarized the distinctive features of for retinal migraine (1.2.4) versus migraine aura without headache (1.2.2).

Trigeminal Autonomic Cephalalgias

TACs are characterized by unilateral headache along with prominent cranial parasympathetic features (lacrimation, rhinorrhea, conjunctival injection, ptosis, miosis). The two main types that need to be differentiated are cluster headache and paroxysmal hemicrania due to the overlap in the duration of headache attack. The third type is short-lasting unilateral neuralgiform headache attacks, which can present as either short-lasting unilateral neuralgiform headache attacks with conjunctival injection and tearing or short-lasting unilateral neuralgiform headache attacks with cranial autonomic symptoms. They usually present with series of stabs or in a saw-tooth pattern

Table 7
Different types of eye pain associated with trigeminal autonomic cephalgia

Criteria	SUNCT and SUNA	Paroxysmal Hemicrania	Cluster Headache
Pain duration	1–600 s	Shorter, usually 2–30 min per attack	Longer, often 15 min to 3 h per attack
Frequency of attacks	Occurring with a frequency of at least one a day with a mean of around 60 attacks per day	More frequent, often several times a day, up to 20 or more	Less frequent, typically 1–3 attacks per day during a cluster period
Pain intensity	Moderate or severe unilateral head pain, with orbital, supraorbital, temporal and/or other trigeminal distribution	Severe, but usually less intense than cluster headaches	Often described as extremely severe, sometimes called "suicide headaches"
Associated autonomic features	Conjunctival injection and/or lacrimation • Nasal congestion and/or rhinorrhoea • Eyelid oedema • Forehead and facial sweating • Forehead and facial flushing • Sensation of fullness in the ear • Miosis and/or ptosis	Conjunctival injection and/or lacrimation • Nasal congestion liand/or rhinorrhoea • Eyelid oedema • Forehead and facial sweating • Miosis and/or ptosis	Conjunctival injection and/or lacrimation • Nasal congestion and/or rhinorrhoea • Eyelid oedema • Forehead and facial sweating • Miosis and/or ptosis
Response to indomethacin	Does not respond to indomethacin	Typically responds dramatically to indomethacin	Does not respond to indomethacin

Abbreviations: SUNA, short-lasting unilateral neuralgiform headache attacks with cranial autonomic symptoms; SUNCT, short-lasting unilateral neuralgiform headache attacks with conjunctival injection and tearing.

each lasting seconds.[21] **Table 7** provides a summary of the TAC with eye manifestations.

Primary headache should not be considered when it starts close to disease or trauma. Also, if the headache intensity and characteristic acutely change, consider a secondary cause.

Practical Tips for Neurology Clinic

- Manage dry eye in patients with incomplete lid closure (facial nerve palsy),[22] impaired blinking (Parkinson disease),[17] neurotrophic keratitis (eg, multiple sclerosis).[23]
- Consider herpetic zoster keratitis in patients with facial cutaneous herpetic zoster eruption, especially in the presence of Hutchinson sign (involvement of the tip of the nose from trigeminal nasociliary nerve). The use of fluorescein dye on the surface of the eye followed by imaging the surace wirh a simple attachment to a smart phone device for blue light can be used to examine corneal surface irregularities.[24]
- Consider optic nerve function assessment in patients with pain with eye movements and blurred vision, including visual acuity, color vision, red desaturation, brightness comparison between each eye, detection of an RAPD, automated perimetry, and observing the optic nerve structure via fundoscopy and assessment with optical coherence tomography. Emerging technologies for assessment of visual acuity and color vision can now be performed on electronic devices, including smart phones after quick calibration,[25,26] but in general, formal ophthalmologic consultation is recommended. Evolving phone adapter technology is increasing being developed and deployed to reliably capture optic nerve images using smart phones.[27]
- In patients with impaired visual acuity, with doubt, if the origin of such impairment is optic nerve disease or retina, photo stress testing is a quick method that can differentiate between the two sources. Prolonged recovery time is expected in cases of retinal and macular diseases, where pigment bleaching is expected after the photo stress, but not in optic nerve diseases.[28,29]

SUMMARY

The close relationships between the central nervous system and the eye underscore the need for neurologists to possess a comprehensive understanding of the primary and referred causes of eye pain. Several ocular and orbital disorders may manifest as eye pain with or without an abnormal eye examination. Such disorders can be misleading, as their benign appearance might mask more grave underlying conditions, potentially leading to misdiagnoses or delayed treatment. Clinicians should be aware of the specific neurologic or systemic disorders (eg, demyelinating diseases or vascular abnormalities) that might first manifest as eye pain. Formal ophthalmic consultation is recommended for patients presenting with eye pain as the predominant complaint especially when red flags for more serious pathology are present. Specific primary headache syndromes can also present with eye pain and have defined diagnostic criteria.

CLINICS CARE POINTS

- Patients with eye pain can present to neurology clinics, either as first-time patients or as a comorbidity in patients with preexisting neurologic conditions.

- Eye pain can be due to intraocular, intraorbital, or intracranial lesions and can also be referred pain to the eye from the neck.
- Neurologists should consider consultation with an ophthalmologist to perform a complete eye and orbital examination including ocular surface, pupil, lid, motility, intraocular pressure, and optic nerve evaluation.
- Knowledge about ocular conditions in addition to signs and symptoms of these conditions enable neurologists to appropriately triage such patients, avoiding unnecessary imaging and invasive testing.

DISCLOSURE

A.G. Lee is a consultant for Horizon (speaker), AstraZeneca, and Bristol Myers Squibb, as well as the National Football League (NFL), the National Aeronautics and Space Administration (NASA), and the US Department of Justice (DOJ).

REFERENCES

1. Kulenkamp J, McClelland CM, Lee MS. Eye pain in the white and quiet eye. Curr Opin Ophthalmol 2020;31(6):483–8.
2. Bowen RC, Koeppel JN, Christensen CD, et al. The Most Common Causes of Eye Pain at 2 Tertiary Ophthalmology and Neurology Clinics. J Neuro Ophthalmol 2018;38(3):320.
3. Lee AG, Beaver HA, Brazis PW. Painful ophthalmologic disorders and eye pain for the neurologist. Neurol Clin 2004;22(1):75–97.
4. Lee AG, Al-Zubidi N, Beaver HA, et al. An Update on Eye Pain for the Neurologist. Neurol Clin 2014;32(2):489–505.
5. Giacomazzi S, Urits I, Hoyt B, et al. Comprehensive Review and Update of Burning Eye Syndrome. J Patient Cent Res Rev 2021;8(3):255–60.
6. Murthy SI, Das S, Deshpande P, et al. Differential diagnosis of acute ocular pain: Teleophthalmology during COVID-19 pandemic - A perspective. Indian J Ophthalmol 2020;68(7):1371–9.
7. Lee A, Brazis P. The evaluation of eye pain with a normal ocular exam. Semin Ophthalmol 2003;18(4):190–9.
8. Sheppard AL, Wolffsohn JS. Digital eye strain: prevalence, measurement and amelioration. BMJ Open Ophthalmol 2018;3(1):e000146.
9. Yang X, Li X, Lai M, et al. Pain Symptoms in Optic Neuritis. Front Pain Res 2022;3:865032.
10. Agrawal RV, Murthy S, Sangwan V, et al. Current approach in diagnosis and management of anterior uveitis. Indian J Ophthalmol 2010;58(1):11–9.
11. de la Maza MS, Jabbur NS, Foster CS. Severity of Scleritis and Episcleritis. Ophthalmology 1994;101(2):389–96.
12. Chaudhry IA, Elkhamry SM, Al-Rashed W, et al. Carotid Cavernous Fistula: Ophthalmological Implications. Middle East Afr J Ophthalmol 2009;16(2):57–63.
13. Dolman PJ. Grading Severity and Activity in Thyroid Eye Disease. Ophthal Plast Reconstr Surg 2018;34(4S):S34.
14. Kapila AT, Ray S, Lal V. Tolosa–Hunt Syndrome and IgG4 Diseases in Neuro-Ophthalmology. Ann Indian Acad Neurol 2022;25(Suppl 2):S83–90.
15. Şahlı E, Gündüz K. Thyroid-associated Ophthalmopathy. Turk J Ophthalmol 2017;47(2):94–105.

16. Stapleton F, Alves M, Bunya VY, et al. TFOS DEWS II Epidemiology Report. Ocul Surf 2017;15(3):334–65.
17. Borm CDJM, Smilowska K, de Vries NM, et al. The Neuro-Ophthalmological Assessment in Parkinson's Disease. J Park Dis 2019;9(2):427–35.
18. Saad S, Abdelmassih Y, Saad R, et al. Neurotrophic keratitis: Frequency, etiologies, clinical management and outcomes. Ocul Surf 2020;18(2):231–6.
19. Headache Classification Committee of the International Headache Society (IHS) The International Classification of Headache Disorders, 3rd edition. Cephalalgia Int J Headache. 2018;38(1):1-211.
20. Viana M, Tronvik EA, Do TP, et al. Clinical features of visual migraine aura: a systematic review. J Headache Pain 2019;20(1):64.
21. Cohen AS, Matharu MS, Goadsby PJ. Short-lasting unilateral neuralgiform headache attacks with conjunctival injection and tearing (SUNCT) or cranial autonomic features (SUNA)—a prospective clinical study of SUNCT and SUNA. Brain 2006;129(10):2746–60.
22. Stew B, Williams H. Modern management of facial palsy: a review of current literature. Br J Gen Pract 2013;63(607):109–10.
23. Versura P, Giannaccare G, Pellegrini M, et al. Neurotrophic keratitis: current challenges and future prospects. Eye Brain 2018;10:37–45.
24. Puthalath AS, Gupta N, Samanta R, et al. Cobalt blue light unit filter - A smartphone attachment for blue light photography. Indian J Ophthalmol 2021;69(10):2841–3.
25. Pathipati AS, Wood EH, Lam CK, et al. Visual acuity measured with a smartphone app is more accurate than Snellen testing by emergency department providers. Graefes Arch Clin Exp Ophthalmol 2016;254(6):1175–80.
26. Suo L, Ke X, Zhang D, et al. Use of Mobile Apps for Visual Acuity Assessment: Systematic Review and Meta-analysis. JMIR MHealth UHealth 2022;10(2):e26275.
27. LaMonica LC, Bhardwaj MK, Hawley NL, et al. Remote Screening for Optic Nerve Cupping Using Smartphone-based Nonmydriatic Fundus Photography. J Glaucoma 2021;30(1):58.
28. Brandl C, Zimmermann ME, Herold JM, et al. Photostress Recovery Time as a Potential Predictive Biomarker for Age-Related Macular Degeneration. Transl Vis Sci Technol 2023;12(2):15.
29. Glaser JS, Savino PJ, Sumers KD, et al. The photostress recovery test in the clinical assessment of visual function. Am J Ophthalmol 1977;83(2):255–60.

Temporomandibular Disorders, Bruxism and Headaches

Marcela Romero-Reyes, DDS, PhD[a,b,]*, Jennifer P. Bassiur, DDS[c,d]

KEYWORDS

- TMDs • TMJ • Headache • Migraine • Orofacial pain • Bruxism • Comorbidity
- Overlapping

KEY POINTS

- TMDs are highly prevalent and may exacerbate a primary headache disorder.
- The neurologist/physician needs to be aware of the presence of TMDs in a headache patient.
- Collaboration with a dentist specialized in orofacial pain is key to optimize patient outcomes.

INTRODUCTION

Primary headache disorders and temporomandibular disorders (TMDs) are conditions of different etiologies and pathophysiologies that share the trigeminal system in their mechanisms.[1] Both conditions are highly prevalent in the population and cause considerable burden.[2–5]

TMDs are the most common orofacial pains of nondental origin.[6,7] They are a constellation of musculoskeletal and neuromuscular conditions involving the temporomandibular joint (TMJ), the muscles of mastication, and their associated structures.[8] TMDs can be a source of headache symptomatology recognized as a secondary headache in the International Classification of Headache Disorders, third edition (ICHD-3) and the Diagnostic Criteria for Temporomandibular Disorders (DC/TMD).[9,10] Different types of headaches such as migraine, chronic daily headache, tension-type headache, and cervicogenic headache can be present with TMDs.[11–13] TMDs often co-occur, particularly

[a] Brotman Facial Pain Clinic, University of Maryland, School of Dentistry; [b] Department of Neural and Pain Sciences, University of Maryland, Baltimore, School of Dentistry, 650 West Baltimore Street, Room 8253, Baltimore, MD 21201, USA; [c] Center for Oral, Facial & Head Pain, College of Dental Medicine, Columbia University Medical Center; [d] Division of Oral & Maxillofacial Surgery, 620 West 168th Street, P & S Box 20, New York, NY 10032, USA
* Corresponding author. Department of Neural and Pain Sciences, University of Maryland, Baltimore School of Dentistry, 650 West Baltimore Street, 8th Floor South, Baltimore, MD 21201.
E-mail address: mromero@umaryland.edu

Neurol Clin 42 (2024) 573–584
https://doi.org/10.1016/j.ncl.2023.12.010
0733-8619/24/© 2024 Elsevier Inc. All rights reserved.
neurologic.theclinics.com

with migraine, as a comorbidity with significant clinical implications and the potential to exacerbate overall symptomatology and make management more challenging.[1,14,15] Therefore, it is of vital importance that the headache physician is aware of the potential contributing factors of the presence of TMDs in a headache patient. In addition, it is important to recognize the need for dialogue with dentistry, particularly the orofacial pain specialist, as a key team member to optimize management outcomes.

Temporomandibular Disorders

Of all the orofacial pains, temporomandibular Disorders (TMDs) are the most prevalent chronic orofacial pain conditions.[16] It is important to clarify that TMDs or TMD is not a clinical diagnosis or a specific disorder. TMDs include a group of over 30 musculoskeletal diagnoses that are classified into TMJ, muscle disorders, and headache attributed to TMDs.[8,10] Furthermore, not all TMDs are painful. According to the DC/TMD, the most common painful TMDs include arthralgia, myogenous disorders, myalgia, and myofascial pain, and headaches attributed to TMDs.[10] Overall, the most common and painful TMDs are myalgia and myofascial pain.[17,18] The intra-articular disorders include disc displacement with reduction, disc displacement without reduction, degenerative joint disease, and TMJ subluxation, which are the most common.[10] The TMJ disc displacement with reduction presents a clicking joint sound that indicates an incoordination of the disc-condyle relationship. It is usually not painful, very often presenting in the general population and does not normally require treatment.[8,19,20] Management is indicated when pain and disfunction are present.

The overall symptomatology that the patient reports with these disorders is localized in the face and jaw, including the temples and the preauricular area, and sometimes it can even be felt as an earache. However, pain can also be referred intraorally and other areas beyond the muscle boundaries, such as in the case of myofascial pain[21,22] that may complicate finding the primary pain source (**Fig. 1**). Pain and dysfunction are

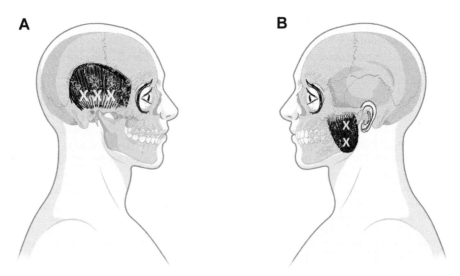

Fig. 1. Myofascial pain presents trigger points that spread beyond the location of palpation within the muscle and beyond its boundaries. (A) Temporalis muscle. (B) Masseter muscle. Palpation may replicate headache symptomatology in headache secondary/attributed to temporomandibular disorders (TMDs). "X" in yellow: trigger point; pattern in green: referral pattern. (Created with BioRender.com.).

present during normal mandibular function that includes chewing, eating, talking, opening wide, presenting limitation of range of motion, and yawning. In addition, sometimes TMJ noises such as popping, clicking, or crepitus are reported.[8,23]

TMDs present an annual incidence rate of the first onset of symptomatology of 3.9%,[5,24] and as with migraine, they are more frequent in women and their prevalence ranges from young to middle-aged adults.[25,26] Regarding their pathophysiology, there are many factors that contribute to the onset, perpetuation, and progression of TMDs. Thanks to the Orofacial Pain Prospective Evaluation and Risk Assessment (OPPERA) studies, we have a better understanding of the complexity of TMDs, establishing their multifactorial nature within a biopsychosocial context,[17,27] where different psychological domains, domains related to pain sensitivity and perception, genetic and epigenetic factors, and overlapping pain and comorbid conditions play a significant role.[5,28,29] Calcitonin gene-related peptide (CGRP), a key neuropeptide in migraine pathophysiology and established therapeutic target, is also involved in TMDs pathogenesis.[30–32]

Long term follow-up studies have demonstrated that TMDs are often self-limiting and improve overtime, where symptomatology remits and patients cope and adapt.[29,33] However, for some patients this is not the case and it can greatly affect their quality of life[4,28] and therefore, there is a significant need to continue to support education and research in TMDs.[16]

Management is evidence-based, conservative, and reversible[8,34] and needs to be customized according to diagnosis where there is an emphasis on patient education and self-help, with the goal of reducing fear and empowering a sense of control over symptomatology. This includes awareness of comorbidities and possible contributing factors, such as parafunctional behaviors (eg, bruxism), educating the patient to rest the masticatory system with avoidance of chewy, crunchy, and hard foods and chewing gum, in addition to some physical therapy modalities.[35] Moreover, pharmacologic management can also be included in the treatment plan such as oral medications, trigger point injection therapy, as well as minimally invasive approaches, such as intra-articular injections, and surgical interventions (eg, arthrocentesis), when indicated (**Box 1**).[35,36] It is important to mention that the use of botulinum toxin (BTX) is not standard of care nor Food and Drug Administration (FDA) approved in the management of TMDs. It could be helpful in patients with significant bruxism and myogenous

---

Box 1
Basic management program of temporomandibular disorders

Nonpharmacological	Pharmacologic
Patient education about TMDs and their specific diagnosis	Medications: May include analgesics, anti-inflammatories, muscle relaxants, antidepressants.
Self-care program: Tailored to patient needs. May include physical therapy modalities, jaw relaxation and rest (eg,; avoidance of hard, chewy foods), exercises, and awareness of parafunctional behaviors.	Muscular trigger point injection therapy TMJ injections when indicated.
Stabilization oral appliance	
Physical therapy (craniofacial and cervical therapeutics)	
Cognitive behavioral interventions	
Surgical intervention only when indicated (arthrocentesis/arthroscopic procedure)	

Abbreviations: TMD, temporomandibular disorder; TMJ, temporomandibular joint.

TMD and is only reserved for cases refractory to conventional therapy.[1,36,37] Other nonpharmacological management may include oral appliances (eg, stabilization splint), in addition to a multidisciplinary care team that includes physical therapy (craniofacial and cervical therapeutics) and behavioral approaches, such as cognitive behavioral therapy, to help address the biopsychosocial framework and together accomplish the goal of reducing pain and restoring function.[8,36]

Temporomandibular Disorders and Headache

TMDs can be comorbid with primary headache disorders but can also present headache symptomatology per se. TMDs are a source of secondary headache described in the ICHD-3 and the DC/TMD as headache attributed to TMD,[9,10] with a variable prevalence among studies, from 5.7% to 29.3%.[38,39] Furthermore, it is important to clarify that headache attributed to TMD does not present migraine features. The diagnostic criteria are very clear in their definition accounting for a headache that appears in temporal relation with a TMD that usually is localized in the temple area ipsilateral to the area of the TMD but can also be present bilaterally. Symptomatology can be provoked during examination while palpating the muscles of mastication (see **Fig. 1**) (eg, temporalis, masseter muscles), replicating the familiar headache symptomatology reported, as well as aggravated or provoked by functional (opening mouth wide, chewing) or parafunctional jaw motion (bruxism).[8–10] This headache may be confused with tension-type headache since their characteristics are similar and more so when is present with pericranial tenderness. In addition, is important to recognize that both headaches may be present in the same patient.[9] However, it has been shown that headache attributed to TMDs is more likely in migraineurs (70.1%) than in tension-type headache (54.1%).[40]

Migraine is the most prevalent primary headache in the TMD population, and this comorbidity has significant clinical implications.[1,41,42] The presence of a painful TMD is determinant in the exacerbation of the migraine phenotype, since it contributes to central sensitization and allodynia, which are markers of the transformation to a more chronic form.[31,43,44] On the other hand, evidence has shown migraine to be a significant predictor of first-onset TMD.[45] Therefore, as a comorbidity they potentially exacerbate and perpetuate each other.[1] Furthermore, the presence of TMDs in headache sufferers may cause important disability. In a recent study, the prevalence of TMDs in a headache cohort was reported to be 56.1% where 40.4% presented psychological burden. Noteworthy, patients with TMDs combined with migraine and tension-type headache had significantly higher prevalence of depression,[46] emphasizing even more the significant implications of this comorbidity for the quality of life of the patient.

Bruxism

Oral parafunctional behaviors relate to an oral habit that is not associated with speech, deglutition, or mastication and includes thumb sucking, nail biting, lip biting, and bruxism.[47] Bruxism is recognized as a group of oral parafunctional behaviors defined as repetitive muscles of mastication activity characterized by the clenching or grinding of teeth, as well as by the bracing or thrusting of the mandible, either awake or during sleep.[48] Its prevalence varies between studies from 22% to 30% for awake bruxism (AB) and 8% to 15% from sleep bruxism (SB) in the adult population.[49] The etiology and pathophysiology of this behavior appears to be multifactorial and centralized,[50] and this is supported by the fact that different central acting classes of medications, stimulants, and addictive substances, as well as acute neurologic illnesses induce it.[51,52] In healthy individuals, bruxism should not be considered as a disorder per se but as muscle behavior that can be harmless, protective, or at risk for clinical consequences.[50]

It is important to be aware that bruxism may not cause TMD symptomatology in all individuals, but in some, it may perpetuate, exacerbate, and even initiate TMD symptoms.[50,53–55] However, the relationship between TMD and bruxism is still yet to be clarified. Studies based on self-report and questionnaires about SB have found a positive association with TMD pain. Instrumental studies using electromyography and polysomnography found either a lower level or a negative association.[56–58] In addition, an important bias is patient beliefs. It was shown that 53.8% of patients with AB and 66.7% of patients with SB attributed their bruxism as a cause of TMD pain.[59] More research is necessary to discern causality.

Bruxism has been implicated in headache disorders. The presence of painful TMDs and SB can increase the risk of episodic tension-type headache and episodic and chronic migraine.[60] There also appears to be an association with AB, although this is data from a self-report study, with no clear headache-type diagnosis.[61] A recent systematic review reported that patients with AB had more chance of presenting tension-type headache but the association with either AB and SB and migraine is yet to be determined.[62] Better designed studies are needed to draw more solid conclusions.

The Nociceptive Trigeminal Inhibition Tension Suppression System (NTI) is a partial coverage device or anterior bite stop which generally covers only the 2 upper or lower incisors. There is evidence that it may be helpful in bruxism[63] but more randomized control trials are necessary to solidify conclusions. In a recent study that assessed the input of nocturnal clenching in chronic migraine, the use of this device improved HIT-6 scores in these patients.[64] However, it is important to highlight that the use of an NTI has the potential to lead to complications particularly related to teeth (eg, mobility, local bone loss, sensitivity) and occlusion, such as the development of an appliance-induced malocclusion (eg, anterior open bite), with inappropriate use.[63]

DISCUSSION

The identification of chronic overlapping painful conditions is of critical clinical importance. Their presence has additive effects that increase the facilitation of sensitization and therefore the exacerbation of the overall pain experience that may render management more challenging.[65,66] This feedback cycle of overlapping painful conditions is well represented when TMDs, headache secondary to TMDs, and comorbidity with migraine, may be present in an individual. This presentation has been associated with greater chronic pain indicators including somatization, higher central sensitization markers, and disability scores.[67]

The most common TMDs are myogenous, highlighted by myofascial pain[17,18] and evidence has shown that the presence of myofascial pain is associated with the risk of transformation from acute to a chronic state in TMDs.[68] Headache attributed to TMDs is highly prevalent in patients with chronic myofascial TMDs.[38,40] It is known that the presence of TMDs increases the prevalence of migraine,[12,14,41] leading to a higher headache disability,[69,70] in addition to contributing to sensitization and potentially aiding in the progression to a chronic migraine state.[43,44] This exacerbated phenotype seen in patients was shown in a preclinical comorbid TMD/migraine model. Masseteric complete Freund's adjuvant (CFA) injection–induced inflammation, used as a surrogate for myogenous TMD, in combination with slow infusion of CGRP, used as a migraine trigger, exacerbated migraine like neuronal activation and sensitization of trigeminal neurons.[31] Moreover, in the same model, masseteric allodynia and hyperalgesia alone, induced trigeminovascular activation and sensitization, without dural stimulation or CGRP infusion.[31] Together, these data begin to explain the overlap of TMDs with headache disorders, primarily with migraine and the possible interactions and contributions either as comorbid disorders or by mediating a secondary headache.[1]

Management in this patient population can be challenging and unfortunately there are no current standardized protocols that target overlapping mechanisms.[1] Studies have suggested that both conditions need to be treated independently, particularly for migraine to improve.[15,71] TMD management includes pharmacologic and nonpharmacological approaches.[36] One in particular, is the use of passive oral stabilization appliances or nightguards that can be included as a part of the management plan for myogenous and arthrogenous TMDs.[8] There is still controversy about their therapeutic effects, but studies support their benefits[72,73] and the use of this modality has been already explored in comorbid patients. A systematic review and meta-analysis reported that the use of maxillary stabilization full-arch coverage appliances may decrease headache frequency and severity in TMD comorbid with tension-type headache and TMD comorbid with migraine but highlighted on the necessity for better quality studies.[74] In another study that explored management in TMD and migraine comorbidity, the use of propranolol, a migraine preventive, in conjunction with the use of a stabilization appliance proved to be beneficial for both.[4,5]

The protocol of care needs to integrate migraine/headache management and TMDs therapeutic approaches.[1] The clinician needs to recognize the importance of the assessment for the possibility of TMD in a headache patient. The TMD examination, performed by a dentist, particularly an orofacial pain specialist, requires a detailed examination of the muscles of mastication and the TMJ to assess symptomatology, dysfunction, potential contributing factors such as parafunctional behaviors or other comorbidities, and to identify the arthrogenous and/or myogenous diagnosis. However, in the medical setting, the physician can discuss TMDs with the patient and screen for TMDs[75] with a brief questionnaire to aid in the recognition of symptomatology (**Box 2**).

Due to the complexity of TMDs and headache disorders, especially migraine, and for the potential of an exacerbated phenotype that they present when overlapping, a multidisciplinary approach to care is vital. This care integrates medicine, dentistry, and other allied health professionals, including physical therapy, sleep medicine, and pain psychology. Orofacial pain is a newly recognized specialty in dentistry that involves the diagnosis, treatment, and management of pain disorders of the jaw,

---

Box 2
Brief temporomandibular disorders screener questionnaire

Do you feel pain, soreness around your face, temple areas, or jaw?

Do you experience pain or jaw stiffness when you wake up in the morning?

Do you experience pain or discomfort while you are chewing, talking, opening your mouth, yawning, or during any other jaw movement?

Do you chew gum and/or hard foods (hard candy, nuts)?

Are you aware of clenching/bruxing?

Question about possible contribution to headache

Have you experienced that your jaw pain symptoms are making your headache more frequent and/or worse?

mouth, face, head, and neck and is committed to evidence-based understanding, prevention, and management of orofacial pain disorders, as well as to improve access to interdisciplinary care.[76] The orofacial pain specialist is a great ally to the medical professional, particularly neurology/headache medicine, for the support and care of this patient population. Expertise working together will provide the best outcomes for these patients that is greatly needed.

SUMMARY

Primary headache disorders and TMDs are highly prevalent in the population and greatly impact the quality of life. TMDs can present headache symptomatology as a secondary headache as well as being comorbid with a primary headache, particularly migraine. Together they may act as overlapping painful conditions, exacerbating the overall pain experience and pain progression, and make management even more challenging. Therefore, it is crucial to identify the presence of TMDs in headache patients to optimize patient outcomes. Collaboration with an orofacial pain specialist is vital. TMDs are multifactorial and parafunctional behaviors such as bruxism may have a role in some patients, and regarding headache, they may also be a contributing factor but more research to identify mechanisms and causality is needed.

CLINICS CARE POINTS

> - Headache symptomatology is present in TMDs as a secondary headache.
> - Migraine is the most prevalent primary headache observed in patients with TMDs and their comorbidity presents important clinical implications.
> - The presence of painful overlapping conditions such as TMDs, headache secondary to TMDs, and migraine (TMDs comorbid with migraine) may exacerbate the overall pain experience and complicate management.
> - The screening for the potential presence of TMDs in a headache patient is essential to optimize patient outcomes.
> - Parafunctional behaviors such as bruxism may contribute to TMDs and headache, but more research is necessary to clarify relationships.
> - Dialogue and collaboration with a dentist specialized in orofacial pain is essential to improve patient outcomes.

DISCLOSURE

The authors have nothing to disclose.

REFERENCES

1. Romero-Reyes M, Klasser G, Akerman S. An Update on Temporomandibular Disorders (TMDs) and Headache. Curr Neurol Neurosci Rep 2023. https://doi.org/10.1007/s11910-023-01291-1.
2. Facial Pain. National Institute of Dental and Craniofacial Research Updated July, 2018. Available at: http://www.nidcr.nih.gov/DataStatistics/FindDataByTopic/FacialPain/. Accessed January 7, 2024.
3. Global, regional, and national burden of migraine and tension-type headache, 1990-2016: a systematic analysis for the Global Burden of Disease Study 2016. Lancet Neurol 2018;17(11):954–76.

4. Pigozzi LB, Pereira DD, Pattussi MP, et al. Quality of life in young and middle age adult temporomandibular disorders patients and asymptomatic subjects: a systematic review and meta-analysis. Health Qual Life Outcome 2021;19(1):83.

5. Slade GD, Ohrbach R, Greenspan JD, et al. Painful Temporomandibular Disorder: Decade of Discovery from OPPERA Studies. J Dent Res 2016;95(10): 1084–92.

6. Durham J, Newton-John TR, Zakrzewska JM. Temporomandibular disorders. Bmj 2015;350:h1154.

7. Kapos FP, Exposto FG, Oyarzo JF, et al. Temporomandibular disorders: a review of current concepts in aetiology, diagnosis and management. Oral Surg 2020; 13(4):321–34.

8. Klasser G, Romero Reyes M. Orofacial pain guidelines for assessment, diagnosis, and management. 7th edition. Chicago, IL: Quintessence Publishing; 2023.

9. Headache Classification Committee of the International Headache Society (IHS) The International Classification of Headache Disorders, 3rd edition. Cephalalgia 2018;38(1):1-211.

10. Schiffman E, Ohrbach R, Truelove E, et al. Diagnostic Criteria for Temporomandibular Disorders (DC/TMD) for Clinical and Research Applications: recommendations of the International RDC/TMD Consortium Network* and Orofacial Pain Special Interest Group†. Journal of oral & facial pain and headache 2014; 28(1):6–27.

11. Goncalves DA, Camparis CM, Speciali JG, et al. Temporomandibular disorders are differentially associated with headache diagnoses: a controlled study. Clin J Pain 2011;27(7):611–5.

12. Réus JC, Polmann H, Souza BDM, et al. Association between primary headaches and temporomandibular disorders: A systematic review and meta-analysis. J Am Dent Assoc 2022;153(2):120–31.e6.

13. Greenbaum T, Dvir Z, Emodi-Perlman A, et al. The association between specific temporomandibular disorders and cervicogenic headache. Musculoskeletal science & practice 2021;52:102321.

14. Yakkaphan P, Smith JG, Chana P, et al. Temporomandibular disorder and headache prevalence: A systematic review and meta-analysis. Cephalalgia Reports 2022;5. 25158163221097352.

15. Goncalves DA, Camparis CM, Speciali JG, et al. Treatment of comorbid migraine and temporomandibular disorders: a factorial, double-blind, randomized, placebo-controlled study. J Orofac Pain 2013;27(4):325–35.

16. National Academies of Sciences E, Medicine, Health, et al. The National Academies Collection: Reports funded by National Institutes of Health. In: Yost O, Liverman CT, English R, et al, eds. Temporomandibular disorders: Priorities for research and care. National Academies Press (US) Copyright 2020 by the National Academy of Sciences. All rights reserved.; 2020.

17. List T, Jensen RH. Temporomandibular disorders: Old ideas and new concepts. Cephalalgia 2017;37(7):692–704.

18. Kuć J, Szarejko KD, Gołębiewska M. The Prevalence and Overlaps of Temporomandibular Disorders in Patients with Myofascial Pain with Referral-A Pilot Study. Int J Environ Res Publ Health 2021;(18):18. https://doi.org/10.3390/ijerph18189842.

19. Poluha RL, Canales GT, Costa YM, et al. Temporomandibular joint disc displacement with reduction: a review of mechanisms and clinical presentation. J Appl Oral Sci : revista FOB 2019;27:e20180433.

20. Scapino RP. The posterior attachment: its structure, function, and appearance in TMJ imaging studies. Part 2. J Craniomandib Disord 1991;5(3):155–66.

21. Graff-Radford SB. Myofascial pain: diagnosis and management. Review. Curr Pain Headache Rep 2004;8(6):463–7.

22. David G Simmons JGT, Simmons LS. 2nd edition. Myofascial pain and dysfunction: the trigger point Manual, vol. 1. LWW; 1998. p. 1056. Upper Half of Body.

23. Romero-Reyes M, Uyanik JM. Orofacial pain management: current perspectives. Review. J Pain Res 2014;7:99–115.

24. Slade GD, Bair E, Greenspan JD, et al. Signs and symptoms of first-onset TMD and sociodemographic predictors of its development: the OPPERA prospective cohort study. J Pain : official journal of the American Pain Society 2013;14(12 Suppl):T20–32 e1-3.

25. Slade GD, Bair E, By K, et al. Study methods, recruitment, sociodemographic findings, and demographic representativeness in the OPPERA study. J Pain 2011;12(11 Suppl):T12–26.

26. Slade G DJ. Prevalence, impact and cost of treatment for temporomandibular disorders.Paper commissioned by the Committee on Temporomandibular Disorders (TMDs): From Reserach Discoveries to Clinical Treatment.(Appendix C), in Temporomandibular disorders: Priorities for research and care. 2020.

27. Klasser GD, Abt E, Weyant RJ, et al. Temporomandibular disorders: current status of research, education, policies, and its impact on clinicians in the United States of America. Quintessence international (Berlin, Germany : 1985). 2022; 0(0):1–20.

28. Bair E, Gaynor S, Slade GD, et al. Identification of clusters of individuals relevant to temporomandibular disorders and other chronic pain conditions: the OPPERA study. Pain 2016;157(6):1266–78.

29. Fillingim RB, Slade GD, Greenspan JD, et al. Long-term changes in biopsychosocial characteristics related to temporomandibular disorder: findings from the OPPERA study. Pain 2018;159(11):2403–13.

30. Romero-Reyes M, Pardi V, Akerman S. A potent and selective calcitonin generelated peptide (CGRP) receptor antagonist, MK-8825, inhibits responses to nociceptive trigeminal activation: Role of CGRP in orofacial pain. Exp Neurol 2015;271:95–103.

31. Akerman S, Romero-Reyes M. Preclinical studies to dissect the neural mechanism for the comorbidity of migraine and temporomandibular disorders (TMD): the role of CGRP. Br J Pharmacol 2020. https://doi.org/10.1111/bph.15263.

32. Cady R, Glenn J, Smith K, et al. Calcitonin gene-related peptide promotes cellular changes in trigeminal neurons and glia implicated in peripheral and central sensitization. Mol Pain 2011;7(1):94.

33. Kapos FP, Look JO, Zhang L, et al. Predictors of Long-Term Temporomandibular Disorder Pain Intensity: An 8-Year Cohort Study. Journal of oral & facial pain and headache 2018;32(2):113–22.

34. Greene CS, American Association for Dental R. Diagnosis and treatment of temporomandibular disorders: emergence of a new care guidelines statement. Oral Surg Oral Med Oral Pathol Oral Radiol Endod 2010;110(2):137–9.

35. Graff-Radford SB, Bassiur JP. Temporomandibular disorders and headaches. Neurol Clin 2014;32(2):525–37.

36. Romero-Reyes M, Arman S, Teruel A, et al. Pharmacological Management of Orofacial Pain. Drugs 2023. https://doi.org/10.1007/s40265-023-01927-z.

37. Delcanho R, Val M, Guarda Nardini L, et al. Botulinum Toxin for Treating Tempo-romandibular Disorders: What is the Evidence? Journal of oral & facial pain and headache 2022;36(1):6–20.

38. Vivaldi D, Di Giosia M, Tchivileva IE, et al. Headache attributed to TMD Is Asso-ciated With the Presence of Comorbid Bodily Pain: A Case-Control Study. Head-ache J Head Face Pain 2018;58(10):1593–600.

39. van der Meer HA, Speksnijder CM, Engelbert RHH, et al. The Association Be-tween Headaches and Temporomandibular Disorders is Confounded by Bruxism and Somatic Symptoms. Clin J Pain 2017;33(9):835–43.

40. Tchivileva IE, Ohrbach R, Fillingim RB, et al. Clinical, psychological, and sensory characteristics associated with headache attributed to temporomandibular disor-der in people with chronic myogenous temporomandibular disorder and primary headaches. J Headache Pain 2021;22(1):42.

41. Franco AL, Goncalves DA, Castanharo SM, et al. Migraine is the most prevalent primary headache in individuals with temporomandibular disorders. J Orofac Pain 2011;24(3):287–92.

42. Gonçalves DA, Speciali JG, Jales LC, et al. Temporomandibular symptoms, migraine, and chronic daily headaches in the population. Neurology 2009; 73(8):645–6.

43. Grossi D, Lipton R, Bigal M. Temporomandibular disorders and migraine chron-ification. Curr Pain Headache Rep 2009;13(4):314–8.

44. Bevilaqua-Grossi D, Lipton RB, Napchan U, et al. Temporomandibular disorders and cutaneous allodynia are associated in individuals with migraine. Cephalalgia 2010;30(4):425–32.

45. Tchivileva IE, Ohrbach R, Fillingim RB, et al. Temporal change in headache and its contribution to the risk of developing first-onset temporomandibular disorder in the Orofacial Pain: Prospective Evaluation and Risk Assessment (OPPERA) study. Pain 2017;158(1):120–9.

46. Ballegaard V, Thede-Schmidt-Hansen P, Svensson P, et al. Are headache and temporomandibular disorders related? A blinded study. Cephalalgia 2008; 28(8):832–41.

47. Mehta NR, Scrivani SJ, Spierings ELH. 31 - Dental and facial pain. In: Benzon HT, Rathmell JP, Wu CL, et al, editors. Practical management of pain. 5th edition. Phil-adelphia, PA: Mosby; 2014. p. 424–40.e3.

48. Lobbezoo F, Ahlberg J, Raphael KG, et al. International consensus on the assess-ment of bruxism: Report of a work in progress. J Oral Rehabil 2018;45(11): 837–44.

49. Manfredini D, Winocur E, Guarda-Nardini L, et al. Epidemiology of bruxism in adults: a systematic review of the literature. J Orofac Pain 2013;27(2): 99–110.

50. Manfredini D, Colonna A, Bracci A, et al. Bruxism: a summary of current knowl-edge on aetiology, assessment and management. Oral Surgery 2020;13(4): 358–70.

51. de Baat C, Verhoeff MC, Ahlberg J, et al. Medications and addictive substances potentially inducing or attenuating sleep bruxism and/or awake bruxism. J Oral Rehabil 2021;48(3):343–54.

52. Burke D, Seitz A, Aladesuru O, et al. Bruxism in Acute Neurologic Illness. Curr Pain Headache Rep 2021;25. https://doi.org/10.1007/s11916-021-00953-4.

53. Glaros AG, Burton E. Parafunctional clenching, pain, and effort in temporoman-dibular disorders. J Behav Med 2004;27(1):91–100.

54. Glaros AG, Forbes M, Shanker J, et al. Effect of parafunctional clenching on temporomandibular disorder pain and proprioceptive awareness. Cranio : J Cranio-Mandibular Pract 2000;18(3):198–204.

55. Ohrbach R, Fillingim RB, Mulkey F, et al. Clinical findings and pain symptoms as potential risk factors for chronic TMD: descriptive data and empirically identified domains from the OPPERA case-control study. J Pain 2011;12(11 Suppl):T27–45.

56. Raphael KG, Janal MN, Sirois DA, et al. Validity of self-reported sleep bruxism among myofascial temporomandibular disorder patients and controls. J Oral Rehabil 2015;42(10):751–8.

57. Raphael KG, Sirois DA, Janal MN, et al. Sleep bruxism and myofascial temporomandibular disorders: a laboratory-based polysomnographic investigation. J Am Dent Assoc 2012;143(11):1223–31.

58. Manfredini D, Lobbezoo F. Sleep bruxism and temporomandibular disorders: A scoping review of the literature. J Dent 2021/08/01/2021;111:103711. https://doi.org/10.1016/j.jdent.2021.103711.

59. van der Meulen MJ, Ohrbach R, Aartman IH, et al. Temporomandibular disorder patients' illness beliefs and self-efficacy related to bruxism. J Orofac Pain 2010;24(4):367–72.

60. Fernandes G, Franco AL, Goncalves DA, et al. Temporomandibular disorders, sleep bruxism, and primary headaches are mutually associated. J Orofac Pain 2013;27(1):14–20.

61. Silva TB, Ortiz FR, Maracci LM, et al. Association among headache, temporomandibular disorder, and awake bruxism: A cross-sectional study. Headache 2022;62(6):748–54.

62. Réus JC, Polmann H, Mendes Souza BD, et al. Association Between Primary Headache and Bruxism: An Updated Systematic Review. Journal of oral & facial pain and headache 2021;35(2):129–38.

63. Stapelmann H, Türp JC. The NTI-tss device for the therapy of bruxism, temporomandibular disorders, and headache - where do we stand? A qualitative systematic review of the literature. BMC Oral Health 2008;8:22.

64. Blumenfeld AM, Boyd JP. Adjunctive treatment of chronic migraine using an oral dental device: overview and results of a randomized placebo-controlled crossover study. BMC Neurol 2022;22(1):72.

65. Greenspan JD, Slade GD, Rathnayaka N, et al. Experimental Pain Sensitivity in Subjects with Temporomandibular Disorders and Multiple Other Chronic Pain Conditions: The OPPERA Prospective Cohort Study. Journal of oral & facial pain and headache 2020;34(Suppl):s43–56.

66. Ohrbach R, Sharma S, Fillingim RB, et al. Clinical Characteristics of Pain Among Five Chronic Overlapping Pain Conditions. Journal of oral & facial pain and headache 2020;34(Suppl):s29–42.

67. Vale Braido GVD, Svensson P, Dos Santos Proença J, et al. Are central sensitization symptoms and psychosocial alterations interfering in the association between painful TMD, migraine, and headache attributed to TMD? Clin Oral Invest 2023;27(2):681–90.

68. Sabsoob O, Elsaraj SM, Gornitsky M, et al. Acute and Chronic Temporomandibular Disorder Pain: A critical review of differentiating factors and predictors of acute to chronic pain transition. J Oral Rehabil 2022;49(3):362–72.

69. Mitrirattanakul S, Merrill RL. Headache impact in patients with orofacial pain. J Am Dent Assoc 2006;137(9):1267–74.

70. Ashraf J, Zaproudina N, Suominen AL, et al. Association Between Temporomandibular Disorders Pain and Migraine: Results of the Health 2000 Survey. Journal of oral & facial pain and headache 2019;33(4):399–407.

71. Gonçalves DG, Camparis C, Franco A, et al. How to Investigate and Treat: Migraine in Patients with Temporomandibular Disorders. Curr Pain Headache Rep 2012/08/01 2012;16(4):359–64.

72. Klasser GD, Greene CS. Oral appliances in the management of temporomandibular disorders. Review. Oral Surg Oral Med Oral Pathol Oral Radiol Endod 2009; 107(2):212–23.

73. Menchel HF, Greene CS, Huff KD. Intraoral appliances for temporomandibular disorders: what we know and what we need to know. Frontiers of Oral and Maxillofacial Medicine 2021;3.

74. Manrriquez SL, Robles K, Pareek K, et al. Reduction of headache intensity and frequency with maxillary stabilization splint therapy in patients with temporomandibular disorders-headache comorbidity: a systematic review and meta-analysis. Journal of dental anesthesia and pain medicine 2021;21(3):183–205.

75. Gonzalez YM, Schiffman E, Gordon SM, et al. Development of a brief and effective temporomandibular disorder pain screening questionnaire: reliability and validity. J Am Dent Assoc 2011;142(10):1183–91.

76. (AAOP) AAoOP. AAOP. Orofacial Pain specialty. Available at: https://aaop.org/specialty/.

Trigeminal and Glossopharyngeal Neuralgia

Anthony K. Allam, BBA, M. Benjamin Larkin, MD, PharmD,
Himanshu Sharma, MD, PhD, Ashwin Viswanathan, MD*

KEYWORDS

- Secondary headaches • Trigeminal neuralgia • Glossopharyngeal neuralgia
- Surgical treatment • Pharmacologic treatment

KEY POINTS

- Trigeminal neuralgia and glossopharyngeal neuralgia are debilitating forms of paroxysmal craniofacial pain and are diagnosed primarily based on history and physical examination.
- First-line therapy for both conditions is pharmacotherapy of which carbamazepine has been the most effective and remains the drug of choice.
- Alternative medications are available for patients unable to tolerate the side effects of carbamazepine.
- Interventional treatments should be considered early in medically refractory cases.

INTRODUCTION

Trigeminal neuralgia (TN) and glossopharyngeal neuralgia (GPN) are two of the most common craniofacial neuralgias that result in severe and often debilitating pain that can significantly impact an individual's quality of life. This article summarizes each condition's characteristics, pathophysiology, and current pharmacotherapeutic and surgical interventions available for managing and treating these conditions.

Trigeminal Neuralgia

Background and epidemiology

TN is rare within the general population, with an overall prevalence of less than 0.1%.[1,2] It remains one of the most frequently diagnosed facial pain syndromes among older adults (>50 years) with an annual incidence of 4 to 13 per 100,000 individuals and is more frequently seen in women than men (1.5–1.7 to 1).[1,3,4] The location of pain is divided based on the three distributions of the trigeminal nerve: V1

Department of Neurosurgery, Baylor College of Medicine, Houston, TX, USA
* Corresponding author. Neurosurgery Department, Baylor College of Medicine, 7200 Cambridge Street Suite 9B, Houston, TX 77030.
E-mail address: ashwinv@bcm.edu

Neurol Clin 42 (2024) 585–598
https://doi.org/10.1016/j.ncl.2023.12.011
0733-8619/24/© 2024 Elsevier Inc. All rights reserved.

(ophthalmic), V2 (maxillary), and V3 (mandibular). The symptoms classically present as recurrent unilateral electric shock-like pains that are brief with an abrupt onset/termination followed by a refractory period in which a new attack cannot occur. Attacks are triggered by innocuous stimuli and tend to occur more frequently on the right side of the face.[5,6] However, attacks may also result from strong somatosensory stimulation outside the trigeminal nerve distribution, such as bright lights or loud sounds.

Approximately, 36% to 42% of patients exhibit pain in one distribution alone, with the nasolabial fold or chin, V2/V3, being particularly susceptible and representing the most common distributions. In 35% of patients, pain is found in both V2 and V3 distributions, whereas 14% of patients will experience pain in all three distributions.[4,6–11] More recently, however, it has been understood that up to 30% of patients may present with continuous pain of moderate intensity within the same distribution as the affected nerve division.[12]

TN does not frequently present with sensory deficits on gross physical examination; however, advanced sensory testing (ie, quantitative sensory testing) can elicit subtle findings.[13,14] Autonomic symptoms were traditionally not considered a part of TN; however, recent work has shown that autonomic symptoms, particularly lacrimation and rhinorrhea, can occur in TN patients.[15,16] These autonomic symptoms can make the diagnosis of TN more challenging given the overlap of symptoms with short-lasting unilateral neuralgiform headaches with autonomic signs.[8,17]

PATHOPHYSIOLOGY

The exact cause of TN remains unknown. However, the prevailing pathophysiologic theory attributes TN pain to peripheral and central nerve dysfunction. Numerous studies concur that focal demyelination of primary trigeminal afferents near the entry of the trigeminal root into the pons (dorsal root entry zone) is involved in the pathophysiological mechanism of TN.[18–21] In particular, the transition from oligodendrocyte to Schwann cell myelination within the proximal 25% of the trigeminal nerve is particularly susceptible to insult, representing a *locus minoris resistentiae*.[22] In addition, animal models and patient biopsies have suggested that these ectopic action potentials may result from dysregulation within voltage-gated sodium channels (Na_v),[23,24] specifically the upregulation of $Na_v1.3$ and $Na_v1.1$ channels and the downregulation of the $Na_v1.7$ channel.[24–27] It is these dysfunctional sensory transmissions, due to the collective up-and-down summation among the aforementioned sodium channels that are thought to be the source for the propagation of numerous amplified ectopic action potentials and the overall functional hyperexcitability responsible for the characteristic shock-like symptoms that patients experience.[24,28–30]

Diagnosis

In 2004, the International Headache Society (IHS) established a set of guidelines for the diagnosis of TN.[31,32] These guidelines were updated in 2018 with the 3rd edition of the International Classification of Headache Disorders (ICHD-3).[12] It is now divided into three main categories: classical, secondary/symptomatic, and idiopathic.[12] The diagnosis of TN is primarily made clinically; thus, a proper and thorough patient history remains of the utmost importance.

Diagnostic criteria

A. Recurrent unilateral facial pain in one or more distributions of the trigeminal nerve with no radiation beyond and fulfilling criteria B and C
B. Pain has the following characteristics:

1. Lasts from a fraction of a second to 2 minutes
2. Severe intensity
3. Electric shock-like, shooting, stabbing, or sharp in quality
C. Precipitated by innocuous stimuli within the affected trigeminal distribution
D. It is not accounted for by another ICHD-3 diagnosis.[12]

In addition to the criteria above, classical TN (CTN) must demonstrate neurovascular compression (NVC) of the trigeminal nerve root. This is most commonly caused by the superior cerebellar artery.[21,33] This compression is thought to cause hyperexcitability within the nerve secondary to subsequent focal demyelination. Associated morphologic changes and vascular compression may be seen with routine three-dimensional MRI reconstruction sequences such as constructive interference in steady state, fast imaging employing steady-state acquisition, fast inflow with a steady-state procession, and spoiled gradient-recalled.[34–36] However, vascular compression is also frequently seen in normal individuals; therefore, signs of NVC without corresponding TN symptoms are quite common.[37]

For the diagnosis of secondary TN, in addition to the above criteria, there must be a separate causative comorbid condition that explains the painful symptoms. Unlike CTN, secondary TN typically demonstrates no refractory period. In approximately 15% of cases, diagnostic imaging, such as CT or MRI, can help identify a structural lesion.[38] Within secondary TN, there are three sub-diagnoses: TN attributed to multiple sclerosis (TN-MS), TN attributed to space-occupying lesions, and TN attributed to other causes. The most common of these is TN-MS, with a 20-fold increased risk of developing TN, accounting for nearly up to 8% of all diagnosed MS patients developing TN throughout the disease course.[8,39–41] The other causes of secondary TN include skull-base bone deformities, connective tissue diseases, arteriovenous malformations, dural arteriovenous fistulae, and genetic causes of neuropathy.[12] It has long been known that familial versions of TN exist, with an estimated prevalence of approximately 1% to 2% in patients diagnosed with TN.[42–44] However, recent studies have shown that the prevalence of familial TN may be as high as 15.3%.[4,45] Bilateral TN has shown a higher familial association of approximately 17%, suggesting a more substantial hereditary component in this subpopulation.[45] However, as a whole, familial cases of TN tend to have significantly higher occurrences of right-sided pain and earlier onset of TN compared with sporadic cases.[46]

Finally, idiopathic TN is considered a diagnosis of exclusion and therefore diagnosed when the criterion for TN is met, but neither classical nor secondary TN can be diagnosed based on MRI and electrophysiological tests.

MANAGEMENT AND TREATMENT OF TRIGEMINAL NEURALGIA

Pharmacologic agents remain the first-line treatment for TN regardless of etiology. Surgical or interventional procedure modalities should be considered only when either pharmacologic measures are contraindicated or the pain becomes refractory to medical therapy.

Pharmacologic Management Options

Carbamazepine is the only FDA-approved medication for the treatment of TN. However, several other neuroleptics, muscle relaxants, and anticonvulsant medications, either alone or in conjunction with one another, have demonstrated varying degrees of success and are frequently prescribed off-label for pain management (**Table 1**).[47,48]

Carbamazepine

Carbamazepine is a sodium channel blocker and is the most commonly prescribed first-line medication for managing TN symptoms.[49–52] Since Blom's first

Table 1
Medical treatment of trigeminal neuralgia: commonly used medications

Medication	Maintenance Dosage (mg/d)	Duration to Relief (days)	Common Side Effects
Carbamazepine	200–1600	1–2 d	Leukopenia, aplastic anemia, drowsiness, ataxia
Oxcarbazepine	300–1200	1–2 d	Changes in vision, difficulty walking
Lamotrigine	200–400	1–2 d	Changes in vision, Stevens–Johnson syndrome
Baclofen	50–80	4–5 d	Confusion, withdrawal symptoms
Phenytoin	200–300	1–2 d	Confusion, decreased coordination
Gabapentin	1800–3600	1–3 wk	Unsteadiness, rolling eye movements
Pregabalin	150–600	1–2 wk	Swelling, blurred vision
Sumatriptan	50–100	15–60 min	Dizziness, tiredness, pressure in the chest, neck, jaw, or throat
Levetiracetam	1000–4000	1–2 h	Nasopharyngitis, sleepiness, headaches, irritability
Topiramate	100–400	1–4 wk	Dizziness, somnolence, cognitive impairment, and weight loss

implementation for TN in 1962, it has been the most extensively studied and validated medication, with level A evidence, for the treatment of TN.[53] Initial dosage is generally 100 to 200 mg twice a day, which is gradually escalated (100 mg every other day up to 1600 mg) to avoid adverse reactions until the pain is relieved or side effects occur.[54]

However, the general use of carbamazepine is limited by its adverse effects. Minor effects include general side effects, such as ataxia, dizziness, memory problem, disturbed sleep, drowsiness, rash, nausea, and vomiting, and electrolyte or hematologic disorders, such as hyponatremia, leukopenia, and aplastic anemia.[54,55] Routine blood sampling is necessary to monitor cell count and organ function. Among severe adverse events, Stevens–Johnson syndrome and toxic epidermal necrolysis are the two most severe.

Oxcarbazepine

Oxcarbazepine is a derivative of carbamazepine with a similar mechanism of action but is associated with improved pharmacodynamic and side-effect profiles. Oxcarbazepine has been shown to have a similar efficacy to carbamazepine even in patients in whom carbamazepine was ineffective.[56] However, this medication has less evidence (level B evidence) for its use than carbamazepine and is generally considered a second-line treatment option.[49,55] Daily dosages start at 150 mg per day and are increased slowly (150 mg per day) to an optimal maintenance dose, typically 300 to 1200 mg per day.[54]

Other Medications

The following medications are supported by randomized controlled trials (level C evidence), but further studies are needed before they can be used as first- or second-line medications: baclofen, lamotrigine, gabapentin ± ropivacaine, pimozide, phenytoin, tizanidine, botulinum toxin A, sumatriptan, and lidocaine. Some medications have shown limited evidence for their use in small lower evidence studies. These include pregabalin, topiramate, levetiracetam, and vixotrigine.

Surgical and Radiosurgical Treatment Options

There are no specific guidelines for selecting and timing surgical interventions for TN. However, in general, it should be considered after the patient has either been unable to tolerate the side effects of medication or failed an adequate medication management trial period.[57] In addition, the patient's age, general health, surgeon's level of expertise, and available facilities may further influence the consideration and timing of any intervention.

Microvascular Decompression

Microvascular decompression (MVD) is the primary surgical treatment for patients suffering from CTN caused by NVC. MVD aims to separate the trigeminal nerve root from the blood vessel(s) that are in contact with the root entry zone. This is done through a retrosigmoid craniotomy to access the trigeminal nerve root within the posterior cranial fossa. Although this procedure is the most invasive technique for treating TN, it provides the lowest rate of pain recurrence and the highest patient satisfaction.[58]

In one of the most extensive MVD series, Barker and colleagues reviewed more than 1100 patients over 20 years.[59] At the 10-year evaluation, 70% of patients were pain-free and 4% required continued medications. Approximately 30% of patients experienced symptom recurrence, and 11% required a second operation. Other studies have demonstrated similar findings, with 62% to 89% of patients with CTN remaining pain-free at 3 to 11 years.[49,60-63] Most recurrences are within 2 years postoperatively, but on average, there is a 4% recurrence rate per year.[64]

Complications from an MVD are rare with morbidity ranging from 0.3% to 3% and mortality from 0.2% to 0.5%. Complications can include cerebral spinal fluid leak, aseptic meningitis, cerebral infarcts, hematomas, unilateral hearing loss, facial weakness, and facial sensory loss.[49,59]

Ablative Techniques

Three percutaneous ablative techniques are commonly used to treat medically refractory TN: radiofrequency ablation rhizotomy (RFA), percutaneous glycerol rhizotomy (PGR), and balloon microcompression (BMC). Typically, these procedures are done with monitored anesthesia care with only BMC requiring general anesthesia. All three techniques rely on accurate cannulation of the trigeminal cistern through the medial portion of the foramen ovale. The entry point is defined by identifying specific anatomic landmarks, described initially by Hartel.[65] This point is 2.5 cm lateral to the corner of the mouth and 1 cm inferior with a trajectory aimed toward a point 3 cm anterior to the ipsilateral external auditory meatus and in the plane of the midpupillary line.

Radiofrequency Ablation

RFA involves inserting an electrode through the foramen ovale into the trigeminal ganglion and thermally ablating the afferent fibers. The initial placement of the probe is determined based on the dermatomal distribution of pain as well as the relationship of the cannula to the clival line with the use of intraoperative fluoroscopy. To ensure that the desired distributions of the trigeminal nerve are being targeted and to decrease the occurrence of adverse events, the patient is awoken to perform sensory test stimulation (100 Hz, 1 millisecond pulse width, 0.1–0.5 V amplitude). Once a location is confirmed, the patient is placed back under general anesthesia for the ablation, typically consisting of two lesions performed at 70 to 80°C for 90 seconds. However, the lesion temperature and duration can vary based on operator experience. Furthermore, patients should be counseled that facial numbness is an expected outcome of the procedure.

Results with RFA are good, with almost 100% of patients reporting immediate pain-free rates in multiple large series.[8,66,67] Recurrence rates in these trials range between 25% and 45% after a single session but drop to almost zero after multiple sessions. A recent pooled analysis revealed that 26% to 82% of patients are pain-free at 4 to 11 years after RFA.[60] Complications include reduced corneal reflex in up to 20% of cases and, less frequently, masseter muscle weakness or dysesthesias.

Patients with secondary TN resultant from multiple sclerosis have also shown promising results, with approximately 70% of patients pain-free after 5 years.[68]

Percutaneous Glycerol Rhizotomy

Hakanson first described the technique of PGR.[69] The technique follows a similar pattern to an RFA ablation in obtaining access to the trigeminal cistern. A cisterno-gram is then performed to estimate the volume of the trigeminal cistern. Afterward, the appropriate volume of glycerol is slowly injected, whereas the patient remains seated for 1 to 2 hours. Like RFA, this technique is effective for both classic and secondary TN. Although, unlike RFA, the effect can take up to 2 weeks to provide relief. Initial pain relief has been reported in approximately 90% of patients in the first 2 months, 60% at 1 year, 50% at 3 years, and 19% to 58% at 4 to 11 years.[60,70,71] Complications are similar to those for RFA and occur in approximately 11% of cases.[72]

Balloon Microcompression

Balloon compression is performed under general anesthesia. The foramen ovale is similarly accessed; however, the procedure requires a larger cannula (14 gauge) through which a No 4 Fogarty micro-balloon is placed and inflated to an intraluminal pressure of 1200 to 1500 mm Hg for 1 to 2 minutes. This results in dural stretching, direct compression of the trigeminal ganglion, and a lesion to afferent fiber while sparing small unmyelinated fibers involved in the corneal reflex. Immediate pain relief is often experienced in 85% to 99% of patients, others within 1 to 2 days following the procedure, with 50% to 80% remaining pain-free at 4 to 11 years.[60,73–75] Complication rates in these studies are also low and range from 4% to 8%. Balloon compression is generally the favored technique for V1 TN pain as this procedure spares the corneal reflex.

STEREOTACTIC RADIOSURGERY

Stereotactic radiosurgery (SRS) has been solidified as an alternative treatment modality for the treatment of TN. Although other methods of radiosurgery exist, the two main methods are Gamma Knife (Elekta, Atlanta, GA), which consists of multiple beams of simultaneous radiation used to create an isolated treatment area and CyberKnife (Accuray, Sunnyvale, CA), where a single radiation beam is instead maneuvered in three-dimensional space to create the targeted lesion.

Gamma Knife Radiosurgery (GKRS) uses radiation (75–85 Gy) from a cobalt-60 gamma emission source to target the root entry zone of the trigeminal nerve root and can be used in patients with or without vascular compression. Owing to the destructive nature of radiosurgery, patients may endorse some sensory loss following the procedure. Although higher doses (90 Gy) typically provided better pain relief outcomes, it is also associated with higher rates of dysesthesias.[49,61,76]

Pain relief, on average, is delayed by 1 month, but pooled analyses demonstrate that the proportion of patients with pain relief increases, peaking at 24 months.[8,77–79] The percentage of patients with continued pain decreases from this point, though 30% to 66% of patients will continue to be pain-free for 4 to 11 years.[60]

CyberKnife has also been shown to be efficacious in treating TN. The optimal treatment parameters were a maximal median dose of 78 Gy and a 6 mm median length of the treated nerve.[80] Similar to GKRS, 70% to 88% of patients had excellent pain relief within 7 to 14 days.[80,81] But, similar to other GKRS, this proportion decreased to approximately 50% at 2 years. The rate of complications was 18%, and nearly 50% of patients experienced facial numbness.[80,81]

Comparison studies between Gamma Knife and MVD have found MVD to be significantly better with more extended periods of pain relief and lower recurrence rates (70%–74% relief at 10 years; 18% recurrence at 25 years) compared with GKRS (67% relief at 3 years).[82–85] However, MVD is associated with higher rates of cerebrospinal fluid leak, hearing loss, and persistent diplopia.[83] Thus, because of the less invasive nature of radiosurgery, it is often offered to patients who are ineligible for the more invasive MVD while still offering favorable pain relief.

Glossopharyngeal Neuralgia

Background and epidemiology

GPN is an uncommon facial pain syndrome characterized by paroxysmal pain episodes along the auricular and pharyngeal branches of the glossopharyngeal and vagus nerves. It was first reported in a patient with a cerebellopontine angle tumor by Weisenburg and colleagues.[86]

GPN is characterized by acute, abrupt paroxysms of severe, sharp, stabbing-like unilateral pain in the distribution of the glossopharyngeal nerve. Patients often experience pain in the ear, the base of the tongue, the tonsillar fossa, and beneath the angle of the jaw. If vagal branches are also affected, patients may experience cough, hoarseness, and parasympathetic events, including bradycardia, asystole, syncopal episodes, and convulsions. This condition is often referred to as vago-GPN.[87] The constellation of symptoms makes the diagnosis confusing, and patients are frequently misdiagnosed with either TN, nervus intermedius neuralgia, or superior laryngeal neuralgia.[88]

The incidence of GPN within the general population is far less than TN and is estimated to be only 0.2 to 0.9 per 100,000 patients.[3,89,90] Patients are typically older than 50 years at the time of presentation and differs from TN, as patients with GPN presents more frequently with symptoms on the left side with a ratio of 3:2.[91,92] Furthermore, a quarter of presenting patients will have bilateral presentations with the disease equally affecting males and females.[90,93]

Diagnosis

The IHS diagnostic guidelines divide GPN into three categories: classical, secondary, or idiopathic.[12] GPN is also clinically diagnosed; thus, a good history and physical examination are needed to rule out other potential causes for the patient's symptoms. It is essential to localize the exact distribution of pain to differentiate patients with TN, GPN, superior laryngeal neuralgia, and nervus intermedius neuralgia.

Diagnostic Criteria[12]:

A. Recurring paroxysmal attacks of unilateral pain in the distribution of the glossopharyngeal nerve and fulfilling criterion B

B. Pain has all the following characteristics:

    1. Lasting from a few seconds to 2 minutes

2. Severe intensity
3. Electric shock-like, shooting, stabbing, or sharp in quality
4. Precipitated by swallowing, coughing, talking, or yawning
C. Not better accounted for by another ICHD-3 diagnosis

In addition to the criteria above, classical GPN is diagnosed when NVC of the glossopharyngeal nerve root is seen either through MRI or intraoperatively. Conversely, a diagnosis of secondary GPN is made when an underlying disease known to cause the above symptoms are discovered and includes neck trauma, multiple sclerosis, tonsillar/regional tumors, cerebellopontine angle tumors, and Arnold-Chiari malformations. Finally, idiopathic GPN is an exclusionary diagnosis when no signs of NVC or a secondary disease process that can explain GPN are seen. Although GPN usually fails to exhibit sensory changes within the affected nerve distribution, mild deficits can be seen in some cases.[12] Other disease processes should be considered when either major sensory deficits are seen or the gag reflex is affected.[12]

MANAGEMENT AND TREATMENT OF GLOSSOPHARYNGEAL NEURALGIA

Owing to the relative rarity and similar presentation of GPN to TN, many medical treatments for TN are also used for treating GPN. The first-line medication includes carbamazepine and oxcarbazepine.[94]

Similarly, patients who are refractory to medical management can undergo destructive and nondestructive surgical interventions, including percutaneous radiofrequency ablation, ultrasound-guided nerve blocks, SRS, and MVD.[95–99] In a study by Liu and colleagues, 12 patients with GPN received an ultrasound-guided nerve block. Immediate pain relief occurred in 83.3% of patients and 33.3% at 18 months.[98] Using RFA, Wang and colleagues treated 71 patients with treatment-resistant GPN, providing immediate pain relief in 78.8% of patients at discharge and 43.0% 10 years later.[97] SRS with Gamma Knife has also reported good results for treating GPN in several case series, with nearly 90% of patients achieving significant pain relief.[96,100–103] MVD with and without rhizotomy for classical GPN has been shown in several studies to have equally good long-term pain-free outcomes (>80%–90%) and a low rate of complications (dysphagia or hoarseness).[104–108]

SUMMARY

Accurate diagnosis and treatment are crucial for improving patient outcomes. TN and GPN are painful conditions which, though rare, are often debilitating to those affected. Medical therapy remains the first-line treatment of both, but minimally invasive, surgical, and radiosurgical modalities are often effective options for patients who remain refractory to medical treatment.

CLINICS CARE POINTS

- Before a diagnosis of trigeminal or glossopharyngeal neuralgia is made, it is important to consider and exclude all alternative diagnoses.
- Carbamazepine is a first-line treatment for both trigeminal and glossopharyngeal neuralgia.
- Surgical treatments for trigeminal and glossopharyngeal neuralgia are considered pain becomes refractory to medical management.

DISCLOSURE

None. The authors have no granting organizations or grant numbers, contract numbers, or other financial or material support sources to disclose.

REFERENCES

1. MacDonald BK, Cockerell OC, Sander JW, et al. The incidence and lifetime prevalence of neurological disorders in a prospective community-based study in the UK. Brain 2000;123(Pt 4):665–76.
2. Cruccu G, Truini A. Refractory Trigeminal Neuralgia. CNS Drugs 2013; 27(2):91–6.
3. Katusic S, Williams DB, Beard CM, et al. Epidemiology and clinical features of idiopathic trigeminal neuralgia and glossopharyngeal neuralgia: similarities and differences, Rochester, Minnesota, 1945-1984. Neuroepidemiology 1991; 10(5–6):276–81.
4. Katusic S, Beard CM, Bergstralh E, et al. Incidence and clinical features of trigeminal neuralgia, Rochester, Minnesota, 1945-1984. Ann Neurol 1990;27(1): 89–95.
5. Ghislain B, Rabinstein AA, Braksick SA. Etiologies and Utility of Diagnostic Tests in Trigeminal Neuropathy. Mayo Clin Proc 2022;97(7):1318–25.
6. Maarbjerg S, Gozalov A, Olesen J, et al. Trigeminal neuralgia–a prospective systematic study of clinical characteristics in 158 patients. Headache 2014; 54(10):1574–82.
7. Haviv Y, Khan J, Zini A, et al. Trigeminal neuralgia (part I): Revisiting the clinical phenotype. Cephalalgia 2016;36(8):730–46.
8. Maarbjerg S, Benoliel R. The changing face of trigeminal neuralgia—A narrative review. Headache J Head Face Pain 2021;61(6):817–37.
9. Benoliel R, Zadik Y, Eliav E, et al. Peripheral painful traumatic trigeminal neuropathy: clinical features in 91 cases and proposal of novel diagnostic criteria. J Orofac Pain 2012;26(1):49–58. http://www.ncbi.nlm.nih.gov/pubmed/ 22292140.
10. Siqueira SR, Teixeira MJ, Siqueira JT. Clinical characteristics of patients with trigeminal neuralgia referred to neurosurgery. Eur J Dermatol 2009;3(3):207–12. http://www.ncbi.nlm.nih.gov/pubmed/19756195.
11. Rasmussen P. Facial pain. II. A prospective survey of 1052 patients with a view of: character of the attacks, onset, course, and character of pain. Acta Neurochir 1990;107(3–4):121–8.
12. Vincent M, Wang S jiun. Headache Classification Committee of the International Headache Society (IHS) The International Classification of Headache Disorders, 3rd edition. Cephalalgia. 2018;38(1):1-211.
13. Younis S, Maarbjerg S, Reimer M, et al. Quantitative sensory testing in classical trigeminal neuralgia-a blinded study in patients with and without concomitant persistent pain. Pain 2016;157(7):1407–14.
14. Maier C, Baron R, Tölle TR, et al. Quantitative sensory testing in the German Research Network on Neuropathic Pain (DFNS): somatosensory abnormalities in 1236 patients with different neuropathic pain syndromes. Pain 2010;150(3): 439–50.
15. Rasmussen P. Facial pain. IV. A prospective study of 1052 patients with a view of: precipitating factors, associated symptoms, objective psychiatric and neurological symptoms. Acta Neurochir 1991;108(3–4):100–9.

16. Simms HN, Honey CR. The importance of autonomic symptoms in trigeminal neuralgia. Clinical article. J Neurosurg 2011;115(2):210–6.

17. Benoliel R, Sharav Y. Trigeminal neuralgia with lacrimation or SUNCT syndrome? Cephalalgia 1998;18(2):85–90.

18. Rappaport ZH, Govrin-Lippmann R, Devor M. An electron-microscopic analysis of biopsy samples of the trigeminal root taken during microvascular decompressive surgery. Stereotact Funct Neurosurg 1997;68(1–4 Pt 1):182–6.

19. Lutz J, Thon N, Stahl R, et al. Microstructural alterations in trigeminal neuralgia determined by diffusion tensor imaging are independent of symptom duration, severity, and type of neurovascular conflict. J Neurosurg 2016;124(3):823–30.

20. Obermann M, Yoon MS, Ese D, et al. Impaired trigeminal nociceptive processing in patients with trigeminal neuralgia. Neurology 2007;69(9):835–41.

21. Maarbjerg S, di Stefano G, Bendtsen L, et al. Trigeminal neuralgia – diagnosis and treatment. Cephalalgia 2017;37(7):648–57.

22. Peker S, Kurtkaya Ö, Üzün İ, et al. Microanatomy of the Central Myelin-Peripheral Myelin Transition Zone of the Trigeminal Nerve. Neurosurgery 2006; 59(2):354–9.

23. Gambeta E, Chichorro JG, Zamponi GW. Trigeminal neuralgia: An overview from pathophysiology to pharmacological treatments. Mol Pain 2020;16. 174480692090189.

24. Chen Q, Yi DI, Perez JNJ, et al. The Molecular Basis and Pathophysiology of Trigeminal Neuralgia. Int J Mol Sci 2022;23(7):3604.

25. Liu M, Zhong J, Xia L, et al. The expression of voltage-gated sodium channels in trigeminal nerve following chronic constriction injury in rats. Int J Neurosci 2019; 129(10):955–62.

26. Siqueira SRDT, Alves B, Malpartida HMG, et al. Abnormal expression of voltage-gated sodium channels Nav1.7, Nav1.3 and Nav1.8 in trigeminal neuralgia. Neuroscience 2009;164(2):573–7.

27. Xu W, Zhang J, Wang Y, et al. Changes in the expression of voltage-gated sodium channels Nav1.3, Nav1.7, Nav1.8, and Nav1.9 in rat trigeminal ganglia following chronic constriction injury. Neuroreport 2016;27(12):929–34.

28. Love S, Coakham HB. Trigeminal neuralgia: pathology and pathogenesis. Brain 2001;124(Pt 12):2347–60.

29. Rasminsky M. Ectopic generation of impulses and cross-talk in spinal nerve roots of ?dystrophic? mice. Ann Neurol 1978;3(4):351–7.

30. Amir R, Devor M. Functional cross-excitation between afferent A- and C-neurons in dorsal root ganglia. Neuroscience 1999;95(1):189–95.

31. Headache Classification Subcommittee of the International Headache Society. The International Classification of Headache Disorders: 2nd edition. Cephalalgia. 2004;24 Suppl 1:9-160.

32. Headache Classification Committee of the International Headache Society (IHS). The International Classification of Headache Disorders, 3rd edition (beta version). Cephalalgia 2013;33(9):629–808.

33. Nurmikko TJ, Eldridge PR. Trigeminal neuralgia–pathophysiology, diagnosis and current treatment. Br J Anaesth 2001;87(1):117–32.

34. Zeng Q, Zhou Q, Liu Z, et al. Preoperative detection of the neurovascular relationship in trigeminal neuralgia using three-dimensional fast imaging employing steady-state acquisition (FIESTA) and magnetic resonance angiography (MRA). J Clin Neurosci 2013;20(1):107–11.

35. Yoshino N, Akimoto H, Yamada I, et al. Trigeminal neuralgia: evaluation of neuralgic manifestation and site of neurovascular compression with 3D CISS MR imaging and MR angiography. Radiology 2003;228(2):539–45.
36. Meaney JF, Miles JB, Nixon TE, et al. Vascular contact with the fifth cranial nerve at the pons in patients with trigeminal neuralgia: detection with 3D FISP imaging. AJR Am J Roentgenol 1994;163(6):1447–52.
37. Peker S, Dinçer A, Necmettin Pamir M. Vascular compression of the trigeminal nerve is a frequent finding in asymptomatic individuals: 3-T MR imaging of 200 trigeminal nerves using 3D CISS sequences. Acta Neurochir 2009;151(9):1081–8.
38. Cruccu G, Gronseth G, Alksne J, et al. AAN-EFNS guidelines on trigeminal neuralgia management. Eur J Neurol 2008;15(10):1013–28.
39. Osterberg A, Boivie J, Thuomas KA. Central pain in multiple sclerosis–prevalence and clinical characteristics. Eur J Pain 2005;9(5):531–42.
40. Foley PL, Vesterinen HM, Laird BJ, et al. Prevalence and natural history of pain in adults with multiple sclerosis: systematic review and meta-analysis. Pain 2013;154(5):632–42.
41. Danesh-Sani SA, Rahimdoost A, Soltani M, et al. Clinical assessment of orofacial manifestations in 500 patients with multiple sclerosis. J Oral Maxillofac Surg 2013;71(2):290–4.
42. Allan W. Familial occurrence of tic douloureux. Arch Neurol Psychiatr 1938;40(5):1019.
43. HARRIS W. Bilateral trigeaiinal tic. its association with heredity and disseminated sclekosis. Ann Surg 1936;103(2):161–72.
44. Fernández Rodríguez B, Simonet C, Cerdán DM, et al. Neuralgia del trigémino clásica familiar. Neurologia 2019;34(4):229–33.
45. Pollack IF, Jannetta PJ, Bissonette DJ. Bilateral trigeminal neuralgia: a 14-year experience with microvascular decompression. J Neurosurg 1988;68(4):559–65.
46. Eide PK. Familial occurrence of classical and idiopathic trigeminal neuralgia. J Neurol Sci 2022;434:120101.
47. IANNONE A, BAKER AB, MORRELL F. Dilantin in the treatment of trigeminal neuralgia. Neurology 1958;8(2):126–8.
48. Jorns TP, Zakrzewska JM. Evidence-based approach to the medical management of trigeminal neuralgia. Br J Neurosurg 2007;21(3):253–61.
49. Cruccu G, Gronseth G, Alksne J, et al. AAN-EFNS guidelines on trigeminal neuralgia management. Eur J Neurol 2008;15(10):1013–28.
50. NICOL CF. A four year double-blind study of tegretol(r)in facial pain. Headache J Head Face Pain 1969;9(1):54–7.
51. Killian JM. Carbamazepine in the Treatment of Neuralgia. Arch Neurol 1968;19(2):129.
52. Campbell FG, Graham JG, Zilkha KJ. Clinical trial of carbazepine (tegretol) in trigeminal neuralgia. J Neurol Neurosurg Psychiatry 1966;29(3):265–7.
53. BLOM S. Trigeminal neuralgia: its treatment with a new anticonvulsant drug (G-32883). Lancet 1962;279(7234):839–40.
54. McMillan R. Trigeminal Neuralgia - A Debilitating Facial Pain. Rev Pain 2011;5(1):26–34.
55. Besi E, Boniface DR, Cregg R, et al. Comparison of tolerability and adverse symptoms in oxcarbazepine and carbamazepine in the treatment of trigeminal neuralgia and neuralgiform headaches using the Liverpool Adverse Events Profile (AEP). J Headache Pain 2015;16:563.

56. Gomez-Arguelles JM, Dorado R, Sepulveda JM, et al. Oxcarbazepine mono-therapy in carbamazepine-unresponsive trigeminal neuralgia. J Clin Neurosci 2008;15(5):516–9.

57. Pollock BE. Surgical management of medically refractory trigeminal neuralgia. Curr Neurol Neurosci Rep 2012;12(2):125–31.

58. Tatli M, Satici O, Kanpolat Y, et al. Various surgical modalities for trigeminal neuralgia: literature study of respective long-term outcomes. Acta Neurochir 2008; 150(3):243–55.

59. Barker FG, Jannetta PJ, Bissonette DJ, et al. The Long-Term Outcome of Micro-vascular Decompression for Trigeminal Neuralgia. N Engl J Med 1996;334(17): 1077–84.

60. Bendtsen L, Zakrzewska JM, Abbott J, et al. European Academy of Neurology guideline on trigeminal neuralgia. Eur J Neurol 2019;26(6):831–49.

61. Gronseth G, Cruccu G, Alksne J, et al. Practice parameter: the diagnostic eval-uation and treatment of trigeminal neuralgia (an evidence-based review): report of the Quality Standards Subcommittee of the American Academy of Neurology and the European Federation of Neurological Societies. Neurology 2008;71(15): 1183–90.

62. Sarsam Z, Garcia-Fiñana M, Nurmikko TJ, et al. The long-term outcome of microvascular decompression for trigeminal neuralgia. Br J Neurosurg 2010; 24(1):18–25.

63. Sindou M, Leston J, Decullier E, et al. Microvascular decompression for primary trigeminal neuralgia: long-term effectiveness and prognostic factors in a series of 362 consecutive patients with clear-cut neurovascular conflicts who under-went pure decompression. J Neurosurg 2007;107(6):1144–53.

64. Burchiel KJ, Clarke H, Haglund M, et al. Long-term efficacy of microvascular decompression in trigeminal neuralgia. J Neurosurg 1988;69(1):35–8.

65. Hartel F. Block anaesthesia and injection of the Gasserian ganglion and the tri-geminal roots. Langenbecks Arch Klin Chir 1912;100:16.

66. Kanpolat Y, Savas A, Bekar A, et al. Percutaneous controlled radiofrequency tri-geminal rhizotomy for the treatment of idiopathic trigeminal neuralgia: 25-year experience with 1,600 patients. Neurosurgery 2001;48(3):524–32 ; discussion 532-4.

67. Taha JM, Tew JM, Buncher CR. A prospective 15-year follow up of 154 consec-utive patients with trigeminal neuralgia treated by percutaneous stereotactic ra-diofrequency thermal rhizotomy. J Neurosurg 1995;83(6):989–93.

68. Kanpolat Y, Berk C, Savas A, et al. Percutaneous controlled radiofrequency rhi-zotomy in the management of patients with trigeminal neuralgia due to multiple sclerosis. Acta Neurochir 2000;142(6):685–9 [discussion 689-90].

69. Hakanson S. Retrogasserian injection of glycerol in the treatment of trigeminal neuralgia and other facial pains. Neurosurgery 1982;10(2):300.

70. Pollock BE. Percutaneous retrogasserian glycerol rhizotomy for patients with idiopathic trigeminal neuralgia: a prospective analysis of factors related to pain relief. J Neurosurg 2005;102(2):223–8.

71. Linderoth B, Håkanson S. Paroxysmal facial pain in disseminated sclerosis treated by retrogasserian glycerol injection. Acta Neurol Scand 1989;80(4): 341–6.

72. Kouzounias K, Lind G, Schechtmann G, et al. Comparison of percutaneous balloon compression and glycerol rhizotomy for the treatment of trigeminal neu-ralgia. J Neurosurg 2010;113(3):486–92.

73. Kouzounias K, Schechtmann G, Lind G, et al. Factors that influence outcome of percutaneous balloon compression in the treatment of trigeminal neuralgia. Neurosurgery 2010;67(4):925–34 [discussion 934].

74. Park SS, Lee MK, Kim JW, et al. Percutaneous balloon compression of trigeminal ganglion for the treatment of idiopathic trigeminal neuralgia : experience in 50 patients. J Korean Neurosurg Soc 2008;43(4):186–9.

75. Skirving DJ, Dan NG. A 20-year review of percutaneous balloon compression of the trigeminal ganglion. J Neurosurg 2001;94(6):913–7.

76. Pollock BE, Phuong LK, Gorman DA, et al. Stereotactic radiosurgery for idiopathic trigeminal neuralgia. J Neurosurg 2002;97(2):347–53.

77. Jawahar A, Wadhwa R, Berk C, et al. Assessment of pain control, quality of life, and predictors of success after gamma knife surgery for the treatment of trigeminal neuralgia. Neurosurg Focus 2005;18(5):E8.

78. Loescher AR, Radatz M, Kemeny A, et al. Stereotactic radiosurgery for trigeminal neuralgia: outcomes and complications. Br J Neurosurg 2012;26(1):45–52.

79. Tuleasca C, Carron R, Resseguier N, et al. Patterns of pain-free response in 497 cases of classic trigeminal neuralgia treated with Gamma Knife surgery and followed up for least 1 year. J Neurosurg 2012;117(Suppl):181–8.

80. Villavicencio AT, Lim M, Burneikiene S, et al. Cyberknife radiosurgery for trigeminal neuralgia treatment: a preliminary multicenter experience. Neurosurgery 2008;62(3):647–55 [discussion 647-55].

81. Lim M, Villavicencio AT, Burneikiene S, et al. CyberKnife radiosurgery for idiopathic trigeminal neuralgia. Neurosurg Focus 2005;18(5):E9.

82. Pollock BE, Schoeberl KA. Prospective comparison of posterior fossa exploration and stereotactic radiosurgery dorsal root entry zone target as primary surgery for patients with idiopathic trigeminal neuralgia. Neurosurgery 2010;67(3):633–8 [discussion 638-9].

83. Linskey ME, Ratanatharathorn V, Peñagaricano J. A prospective cohort study of microvascular decompression and Gamma Knife surgery in patients with trigeminal neuralgia. J Neurosurg 2008;109(Suppl):160–72.

84. Pollock BE. Comparison of posterior fossa exploration and stereotactic radiosurgery in patients with previously nonsurgically treated idiopathic trigeminal neuralgia. Neurosurg Focus 2005;18(5):E6.

85. Sanchez-Mejia RO, Limbo M, Cheng JS, et al. Recurrent or refractory trigeminal neuralgia after microvascular decompression, radiofrequency ablation, or radiosurgery. Neurosurg Focus 2005;18(5):e12.

86. Weisenburg TH. Cerebello-pontile tumor diagnosed for six years as tic douloureux. J Am Med Assoc 1910;LIV(20):1600.

87. Burfield L, Ahmad F, Adams J. Glossopharyngeal neuralgia associated with cardiac syncope. BMJ Case Rep 2016;2016.

88. Blumenfeld A, Nikolskaya G. Glossopharyngeal neuralgia. Curr Pain Headache Rep 2013;17(7):343.

89. Manzoni GC, Torelli P. Epidemiology of typical and atypical craniofacial neuralgias. Neurol Sci 2005;26(Suppl 2):s65–7.

90. Katusic S, Williams DB, Beard CM, et al. Incidence and clinical features of glossopharyngeal neuralgia, Rochester, Minnesota, 1945-1984. Neuroepidemiology 1991;10(5–6):266–75.

91. Rey-Dios R, Cohen-Gadol AA. Current neurosurgical management of glossopharyngeal neuralgia and technical nuances for microvascular decompression surgery. Neurosurg Focus 2013;34(3):E8.

92. Chen J, Sindou M. Vago-glossopharyngeal neuralgia: a literature review of neurosurgical experience. Acta Neurochir 2015;157(2):311–21 [discussion 321].

93. Koopman JSHA, Dieleman JP, Huygen FJ, et al. Incidence of facial pain in the general population. Pain 2009;147(1–3):122–7.

94. Fromm GH. Clinical pharmacology of drugs used to treat head and face pain. Neurol Clin 1990;8(1):143–51. http://www.ncbi.nlm.nih.gov/pubmed/2181262.

95. Isamat F, Ferrán E, Acebes JJ. Selective percutaneous thermocoagulation rhizotomy in essential glossopharyngeal neuralgia. J Neurosurg 1981;55(4):575–80.

96. Yomo S, Arkha Y, Donnet A, et al. Gamma Knife surgery for glossopharyngeal neuralgia. J Neurosurg 2009;110(3):559–63.

97. Wang X, Tang Y, Zeng Y, et al. Long-term outcomes of percutaneous radiofrequency thermocoagulation for glossopharyngeal neuralgia: A retrospective observational study. Medicine 2016;95(48):e5530.

98. Liu Q, Zhong Q, Tang G, et al. Ultrasound-guided glossopharyngeal nerve block via the styloid process for glossopharyngeal neuralgia: a retrospective study. J Pain Res 2019;12:2503.

99. Pagura JR, Schnapp M, Passarelli P. Percutaneous radiofrequency glossopharyngeal rhizotomy for cancer pain. Appl Neurophysiol 1983;46(1–4):154–9.

100. O'Connor JK, Bidiwala S. Effectiveness and safety of Gamma Knife radiosurgery for glossopharyngeal neuralgia. SAVE Proc 2013;26(3):262–4.

101. Williams BJ, Schlesinger D, Sheehan J. Glossopharyngeal neuralgia treated with gamma knife radiosurgery. World Neurosurg 2010;73(4):413–7.

102. O'Connor JK, Bidiwala S. Effectiveness and safety of Gamma Knife radiosurgery for glossopharyngeal neuralgia. SAVE Proc 2013;26(3):262–4.

103. Stieber VW, Bourland JD, Ellis TL. Glossopharyngeal neuralgia treated with gamma knife surgery: treatment outcome and failure analysis. Case report. J Neurosurg 2005;102(Suppl):155–7.

104. Ferroli P, Fioravanti A, Schiariti M, et al. Microvascular decompression for glossopharyngeal neuralgia: a long-term retrospectic review of the Milan-Bologna experience in 31 consecutive cases. Acta Neurochir 2009;151(10):1245–50.

105. Kandan SR, Khan S, Jeyaretna DS, et al. Neuralgia of the glossopharyngeal and vagal nerves: long-term outcome following surgical treatment and literature review. Br J Neurosurg 2010;24(4):441–6.

106. Patel A, Kassam A, Horowitz M, et al. Microvascular decompression in the management of glossopharyngeal neuralgia: analysis of 217 cases. Neurosurgery 2002;50(4):705–10 [discussion 710-1].

107. Sampson JH, Grossi PM, Asaoka K, et al. Microvascular decompression for glossopharyngeal neuralgia: long-term effectiveness and complication avoidance. Neurosurgery 2004;54(4):884–9 [discussion 889-90].

108. Rushton JG, Stevens JC, Miller RH. Glossopharyngeal (vagoglossopharyngeal) neuralgia: a study of 217 cases. Arch Neurol 1981;38(4):201–5.

Cough, Exertional, and Sex Headaches

Monique Montenegro, MD[a], Fred Michael Cutrer, MD[b],*

KEYWORDS

- Cough • Exertional • Sex headache

KEY POINTS

- Cough, exertional, and sex headaches all share similar secondary causes and pathophysiology involving transient increases in intracranial pressure.
- All typically occur in middle age, though headaches associated with sexual activity can have a bimodal distribution.
- All of these secondary headache types have potential life-threatening vascular etiologies which warrant further investigation.

INTRODUCTION

Evaluation of a patient presenting with cough, exertional, or sex headache involves ruling out vascular causes such as subarachnoid hemorrhage, aneurysms, arterial dissection, or reversible cerebral vasoconstrictive syndrome (RCVS), as well as cerebrospinal fluid (CSF) dynamics disorders such as spontaneous intracranial hypotension (SIH) (due to CSF leak or CSF-venous fistula) or posterior fossa obstruction of CSF flow (including Chiari I malformation for cough headache). Diagnostic studies and treatment options for the most common etiologies of these headaches will be described.

INTERNATIONAL CLASSIFICATION OF HEADACHE DISORDERS, THIRD EDITION

Though our foremost aim is to describe the etiology and presentation of secondary cough, exertional, and sex headaches, a review of the International Classification of Headache Disorders third edition (ICHD-3) criteria for the primary equivalents of these headache disorders [see **Boxes 1** and **2**] is valuable if only to define the features of these headaches and to assist in differentiating primary from secondary.

DISCUSSION
Clinical Manifestations of Cough Headaches

Cough headache (also known as Valsalva headache) may be induced by coughing, sneezing, singing, nose-blowing, straining, laughing, crying, lifting, straining, bending,

a General Neurology and Headache Division, University of Minnesota Medical School, Minneapolis, MN, USA; b Mayo Clinic, 200 First Street Southwest, Rochester, MN 55901, USA
* Corresponding author.
E-mail address: Cutrer.michael@mayo.edu

Neurol Clin 42 (2024) 599–614
https://doi.org/10.1016/j.ncl.2023.12.012
0733-8619/24/© 2023 Elsevier Inc. All rights reserved.

neurologic.theclinics.com

Box 1
Primary cough, exertional, and sex headaches — International Classification of Headache Disorders, third edition

Primary cough headache
A. At least 2 headache episodes fulfilling criteria B–D
B. Brought on by and occurring only in association with coughing, straining, and/or other Valsalva maneuver
C. Sudden onset
D. Lasting between 1 second and 2 hours
E. Not fulfilling ICHD-3 criteria for any other headache disorder
F. Not better accounted for by another ICHD-3 diagnosis

Primary exercise/exertional headache
A. At least 2 headache episodes fulfilling criteria B–C
B. Brought on by and occurring only during or after strenuous physical exercise
C. Lasting less than 48 hours
D. Not better accounted for by another ICHD-3 diagnosis

Primary headache associated with sexual activity
A. At least 2 headache episodes of pain in the head and/or neck fulfilling criteria B–D
B. Brought on by and occurring only during sexual activity
C. Either or both of the following:
  1. Increasing in intensity with increasing sexual excitement
  2. Abrupt explosive intensity just before or with orgasm
D. Lasting from 1 minute to 24 hours with severe intensity and/or up to 72 hours with mild intensity
E. Not better accounted for by another ICHD-3 diagnosis

Abbreviation: ICHD-3, International Classification of Headache Disorders, third edition.

---

and stooping. Pain reaches its peak immediately after the onset of these actions. In Pascual and colleagues'[1] prospective study specifically evaluating secondary cough headaches, 40 patients had a primary occipital-suboccipital pain localization but hemicranial and bicranial distributions were also reported. Pain characterization was variable, but most described it as pressing, some as explosive, and some as electric or a mixture of all of these. Usually, other symptoms such as dizziness, unsteadiness, facial and upper limb numbness, vertigo, and syncope which implied posterior fossa localization accompanied these headaches. Only in 7 patients, were associated symptoms absent.[1] Mean age of onset for secondary cough headaches is 39 to 44 (depending on the source) and headaches occur predominantly in males.[1,2] In Chen and colleagues'[3] study, it was found that primary cough headache could last up to 2 hours and secondary headache up to 30 minutes in a study of 83 patients. There are no associated symptoms of nausea, vomiting, conjunctival injection, lacrimation, rhinorrhea, or sinus congestion, and migrainous features of photophobia, phonophobia, and osmophobia are not characteristic.

Etiology of Cough Headaches

International Headache Society (IHS) criteria note that up to 40% of cough headaches are symptomatic of an underlying secondary cause. In Pascual and colleagues'[1] prospective study, 40 out of 68 patients (59%) were found to have secondary cough headaches, typically lasting seconds but with an overall average duration of 5 years (maximum 30 years).

In Symonds'[4] widely cited series of cough headache, etiologies of the 6 patients with secondary cough headache varied from infratentorial meningioma, midbrain cyst bulging into the fourth ventricle, and Paget's disease of the skull with basilar

---

Box 2
Probable primary cough, exertional, and sex headaches—International Classification of Headache Disorders, third edition

Probable primary cough headache
A. Either of the following:
   1. A single headache episode fulfilling criteria B through D
   2. At least 2 headache episodes fulfilling criteria and the and either of criteria C and D
B. Brought on by and occurring only in association with coughing, straining, and/or other Valsalva maneuver
C. Sudden onset
D. Lasting between 1 second and 2 hours
E. Not fulfilling ICHD-3 criteria for any other headache disorder
F. Not better accounted for by another ICHD-3 diagnosis

Probably Exercise/Exertional Headache
A. Either of the following:
   1. At least 2 headache episodes fulfilling criteria B through C
   2. At least 2 headache episodes fulfilling criteria and the and either of criteria B and C
B. Brought on by and occurring only in association with strenuous physical exercise
C. Lasting less than 48 hours
D. Not fulfilling ICHD-3 criteria for any other headache disorder
E. Not better accounted for by another ICHD-3 diagnosis

Probable primary headache associated with sexual activity
A. Either of the following:
   1. A single headache episode fulfilling criteria B-D
   2. At least 2 headache episodes fulfilling criterion B and either but not both of criteria C and D
B. Brought on by and occurring only during sexual activity
C. Either or both of the following:
   1. Increasing in intensity with increasing sexual excitement
   2. Abrupt explosive intensity just before or with orgasm
D. Lasting from 1 minute to 24 hours with severe intensity and/or up to 72 hours with mild intensity
E. Not fulfilling ICHD-3 criteria for any other headache disorder
F. Not better accounted for by another ICHD-3 diagnosis

Abbreviation: ICHD-3, International Classification of Headache Disorders, third edition.

---

impression. In Chen and colleagues'[3] study, additional secondary causes were lung adenocarcinoma to the cerebellum with accompanying hydrocephalus, acute sphenoid sinusitis, and alveolar sarcoma. Medulloblastoma has also been reported.[5]

It was previously thought that Chiari I malformation was the most common cause for secondary cough headaches, however, this assumption has been challenged by the number of patients with cough headache identified with SIH using advanced radiological imaging. These advances have led to better identification of specific causes of SIH including type 1 CSF leaks which consist of a dural tear, type 2 CSF leaks due to meningeal diverticula, and type 3 CSF leaks due to CSF-venous fistulas.[6] It is thought that the pathophysiology behind cough headache is explained by a sudden increase in intracranial pressure causing the cerebellar tonsils to descend into the foramen magnum causing a transient increase in pressure which can occur in both Chiari I malformation and SIH.[7,8]

In Atkinson and colleagues'[9] review of acquired Chiari I due to spontaneous spinal cerebrovascular fluid leakage and chronic intracranial hypotension syndrome, 2 out of 3 patients with acquired Chiari were described as having cough headache and for one of these, cough due to an upper respiratory infection incited the onset of the headaches and presumably also the leak. Chiari I malformation identification is defined by tonsillar descent as a defining feature and this is also present in SIH, but accompanied by whole-brain descent so that multiple areas of that descent can be identified on imaging through Bern imaging criteria.[10]

Chiari I malformation tends to also present with syrinx, which is not a common feature for the presence of SIH. As per IHS criteria, the identification of Chiari I malformation on MRI requires a 5-mm caudal descent of the cerebellar tonsils or 3-mm caudal descent of the cerebellar tonsils and crowding of the subarachnoid space and the craniocervical junction. Clues to Chiari I can be found in compression of CSF spaces posterior and lateral to the cerebellum, decreased height of the supraocciput, increased slope of the tentorium, or kinking of the medulla oblongata.[11] Initiation of headache with cough or Valsalva is one of the diagnostic criteria for Chiari I malformation presented in **Box 3**.

Other less commonly reported etiologies of secondary cough headache are meningitis associated with microfistula between sinuses and the brain resulting in pneumocephalus, or unruptured cerebral aneurysms which progress to involve other neurologic signs such as a third nerve palsy, carotid-cavernous fistula, and bilateral jugular venous valve incompetence.[12–15] Posterior reversible encephalopathy syndrome (PRES), another possible cause of secondary cough headaches, has been described in association with a thunderclap variant.[16] **Box 4** includes the IHS lists criteria for RCVS which can also present as cough headaches. A case of cough headache in the setting of SIH complicated by cerebral venous sinus thrombosis was reported by Ferrante and colleagues.[17,18] The causes of secondary cough headache types discussed in this article are listed in **Box 5**.

Diagnostic Evaluation of Cough Headaches

Distinguishing between primary and secondary headaches is challenging from the history and examination alone, and when confronted with this problem, a modified Valsalva maneuver has been described to differentiate. The examination involves having the patient breathe into a connecting tube of a standard aneroid sphygmomanometer to 60 mm Hg for 10 seconds. If the headache is provoked, testing is positive for secondary cough headache. This test has not been validated but is consistent with

---

Box 3
Headache attributed to Chiari malformation type 1

A. Headache fulfilling criterion C

B. Chiari malformation type 1 (CM1) has been demonstrated

C. Evidence of causation demonstrated by at least 2 of the following:
  1. Either or both of the following:
     a. Headache is developed in temporal relation to the CM1 or led to its discovery
     b. Headache has resolved within 3 months after successful treatment of the CM1
  2. Headache has 1 or more of the following 3 characteristics:
     a. Precipitated by cough or other Valsalva like maneuver
     b. Occipital or suboccipital location
     c. Lasting less than 5 minutes
  3. Headache is associated with other symptoms and/or clinical signs of brainstem, cerebellar, lower cranial nerve, and/or cervical spinal cord dysfunction

D. Not better accounted for by another ICHD-3 diagnosis

Abbreviation: ICHD-3, International Classification of Headache Disorders, third edition.

Box 4
Acute headache attributed to reversible vasoconstrictive syndrome

A. Any new headache fulfilling criterion C

B. RCVS has been diagnosed

C. Evidence of causation demonstrated by either or both of the following:
1. Headache, with or without focal deficits and/or seizures, has led to angiography (with "string of beads" appearance) and diagnosis of RCVS
2. Headache has one or more of the following characteristics:
   a. Thunderclap headache
   b. Triggered by sexual activity, exertion, Valsalva maneuvers, emotion, bathing, and/or showering
   c. Present or recurrent during ≤1 month after onset, with no new significant headache after greater than 1 month

D. Either of the following:
1. Headache has resolved within 3 months of onset
2. Headache has not yet resolved by 3 months from onset have not yet passed

E. Not better accounted for by another ICHD-3 diagnosis

Abbreviations: ICHD-3, International Classification of Headache Disorders, third edition; RCVS, reversible cerebral vasoconstrictive syndrome.

---

the theory of secondary cough headaches pathophysiology which has been described.[19]

Given the numerous possible secondary causes of cough headache, it is prudent to begin diagnostic evaluation with an MRI of the brain with and without contrast to rule out a posterior fossa lesion, subdural hematoma, Chiari I malformation, or signs of SIH. Even if signs of SIH are absent on initial MRI and there is suspicion for a CSF leak, nuclear medicine cisternogram is helpful to rule out a leak. CSF leak is a curable underlying etiology of cough headaches and it is important to determine whether it is present. If suspicion is very high, given a normal MRI, full spine noncontrast MRIs

---

Box 5
Causes of secondary cough headaches[4,11,14,16,58-60]

Arnold-Chiari malformation type I

Spontaneous intracranial hypotension

Carotid or vertebrobasilar diseases

Middle cranial fossa or posterior fossa tumors

Midbrain cyst

Basilar impression

Platybasia

Subdural hematoma

Cerebral aneurysm

Reversible cerebral vasoconstriction syndrome

Posterior reversible encephalopathy syndrome

Encephalitis

Carotid-cavernous fistula

should be obtained to evaluate for epidural fluid collections (denoting a fast leak) and if absent, lateral decubitus digital subtraction myelograms can be obtained with the patient lying on both sides looking for the source of a slow leak. If these studies are unrevealing, magnetic resonance angiography (MRA) of the intracranial vessels may be obtained to evaluate for unruptured cerebral aneurysms. Other studies are considered on a case-by-case basis and other supportive features which are present, for example, conjunctival chemosis, pulsating exophthalmos, or papilledema, would warrant investigation with magnetic resonance venography and MRA, potentially a cerebral angiogram if a carotid cavernous fistula is found. Valsalva maneuver jugular venous ultrasound is not routinely performed. Computerized tomography (CT) scanning is preferred if pneumocephalus is a concern.

When evaluating for congenital abnormalities of the craniovertebral junction such as basilar impression or platybasia, MRI can be used; however, bony elements are less prone to artifact with CT and a combination of 2 imaging techniques may be necessary. Depending on the patient's history of headache onset, dynamic X rays, CT, or MRI scanning may yield the underlying etiology.[20] Vasculature in the posterior fossa may also be involved in disorders of craniovertebral junction and CT angiography (CTA) or MRA may be considered for follow-up identification of these disorders.

Treatment of Secondary Cough Headaches

The treatment of Chiari I malformations is surgical foramen magnum decompression and may be performed in conjunction with duraplasty and/or cerebellar tonsil resection. If syrinx is present, duraplasty is favored. In a recent case series by Farag and Bahra,[21] it was found that in 2 patients diagnosed with Chiari I malformation, a cyclooxygenase-2 inhibitor (specifically etoricoxib) was an effective therapy for up to 3 years. There is 1 case report of Chari I malformation secondary cough, Valsalva, and sneeze headaches responding to propranolol and indomethacin.[22]

If SIH is determined to be the source of cough headaches, treatment may be surgical to repair the leak; however, an epidural blood patch may be utilized preliminarily. If a CSF-venous fistula is found, either surgical or interventional radiology–guided embolization are performed to permanently eliminate the leak. Surgical and neuro-oncologic evaluations are necessary when mass lesions are present in the posterior fossa. Depending on the size of a subdural hematoma, a middle meningeal artery embolization could be considered. Embolization of a carotid-cavernous fistula or clipping of a symptomatic cerebral aneurysm are often necessary. In cases of craniovertebral disorders such as basilar impression and platybasia, surgical referral may be required; however, these disorders can be secondary to connective tissue (osteogenesis imperfecta or Paget's disease) and rheumatologic disorders making surgical treatment potentially less successful.

Summary

Assessing for cough headache is recommended when taking a headache history as the list of causes of secondary cough headache is extensive. With improved imaging modalities, its differential is expanding.

CLINICS CARE POINTS

- Secondary cough headaches typically present in middle-aged males and may occur with any event which induces a Valsalva maneuver.

- Secondary cough headaches are associated with disruptions in CSF dynamics specifically in the posterior fossa, either structurally or as a consequence of vascular influences.
- Investigation into the etiology of cough headaches is fundamental as the causes can range from classically acute vascular etiologies (subdural hematoma and aneurysms) to chronic neoplastic causes (midbrain or posterior fossa lesions).

Clinical Manifestations of Exertional Headaches

In contrast to cough headaches, exertional or exercise headaches are provoked by sustained exercise rather than by brief episodes of Valsalva during, for example, weightlifting. Headaches tend to be throbbing in character, bilateral, and may cause physical activity to be avoided. Headaches tend to last an average of minutes to 48 hours.[23] Localization tends to be frontal, anterior, or temporal.[24] Character is usually described as throbbing and pulsatile. **Boxes 1** and **2** include the criteria for exertional headaches and probable exertional headaches. There is usually an association between migraines and exertional headaches. In the Sjaastad and Bakketeig[24] review of clinical manifestations of exertional headache, 93/202 (46%) patients had migraine and exertional headache overlap. Aggravation with routine activity is a criterion for migraine, so distinguishing between these 2 headache types is important for appropriate investigation into secondary causes. In migraine, there is usually nausea or vomiting, and the headache persists long after exercise has ceased. Unilaterality is also typically not seen in exertional headaches. Migraine type headaches may be induced by nitroglycerin.[11]

Etiology of Exertional Headaches

In Pascual and colleagues'[1] prospective study specifically evaluating secondary exertional headaches, 12 patients averaging 42 years of age with a female predominance had a secondary exertional headache out of a total of 28 patients with any exertional headache. Ten of the 12 were found to have subarachnoid hemorrhage. While one had breast cancer with intracerebral metastasis and another had pansinusitis. Supratentorial and posterior fossa tumors, intracranial and extracranial vascular malformations, third ventricular colloid cysts, and lateral ventricular tumors should also be considered in patients presenting with exertional headaches.[25,26] While not classic, a delayed exertional headache may be associated with SIH.[27] Exertional headache has been associated with a reversible coronary artery vasospasm.[28]

The pathophysiology of exertional headaches has been speculated to be due to increased intra-abdominal pressure which is relayed intracranially via the venous system with distension of pain-sensitive structures.[29] This is similar to the physiology that Williams and colleagues[8] proposed for Valsalva headache. Doepp and colleagues[30] hypothesized that internal jugular venous valve incompetence led to retrograde venous flow during exertion or Valsalva with transient increase of intracranial pressure and demonstrated venous valve incompetence using Doppler techniques in 70% of exertional headache patients and 20% of control patients, lending support to their hypothesis.

Cardiac cephalgia is described in the ICHD-3 and is a recognized presentation of headaches which are usually aggravated by exercise during myocardial ischemia. These are responsive to nitroglycerine. See **Box 6** for IHS criteria.[11] Lipton and colleagues[31] initially described this disorder in 1997, and the pain in these cases was bifrontal, sharp, squeezing, and pressurelike which increased with the duration of exercise. In 27% of cases described, cardiac cephalgia is the only reported event of cardiac ischemia.[32] Cardiac cephalagia is not necessarily exertional but has been noted

---

Box 6
Cardiac cephalgia—International Classification of Headache Disorders, third edition criteria

A. Any headache fulfilling criterion C

B. Acute myocardial ischemia has been demonstrated

C. Evidence of causation demonstrated by at least 2 of the following:
1. Headache has developed in temporal relation to the onset of acute myocardial ischemia
2. Headache has significantly improved or resolved in parallel with improvement or resolution of the myocardial ischemia

D. Headache has at least 2 of the following 4 characteristics:
a. Moderate to severe intensity
b. Accompanied by nausea
c. Not accompanied by photophobia or phonophobia
d. Aggravated by exertion

E. Headache is relieved by nitroglycerin or derivatives of it

F. Not better accounted for by another ICHD-3 diagnosis

Abbreviation: ICHD-3, International Classification of Headache Disorders, third edition.

---

to be in 53.1% of 32 cases in a pooled data analysis by Wei and colleagues.[33,34] Exertional headaches have been described in 1 case without any evidence of cardiac ischemia on cardiac stress testing but present on Sestamibi perfusion testing.[35,36] As previously mentioned, there is overlap between migraine and exertional headache, and exclusion of cardiac cephalgia is required before abortive therapies such as triptans or dihydroergotamine are considered.

Case reports have described other rare causes of exertional headaches including elongation of the styloid process, which usually presents as Eagle's syndrome (classically described as persistent throat pain and globus sensation post-tonsillectomy).[37] Pheochromocytoma has also been described as a secondary cause and presents with elevations in blood pressure and in 1 case report, it presented with pulmonary edema.[38]

Fusiform aneurysms in the vertebral arteries have rarely been associated with exertional headaches.[39] Exertional headache has been associated with varicella-zoster viral vasculopathy.[40] In 1 case report, bilateral transverse sinus stenosis was found to be associated with exertional headache.[41] Secondary causes of exertional or exercise headache are listed in **Box 7**.

Diagnostic Evaluation of Exertional Headaches

The evaluation of exertional headache should include an MRI of the brain with and without contrast and MRA to exclude any mass-occupying lesions or vascular abnormalities, such as aneurysms or RCVS. If a patient presents after 6 hours of initial onset, obtaining a lumbar puncture (LP) evaluating for xanthochromia would be justified. Investigations into SIH could also be considered depending on the overall clinical presentation and if any other headache types are present (orthostatic, cough, or Valsalva-associated). For completeness, in the setting of hypertension, 24-hour urine metanephrines can be obtained. LP is considered if fever or infectious symptoms and a subacute onset accompanied the headaches. Venous MRI can be used to identify venous sinus stenosis.

When suspicion for cardiac cephalgia is high, it is critical to begin with a cardiac stress test, but it may be necessary to obtain stress myocardial perfusion imaging

| Box 7 |
| Causes of secondary exercise/exertional headaches[25–28,37,38,40] |
| Subarachnoid hemorrhage |
| Arterial dissection |
| Reversible vasoconstriction syndrome |
| Cardiac ischemia |
| Intracerebral metastasis |
| Pansinusitis |
| Posterior fossa tumors |
| Third ventricular colloid cyst |
| Intracranial/extracranial vascular malformations |
| Pheochromocytoma |
| Varicella zoster vasculopathy |
| Elongated styloid process |

with Tc-99m sestamibi testing single-photon emission CT to assess for cardiac ischemia as stress testing has been reported less sensitive.[36] Coronary angiography is the gold standard for evaluation of cardiac ischemia.

Therapeutic Options for Secondary Exertional Headaches

The treatment for subarachnoid hemorrhage in the acute period is assessment and observation for the development of acute hydrocephalus and rebleed from the aneurysm. Admission to a neurologic intensive care unit for necessary shunting or treatment with hyperosmolar therapies while awaiting neurosurgery is indicated. For cardiac cephalgia, coronary stenting or bypass is indicated for elimination of the headache, but treatment with nitroglycerin or verapamil may alleviate symptoms in the interim. If RCVS is found to be the cause, permissive hypertension and removal of any provoking medications are most beneficial. Avoidance of selective serotonin reuptake inhibitors and triptans would also be warranted. Coronary vasospasm treated with nitroglycerin by intraarterial injection has shown benefit.[28] In the case of venous sinus stenosis, 1 report treated exertional headache successfully with venous stenting.

Summary

Exertional initiation rather than aggravation can be used to differentiate between true exertional headache and migraine. The sudden onset with no time of initial progression in thunderclap headache helps to distinguish it from exertional headache. Exertional headaches have several serious secondary underlying causes, including subarachnoid hemorrhage, RCVS, and cardiac cephalgia, which necessitate prompt investigation.

CLINICS CARE POINTS

- Secondary exertional headaches typically present in middle-aged females and may overlap with migraine headaches.

- Secondary exertional headaches are associated with a myriad of vascular causes, including aneurysmal bleeds, arterial vasospasm, and cardiac ischemia.
- In patients presenting with exertional headaches, findings can be most evident in the posterior fossa, as they occur in SIH, neoplasm, and colloid cyst of the third ventricle.

Clinical Manifestations of Sex Headaches

The IHS criteria for sex headache (also coital cephalgia, coital headache, orgasmic headache) require that it be induced by sexual activity. The criteria are listed in **Box 1**. In the original IHS criteria, headaches were categorized into 3 different types: type 1 which was usually dull, bilateral aching which increases with sexual excitement, type 2, an explosive headaches with onset during sexual activity,[42] and type 3 was a postural headache occurring after sex. This type is now attributed to SIH in the current ICHD-3 criteria but was previously included in this category prior to ICHD-2.[11] The mean age of onset is 39 years for sex headaches. There is male predominance for sex headache in the literature.[42]

In Frese and colleagues'[42] study of 51 patients, the median duration of pain was 4 hours but it ranged from minutes to 24 hours. It was predominantly occipital, male predominant, and had a bimodal peak age of onset (20–24 years and 35–40 years). Tension-type headache was the most common concurrent headache disorder among their sample. It also was reported to occur with masturbation, nocturnal emission, and dreaming during sleep. It was noted to occur in bouts with an average of 3 months between attacks.[43]

An orgasmic headache can have a thunderclap onset; it can be challenging to differentiate these 2 headache types. In contrast to primary sex headaches, secondary sex headaches caused of subarachnoid hemorrhage would be expected to be accompanied nausea, vomiting, loss of consciousness, and neck stiffness. Symptoms separating primary sex headache from headache in reversible cerebral vasoconstrictive syndrome (RCVS) or middle cerebral artery dissection would include fluctuant neurologic deficits such as visual blurring or cortical vision loss, less likely hemiparesis, aphasia, and seizures.[11,44,45] If the sex headache is recurrent, re-evaluation for thunderclap headaches should occur even though no initial cause is found, as recurrence is 90% sensitive and 99% specific for thunderclap headaches, and a criteria for the diagnosis of RCVS.[11,44]

In sex headaches, muscle contraction in the neck may be important given the tension in the posterior musculature associated with increased sexual excitement, and when coupled with neck extension during intercourse, it may be the inciting factor(s) in some sex headaches.

A possible variant of sex headache has been described in 2 individuals as masturbatory-orgasmic extracephalic pain. This pain was characterized as ice pick–like in both and both had associated spinal pathologies (in one, cervical spondylosis and in the other, tethered cord syndrome).[46]

Etiology of Sex Headaches

Of the 14 patients reported by Pascual and colleagues[2] in the 1996 study, only 1 had secondary sexual headache and this was a 60-year-old male diagnosed with subarachnoid hemorrhage. Yeh and colleagues[47] reviewed 20/30 patients with secondary causes for sex headaches and found that 18 had RCVS, 1 with basilar artery dissection, and another with subarachnoid hemorrhage. Basilar arterial dissection has been associated with sex headache by Delasobera and colleagues[48] as well. It has been estimate that 4% to 12% of sex headaches are due to subarachnoid hemorrhage.[49–51]

Longer duration (greater than 30 minutes to 4 hours) and an episodic course favor RCVS as over primary sex headache.[47] RCVS has been associated with headache during orgasm. Given that sequelae of RCVS include cortical subarachnoid hemorrhage, intracerebral hemorrhage, infarct, and posterior reversible encephalopathy syndrome (PRES), RCVS etiology should be considered if any of these sequelae are found. The criteria for RCVS are given in **Box 4**.

The pathophysiology for secondary sex headache, similarly to cough and exertional headaches, is proposed to be vascular in origin. In Evers and colleagues'[52] study, transcranial Doppler studies of patients with the explosive sex headache subtype showed a significant increase in the cerebral blood flow velocity and decrease in the pulsatility index (assesses resistance in a pulsatile vascular system). Additionally, they reported that systemic blood pressure was higher during physical exertion than other groups included in the study. This study only evaluated patients while using acetazolamide (simulating hypercapnia) and during exercise and so did not include hormonal changes which may contribute to the headaches.[52]

Non-neurologic disorders which may be considered in the evaluation of secondary sex headaches include glaucoma, sinusitis, Cushing's disease, myxedema, pheochromocytoma, and hypoglycemia.[53] Chronic obstructive pulmonary disease and acute anemia may also present in this way. Total occlusion of the abdominal aorta has previously been reported below the renal vessels and aortoiliac bypass produced recovery.[53] Birth control pills have also been described as being associated with sex headaches.[54] Secondary causes of headache associated with sexual activity are included in **Box 8**.

Diagnostic Evaluation of Sex Headaches

When presented with the highly variable association of sex headache with secondary causes, obtaining a noncontrast CT and a CT head angiogram allow for assessment for subarachnoid hemorrhage, infarct, intracerebral hemorrhage, or RCVS in the emergent setting. Hypodensities in the posterior white matter can be used to determine if further confirmatory imaging is needed for underlying etiology such as PRES.

Box 8
Common causes of secondary headache associated with sexual activity[2,47,48,53,61]

Subarachnoid hemorrhage

Intracranial and extracranial arterial dissection

Reversible cerebral vasoconstrictive syndrome (multiple explosive headaches during sexual activity)

Pheochromocytoma

Glaucoma

Sinusitis

Cushing's disease

Myxedema

Hypoglycemia

Chronic obstructive pulmonary disease

Acute anemia

Total occlusion of abdominal aorta

Pineal cyst

If these hypodensities are revealed, a noncontrast MRI of the brain can be obtained, but addition of contrast can also visualize any neurologic etiologies such as mass lesions or enhancement of an infectious process which may contribute to headache presentation. However, in RCVS, consider that imaging may be abnormal in 30% to 80% of cases with PRES.[11] MRI in this etiology may show T2 or T2 fluid-attenuated inversion recovery sequence hyperintensities of the subcortical and cortical regions of the occipito-parietal lobes as well as the cerebellum, brainstem, or frontal regions in more severe presentations (consistent with vasogenic edema).[55]

If imaging is normal, and there continues to be a relapsing course, consider if the CTA or MRA imaging was performed in the first week of symptom onset, as imaging may be normal within this timeline.[56] Angiography will show "string and beads" appearance of focal segmental narrowing of the cerebral arteries. Repeating the imaging at a later date is an option versus considering a formal conventional angiogram for a definitive evaluation.

In order to classify sexual headaches as primary or secondary, Lin and colleagues[57] proposed a composite algorithm of categorizing and diagnosing sexual headaches occurring greater than or equal to 2 times into 4 different groups: primary sexual headache, RCVS, probable RCVS, and other secondary causes. The differentiating diagnostic testing would be an MRI of the brain with and without contrast, MR angiogram, and MR venogram, and if positive for pathologic findings, it would support other causes. If showing vasoconstriction, its reversibility would support RCVS versus another cause. If not showing vasoconstriction, then a strict sexual trigger would determine primary sexual headache, instead of probable RCVS (and CSF studies would be utilized to help determine the cause).[57]

Therapeutic Options for Secondary Sex Headaches

Patients may elect to take a more passive role during intercourse or transient stopping of intercourse. In the case of secondary sex headaches attributed to subarachnoid hemorrhage, acute and neurosurgical management as listed previously in the exertional headache section would apply. When the etiology is RCVS, supportive care is indicated along with permissive hypertension. Calcium channel blockers such as nimodipine or verapamil can be employed for both pain and the management of vasoconstriction. Elimination of any precipitating or aggravating medications such as serotonergic antidepressants, amphetamines, marijuana, triptans, or any other vasoconstrictive medications is indicated. Patients may continue to have headaches of chronic migrainous phenotype even after RCVS is treated.[56]

For intracranial or extracranial dissections, treatment with aspirin and clopidogrel is indicated; however, precise management would be dictated on a case-by-case basis.

If the underlying cause is hydrocephalus, evaluation by neurosurgery for consideration of a shunt is necessary.

Summary

Sex headaches have a variety of phenotypes ranging from gradual onset to thunderclap. In some, the headache can be delayed and be associated with SIH. It is challenging to distinguish primary sex headache from secondary caused by RCVS, as they both require recurrence, occurring with continued sexual activity. Sequelae of RCVS include ischemic infarcts or PRES. Urgent evaluation for these etiologies and management should be executed. Other secondary etiologies may include intracranial and extracranial arterial dissections, non-communicating hydrocephalus, or subarachnoid hemorrhage.

CLINICS CARE POINTS

- Secondary sex headaches are most often present in males, in a bimodal age distribution of early 20s and early middle age.
- Sex headaches can mimic recurrent thunderclap headache and several of the etiologies of thunderclap are in the differential for secondary sex headache.
- Evaluation for RCVS should be performed as patients may be on serotonergic medications for concurrent migraines.

DISCLOSURE

Dr M. Montenegro and Dr F.M. Cutrer have no financial conflicts of interest pertaining the content of the article.

REFERENCES

1. Pascual J, González-Mandly A, Martín R, et al. Headaches precipitated by cough, prolonged exercise or sexual activity: a prospective etiological and clinical study. J Headache Pain 2008;9(5):259–66.
2. Pascual J, Iglesias F, Oterino A, et al. Cough, exertional, and sexual headaches: an analysis of 72 benign and symptomatic cases. Neurology 1996;46(6):1520–4.
3. Chen P, Fuh J, Wang S. Cough headache: a study of 83 consecutive patients. Cephalalgia 2009;29(10):1079–85.
4. Symonds C. Cough headache. Brain 1956;79(4):557–68.
5. Eross EJ, Swanson JW. A Rare Cause of Cough Headache in an Adult. Headache J Head Face Pain 2002;42(5):382.
6. Schievink WI, Maya MM, Jean-Pierre S, et al. A classification system of spontaneous spinal CSF leaks. Neurology 2016;87(7):673–9.
7. Calandre L, Hernandez-Lain A, Lopez-Valdes E. Benign Valsalva's Maneuver-Related Headache: An MRI Study of Six Cases. Headache J Head Face Pain 1996;36(4):251–3.
8. Williams B. Cough Headache due to Craniospinal Pressure Dissociation. Arch Neurol 1980;37(4):226–30.
9. Atkinson JL, Weinshenker BG, Miller GM, et al. Acquired Chiari I malformation secondary to spontaneous spinal cerebrospinal fluid leakage and chronic intracranial hypotension syndrome in seven cases. J Neurosurg 1998;88(2):237–42.
10. Dobrocky T, Grunder L, Breiding PS, et al. Assessing Spinal Cerebrospinal Fluid Leaks in Spontaneous Intracranial Hypotension With a Scoring System Based on Brain Magnetic Resonance Imaging Findings. JAMA Neurol 2019;76(5):580–7.
11. Headache Classification Committee of the International Headache Society (IHS) The International Classification of Headache Disorders, 3rd edition. Cephalalgia 2018;38(1):1-211. doi:10.1177/0333102417738202.
12. Jacome DE, Stamm MA. Malignant cough headache. Headache 2004;44(3):259–61.
13. Smith WS, Messing RO. Cerebral Aneurysm Presenting as Cough Headache. Headache 1993;33(4):203–4.
14. Simić S, Radmilo L, Villar JR, et al. Hemicranial Cough-Induced Headache as a First Symptom of a Carotid-Cavernous Fistula-Case Report. Medicina 2020;56(4):194.

15. Liu H, Cao X, Zhang M, et al. A case report of cough headache with transient elevation of intracranial pressure and bilateral internal jugular vein valve incompetence: A primary or secondary headache? Cephalalgia 2018;38(3):600–3.

16. Maramattom BV. Cough headache as a presenting feature of posterior reversible encephalopathy syndrome (PRES). Clin Med 2021;21(2):e237.

17. Ferrante T, Latte L, Abrignani G, et al. Cough headache secondary to spontaneous intracranial hypotension complicated by cerebral venous thrombosis. Neurol Sci 2012;33(2):429–33.

18. Kato Y, Hayashi T, Sano H, et al. Cough headache presenting with reversible cerebral vasoconstriction syndrome. Internal Medicine 2018;57(10):1459–61.

19. Lane RJM, Davies PTG. Modified Valsalva test differentiates primary from secondary cough headache. J Headache Pain 2013;14(1):31.

20. Pinter NK, McVige J, Mechtler L. Basilar Invagination, Basilar Impression, and Platybasia: Clinical and Imaging Aspects. Curr Pain Headache Rep 2016; 20(8):49.

21. Farag M, Bahra A. Secondary cough headache: Independent course of headache and response to a COX-2 inhibitor. Clin Neurol Neurosurg 2023;227:107646.

22. Buzzi MG, Formisano R, Colonnese C, et al. Chiari-Associated Exertional, Cough, and Sneeze Headache Responsive to Medical Therapy. Headache J Head Face Pain 2003;43(4):404–6.

23. Cutrer FM, DeLange J. Cough, exercise, and sex headaches. Neurol Clin 2014; 32(2):433–50.

24. Sjaastad O, Bakketeig L. Exertional Headache – II. Clinical Features Vaga Study of Headache Epidemiology. Cephalalgia 2003;23(8):803–7.

25. Cutrer FM, Boes CJ. Cough, exertional, and sex headaches. Neurol Clin 2004; 22(1):133–49.

26. Kang K, Kim JH, Kim B-K. Exercise Headache Associated With an Arteriovenous Fistula of the External Carotid Artery. J Clin Neurol 2022;18(1):93.

27. Garcia-Albea E, Cabrera F, Tejeiro J, et al. Delayed postexertional headache, intracranial hypotension and racket sports. J Neurol Neurosurg Psychiatry 1992;55(10):975.

28. Yang Y, Jeong D, Jin DG, et al. A case of cardiac cephalalgia showing reversible coronary vasospasm on coronary angiogram. J Clin Neurol 2010;6(2):99–101.

29. Tinel J. La céphalée a l'effort. Syndrome de distension douloureuse des veines intracraniennes. Medicine (Paris) 1932;13:113–8.

30. Doepp F, Valdueza JM, Schreiber SJ. Incompetence of internal jugular valve in patients with primary exertional headache: a risk factor? Cephalalgia 2008; 28(2):182–5.

31. Lipton RB, Lowenkopf T, Bajwa ZH, et al. Cardiac cephalgia: A treatable form of exertional headache. Neurology 1997;49(3):813–6.

32. Bini A, Evangelista A, Castellini P, et al. Cardiac cephalgia. J Headache Pain 2009;10(1):3–9.

33. Gutiérrez-Morlote J, Pascual J. Cardiac cephalgia is not necessarily an exertional headache: case report. Cephalalgia 2002;22(9):765–6.

34. Wei J, Wang H. Cardiac cephalalgia: case reports and review. Cephalalgia 2008; 28(8):892–6.

35. Sathirapanya P. Anginal Cephalgia: A Serious Form of Exertional Headache. Cephalalgia 2004;24(3):231–4.

36. Cutrer FM, Huerter K. Exertional headache and coronary ischemia despite normal electrocardiographic stress testing. Headache 2006;46(1):165–7.

37. Maggioni F, Marchese-Ragona R, Mampreso E, et al. Exertional Headache as Unusual Presentation of the Syndrome of an Elongated Styloid Process. Headache 2009;49(5):776–9.
38. Paulson GW, Zipf RE Jr, Beekman JF. Pheochromocytoma causing exercise-related headache and pulmonary edema. Ann Neurol 1979;5(1):96–9.
39. Mauri G, Vega P, Murias E, et al. Fusiform aneurysms of the vertebral artery: A hidden cause of exertional headache? Cephalalgia 2012;32(9):715–8.
40. Chen W-H, Peng C-H, Lui C-C, et al. Varicella-zoster virus and exertional headache: Evidence of viral vasculopathy in Valsalva maneuver-related headache syndrome. Neurol Asia 2011;16(4).
41. Donnet A, Dufour H, Levrier O, et al. Exertional Headache: A New Venous Disease. Cephalalgia 2008;28(11):1201–3.
42. Frese A, Eikermann A, Frese K, et al. Headache associated with sexual activity: demography, clinical features, and comorbidity. Neurology 2003;61(6):796–800.
43. Frese A, Rahmann A, Gregor N, et al. Headache Associated With Sexual Activity: Prognosis and Treatment Options. Cephalalgia 2007;27(11):1265–70.
44. Rocha EA, Topcuoglu MA, Silva GS, et al. RCVS2 score and diagnostic approach for reversible cerebral vasoconstriction syndrome. Neurology 2019;92(7): e639–47.
45. Szatmary Z, Boukobza M, Vahedi K, et al. Orgasmic headache and middle cerebral artery dissection. J Neurol Neurosurg Psychiatr 2006;77(5):693–4.
46. Jacome DE. Masturbatory-Orgasmic Extracephalic Pain. Headache J Head Face Pain 1998;38(2):138–41.
47. Yeh Y-C, Fuh J-L, Chen S-P, et al. Clinical features, imaging findings and outcomes of headache associated with sexual activity. Cephalalgia 2010;30(11): 1329–35.
48. Delasobera BE, Osborn SR, Davis JE. Thunderclap Headache with Orgasm: A Case of Basilar Artery Dissection Associated with Sexual Intercourse. The Journal of Emergency Medicine 2012;43(1):e43–7.
49. Turner IM, Harding TM. Headache and sexual activity: a review. Headache 2008; 48(8):1254–6.
50. Lundberg P, Osterman P. The Benign and Malignant Forms of Orgasmic Cephalgia. Headache J Head Face Pain 1974;14(3):164–5.
51. Locksley HB. Natural history of subarachnoid hemorrhage, intracranial aneurysms and arteriovenous malformations: based on 6368 cases in the cooperative study. J Neurosurg 1966;25(3):321–4.
52. Evers S, Schmidt O, Frese A, et al. The cerebral hemodynamics of headache associated with sexual activity. Pain 2003/03/01/2003;102(1):73–8. https://doi.org/10.1016/s0304-3959(02)00341-x.
53. Sands GH, Newman L, Lipton R. Cough, exertional, and other miscellaneous headaches. Med Clin 1991;75(3):733–47.
54. Paulson GW, Klawans HL Jr. Benign Orgasmic Cephalalgia. Headache J Head Face Pain 1974;13(4):181–7.
55. Gao B, Lyu C, Lerner A, et al. Controversy of posterior reversible encephalopathy syndrome: what have we learnt in the last 20 years? J Neurol Neurosurg Psychiatr 2018;89(1):14–20.
56. Singhal AB, Hajj-Ali RA, Topcuoglu MA, et al. Reversible cerebral vasoconstriction syndromes: analysis of 139 cases. Arch Neurol 2011;68(8):1005–12.
57. Lin PT, Wang YF, Fuh JL, et al. Diagnosis and classification of headache associated with sexual activity using a composite algorithm: A cohort study. Cephalalgia 2021;41(14):1447–57.

58. Cough KE. Headache. vol 4. Headache Handbook of clinical neurology. London, UK: Elsevier Science Publishers; 1986.
59. Eross EJ, Swanson JW, Krauss WE, et al. A rare cause of cough headache in an adult. Headache 2002;42(5):382.
60. Mokri B. Spontaneous CSF leaks mimicking benign exertional headaches. Cephalalgia 2002;22(10):780–3.
61. Barranco R, Lo Pinto S, Cuccì M, et al. Sudden and Unexpected Death During Sexual Activity, Due to a Glial Cyst of the Pineal Gland. Am J Forensic Med Pathol 2018;39(2):157–60.

Other Secondary Headaches

Odontogenic Pain and Other Painful Orofacial Conditions

Emma V. Beecroft, BDS, MFDS RCS (Ed & Eng), PG Dip Con Sed[a,b,1,*],
David Edwards, MRes, MSc, MFDTEd, MFDS RCS(Ed), PGDip Con Sed, PGDip Rest Dent RCS(Eng), PGCert MEd Ed, FHEA[a,b,1],
James R. Allison, MFDS RCSEng/ RCPS (Glasg), MDTFEd, FHEA[a,b,1]

KEYWORDS

- Orofacial pain • Odontogenic pain • Persistent idiopathic dentoalveolar pain disorder
- Posttraumatic trigeminal neuropathic pain • Persistent idiopathic facial pain
- Burning mouth syndrome

KEY POINTS

- ICHD-3 does not cover all orofacial pain conditions that may present in the neurology setting.
- The use of ICOP in addition to ICHD-3 will support clinicians in separating orofacial pain conditions from headache conditions.
- Thorough investigation of patients with headache should include examination of the oral cavity.
- Clinicians should be familiar with common oral pathologic conditions that may cause headache presentations and consider referral to oral or dental specialists where appropriate.

INTRODUCTION

Differentiation between headache disorders and orofacial pain conditions can be notoriously difficult. The orofacial region, which consists of the oral cavity and face, represents a significant anatomic region of the head and neck. Wide cranial referral patterns are often displayed for orofacial pain conditions, and the converse is also true, with headache conditions presenting in the orofacial region, at times exclusively.[1] The overlap between orofacial pain and headache conditions has been long been appreciated, with orofacial pain conditions represented in the International Classification of Headache Disorders (ICHD)

[a] School of Dental Sciences, Faculty of Medical Sciences, Newcastle University, Newcastle Upon Tyne, United Kingdom; [b] Newcastle Upon Tyne Hospitals NHS Foundation Trust, Newcastle Upon Tyne, United Kingdom
[1] Equal contribution.
* Corresponding author. School of Dental Sciences, Faculty of Medical Sciences, Newcastle University, Framlington Place, Newcastle upon Tyne, NE2 4BW, United Kingdom.
E-mail address: emma.beecroft@newcastle.ac.uk

Neurol Clin 42 (2024) 615–632
https://doi.org/10.1016/j.ncl.2023.12.013
0733-8619/24/© 2024 Elsevier Inc. All rights reserved.

since its inception in 1988.[2] In subsequent iterations (ICHD-2 in 2004[3] and ICHD-3 in 2018[4]), the classification of these orofacial conditions was developed, reflecting their status as distinct disease entities. Importantly, ICHD-3 was developed to classify and provide explicit diagnostic criteria for *headache* disorders, and as such, classification of orofacial pain conditions within ICHD-3 is not exhaustive.

A comprehensive classification of orofacial pain conditions is available in the International Headache Society's International Classification of Orofacial Pain (ICOP), published in 2020.[1] ICOP was developed to avoid "misdiagnosis and a resultant misdirection of treatment".[1] ICOP groups orofacial pain conditions into broad diagnostic categories, with further specific subtype or subform classifications in the same manner as ICHD-3.[1]

As a comprehensive classification system, ICOP denotes both common and rare disease entities, all of which may occasionally present in the neurology setting. A detailed knowledge of ICOP is not necessary; however, an awareness of the classification and familiarity with its main diagnoses will allow clinicians to identify orofacial pain conditions and differentiate these from headache conditions. **Box 1** gives a high-level overview of classifications within ICOP. This article will focus on the odontogenic pain and other orofacial pain conditions outlined in ICOP. We will outline common presenting features and discuss clinical identification with a view to supporting diagnostic clarity within the neurology setting.

ODONTOGENIC PAIN

Odontogenic pain may broadly be classified as pain from the dental pulp (neurovascular bundle within the tooth) or pain from the supporting structures: periodontium,

---

Box 1
Broad groupings of orofacial pain conditions included in ICOP 2020[1]

1. Orofacial pain attributed to disorders of dentoalveolar and anatomically related structures
   1.1. **Dental/odontogenic pain**
   1.2. Oral mucosal, salivary gland and jaw bone pains

2. Myofascial orofacial pain

3. Temporomandibular joint (TMJ) pain

4. Orofacial pain attributed to lesion or disease of the cranial nerves
   4.1. Pain attributed to lesion or disease of the trigeminal nerve
       4.1.1. Trigeminal neuralgia
       4.1.2. Other trigeminal neuropathic pain
           4.1.2.3. **Posttraumatic trigeminal neuropathic pain**
   4.2. Pain attributed to lesion or disease of the glossopharyngeal nerve

5. Orofacial pains resembling presentations of primary headaches Introduction
   5.1. Orofacial migraine
   5.2. Tension-type orofacial pain
   5.3. Trigeminal autonomic orofacial pain
   5.4. Neurovascular orofacial pain

6. Idiopathic orofacial pain
   6.1. **Burning mouth syndrome (BMS)**
   6.2. **Persistent idiopathic facial pain (PIFP)**
   6.3. **Persistent idiopathic dentoalveolar pain (PIDP)**
   6.4 Constant unilateral facial pain with additional attacks (CUFPA)

Conditions underlined and in bold text are discussed in detail in this article.

alveolar bone, and gingiva. Odontogenic pain is common, affecting 9% to 12% of adults in western populations.[5,6] Symptomatic irreversible pulpitis is reported as the most common and impactful odontogenic pain condition.[7]

Presentation

Symptomatic irreversible pulpitis

Symptomatic irreversible pulpitis originates from inflammation of the dental pulp, resulting in spontaneous pain, or pain that lasts for more than 30 seconds following stimulation, usually with a thermal stimulus, such as a hot or cold drink. Although thermal allodynia is common, mechanical allodynia is less common.[8] Patients often report having used pain-relieving medications, which may or may not partially alleviate their pain, and reports of disturbed sleep and inability to work or perform usual daily activity are common.[7] The pain is usually difficult to localize, with radiation to all 3 divisions of the trigeminal nerve possible, meaning the patient often will not know if the pain is from an upper or lower tooth.

As symptomatic irreversible pulpitis progresses, the inflammatory response affects the surrounding structures including the periapical tissues and alveolar bone, resulting in *symptomatic apical periodontitis*. In addition to symptoms of irreversible pulpitis, mechanical allodynia, presenting as well-localized pain on biting on the affected tooth, now becomes a predominant feature, meaning the patient can now more easily localize the cause.

Other odontogenic causes

If symptomatic irreversible pulpitis is not treated, pulp necrosis will soon follow. Pulp necrosis is not usually painful and so individuals may report a transient, pain-free period. Eventually, the patient may develop an *acute apical abscess.* Although this may be confused with pulpitis, symptoms are quite different (**Table 1**).[8] Pain is usually spontaneous but it is well localized by the patient to a single tooth, and there is no thermal allodynia as the pulp is necrosed. Mechanical allodynia is expected, described as pain on biting, and the tooth may even feel elevated in the socket. Radiation of the pain is sometimes seen, and there is often intraoral or extraoral swelling.

Periodontal (gum) diseases such as *gingivitis* (limited to the gingival tissues) and *periodontitis* (affecting the periodontal ligament and alveolar bone) are very common, affecting more than 3 in 5 adults globally.[9] Periodontitis is usually asymptomatic until advanced, with the most common complaint being loose or mobile teeth. Patients with advanced periodontitis are at risk of developing a *periodontal abscess*, which may present similarly to an acute apical abscess[10]; however, the affected tooth is likely to be mobile and the abscess often presents as a "gum boil" due to the intraoral collection and drainage of pus immediately beside the tooth.

Pathogenesis

Symptomatic irreversible pulpitis

Symptomatic irreversible pulpitis usually results from dental caries (**Fig. 1**). As bacteria penetrate the pulp space, there is a marked inflammatory response, which inevitably overwhelms the defensive capabilities of the pulp, and progressive necrosis ensues. In the initial stages, Aδ nerve fibers, which are located in a plexus around the periphery of the pulp, become stimulated; this typically causes pain, which is sharp in character. As the inflammation progresses, C fibers, which are located more deeply within the pulp, become activated producing pain with a more dull, aching, or throbbing character.

Table 1
Summary of common painful odontogenic conditions

Diagnosis	Type of Pain	Pain Severity	Radiation	Precipitating Factors	Use of Medication	Localization	Disturbed Sleep	Swelling
Symptomatic reversible pulpitis	Sharp, stabbing pain, which occurs on stimulation	Mild–moderate	Not normally	Cold ++ Heat + Lasts <30 s	Not usually taken	Difficult to localize	Rarely	No
Symptomatic irreversible pulpitis	Dull, throbbing, spontaneous, pain worsened by stimulation	Severe	Frequent	Cold[a] + Heat ++ Lasts >30 s	Usually taken and often little benefit	Difficult to localize	Usually	No
Acute apical abscess	Dull, throbbing, spontaneous, pain worsened by stimulation	Moderate– severe	Sometimes	Biting on tooth No pain with hot/cold	Usually taken and offers some benefit	Well localized	Usually	Yes, intraoral or extraoral. May have associated trismus
Periodontal abscess	Dull, throbbing, spontaneous, pain worsened by stimulation	Moderate	Unusual	Biting on tooth Tooth will be mobile	Sometimes taken and offers some benefit	Well localized	Sometimes	Yes, intraoral

[a] In later stages, cold may relieve the pain of symptomatic irreversible pulpitis.

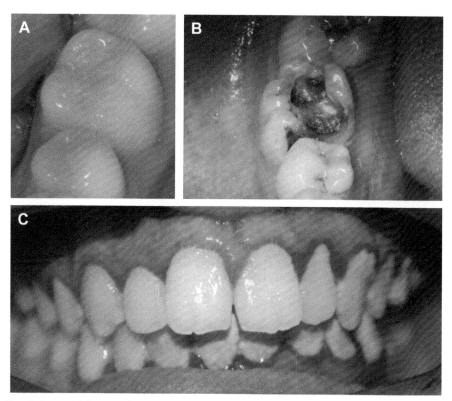

Fig. 1. Intraoral images showing oral health and disease. (*A*) Healthy lower left premolar and molar tooth with healthy supporting tissues; note the integrity of the crowns of the teeth, and the uniform color and texture of gingivae (gums), absence of dental plaque or inflammation. (*B*) Carious (decayed) lower right first molar tooth. (*C*) Gingivitis, visible as clearly demarcated erythema and inflammation at the gingival margins, related to substantial dental plaque deposits.

The marked inflammatory response to bacterial invasion may lead to peripheral sensitization, including nerve sprouting and a reduction in action threshold potential at the level of the tooth, as well as neuroinflammation mediated by satellite cell activation in the trigeminal ganglion.[11–13] Similar mechanisms are seen in the brainstem through the activation of microglia, contributing to central sensitization.[14,15] These changes help to explain the widening of the field of perceived pain experienced by patients, as well as mechanical and thermal allodynia.

Other odontogenic causes
As already outlined, the dental pulp usually becomes necrotic due to dental caries, following the progression of symptomatic irreversible pulpitis. Occasionally however, trauma to the teeth may be the cause of necrosis, which may progress painlessly until acute apical periodontitis occurs; it is always worth asking a patient if they have ever suffered trauma. Nonetheless, a nonvital pulp is an ideal substrate for bacterial colonization, and this ultimately progresses to involve the periapical tissues, culminating in an *acute apical abscess* consisting of opportunistic oral pathogens.[16] In contrast, a *periodontal abscess* is usually seen in patients with significant alveolar bone loss and typically consists of common periodontal pathogens.[17]

Diagnostic Clues

The accurate diagnosis of odontogenic pain is critical, first to differentiate from headache conditions and second to ensure appropriate management, which invariably involves an operative dental intervention. The presenting symptoms described above are usually helpful diagnostically but pain often does not always fit neatly into diagnostic criteria. **Table 1** summarizes the most likely signs and symptoms seen in common odontogenic conditions. Crucially, pain of infective origin (acute apical abscess) is usually well localized, often has associated swelling, and is not made worse by thermal stimuli. In contrast, pain from a mainly inflammatory condition (symptomatic irreversible pulpitis) is usually precipitated by thermal stimuli, is poorly localized, and is rarely associated with swelling.

Further Investigations

In the nondental setting, further investigations may be limited. An extensive history, as outlined in **Table 1** and is usually sufficient to arrive at a reasonable provisional diagnosis. In addition, extraoral examination may identify swelling or trismus, indicative of *acute apical abscess*. Intraoral examination may identify teeth with obvious lost restorations or dental caries (cavities/holes), as demonstrated in **Fig. 1**, which could have led either to *symptomatic irreversible pulpitis* or *pulp necrosis*, and subsequently an *acute apical abscess*. Additionally, *periodontitis*, indicated by visible plaque, gingival inflammation (see **Fig. 1**), gingival recession, and mobile teeth may be apparent on intraoral examination. It may be possible to see swelling in the gingiva adjacent to the painful tooth, suggestive of either a *periodontal abscess* or *acute apical abscess*. If teeth are pressed or percussed, they will be painful in the case of an *acute apical abscess*, and possibly in the presence of a *periodontal abscess*.

Panoramic radiography, such as an orthopantomograph, may help assess the dentition and associated structures (**Fig. 2**). Should radiographic signs indicative of dental disease be identified, referral to an appropriate dental team for management

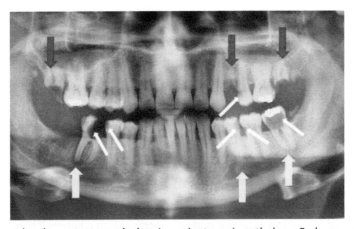

Fig. 2. Dental orthopantomograph showing odontogenic pathology. Red arrows indicate retained tooth roots with loss of coronal tooth tissue. White arrows represent radiolucencies in the crowns of the teeth consistent with dental caries (decay). Yellow arrows show periapical radiolucencies representing widening of the periodontal ligament space or alveolar bone loss often seen in the transition from symptomatic irreversible pulpitis to acute apical abscess.

would be warranted. In the dental setting, electrical and thermal testing of the tooth will distinguish between vital tooth and nonvital teeth.

Advanced *acute apical abscess* may give rise to systemic signs and symptoms such as fever, pyrexia, tachycardia, and tachypnoea. It is also important to check patients' mouth opening (trismus) and swallowing (dysphagia), as well as cellulitis spreading toward the eye or cervical lymphadenopathy, which may suggest progressing infection. Odontogenic infection can cause significant morbidity and mortality if untreated due to sepsis and airway compromise.

Management

Symptomatic irreversible pulpitis

The severity of pain in symptomatic irreversible pulpitis often has a severe impact on patients' quality of life; swift management is therefore essential.[7] Simple analgesia such as non steroidal anti-inflammatiry drugs (NSAIDs) and paracetamol/acetaminophen may offer mild relief, although opioid analgesics are usually of little additional benefit. Systemic antibiotics have no effect in this inflammatory condition[18] and removal of the inflamed pulp through tooth extraction or the initiation of root canal therapy (pulpectomy) is required. Patients presenting to the nondental settings with dental or periodontal pathology on clinical examination should be advised to consult a dental practitioner for the management of their odontogenic condition as a priority.

Other odontogenic causes

An *acute apical abscess* has the potential to develop into a medical emergency, especially where swelling is affecting swallowing or spreads toward the eye. Unlike *symptomatic irreversible pulpitis*, systemic antibiotics are effective for an *acute apical abscess* but should only be used as an adjunct where removal of the cause and surgical drainage of infection cannot be fully or immediately achieved, or where there is systemic involvement. Drainage is achieved through incision of an accessible abscess, tooth extraction, or accessing the pulp space and using endodontic instruments to reach beyond the tooth apex. Should such cases present to the nondental setting, urgent (same day) referral to an appropriate service should be made to ensure the severe odontogenic infection is managed promptly.

PERSISTENT IDIOPATHIC DENTOALVEOLAR PAIN DISORDER

Historic alternative terminology: atypical odontalgia; primary persistent dentoalveolar pain disorder; and phantom tooth pain.

Persistent idiopathic dentoalveolar pain disorder (PIDP) is persistent ($\geq$3 month) unilateral pain in a defined area of the dentoalveolar region in absence of any other demonstrable pathologic condition.[1] Detailed ICOP criteria for PIDP are shown in **Table 2**.

Presentation

Pain symptoms reported by patients are variable, and individuals typically find PIDP difficult to describe. Most commonly, pain is reported as a dull, nagging, pulling, ache.[1,19,20] Other descriptors include pressure, itching, or burning, with pain intensity often reported to be worse during times of stress.[19,20] The pain tends to be poorly localized and may present similarly to odontogenic pain, meaning diagnosis can be confused with symptomatic irreversible pulpitis.[19] Intermittent sharp exacerbations described as electric or stabbing in nature, and sensory symptoms such as tingling and paraesthesia can also present in PIDP leading to other common misdiagnoses such as trigeminal neuralgia, migraine, and facial headache variants.[19]

Table 2
ICOP diagnostic classification for nonodontogenic orofacial pain conditions included in this article[1]

Diagnosis	Diagnostic Criteria

PIDP *(Termed Probable PIDP if all diagnostic but present for <3 mo)*	A. Intraoral dentoalveolar pain fulfilling criteria B and C
	B. Recurring daily for >2 h/d for >3 mo
	C. Pain has both of the following characteristics
	  i. Localized to a dentoalveolar site (tooth or alveolar bone)
	  ii. Deep, dull, pressure-like quality
	D. Clinical and radiographic examinations are normal, and local causes have been excluded
	Somatosensory changes may be present *(PIDP with somatosensory change)* or not present *(PIDP without somatosensory change)* on qualitative or quantitative somatosensory testing

PTTN *(Termed Probable PTTN if all diagnostic criteria except confirmatory diagnostic tests not completed)*	A. Pain within the distribution(s) of one or both trigeminal nerve(s), persisting or recurring for > 3 mo and fulfilling criteria C and D
	B. Both of the following:
	  i. History of a mechanical, thermal, radiation, or chemical injury to the peripheral trigeminal nerve(s)
	  ii. Diagnostic test(s) confirm a lesion of the peripheral trigeminal nerve(s) explaining the pain.
	C. Onset within 6 mo of injury
	D. Associated somatosensory symptoms and/or signs in the same neuroanatomical distribution

PIFP *(Termed Probable PIFP if all diagnostic criteria but present for < 3 mo)*	A. Pain has both of the following characteristics:
	  i. Poorly localized, and not following the distribution of a peripheral nerve
	  ii. Dull, aching, or nagging quality
	B. Clinical and radiographic examinations are normal, and local causes have been excluded.
	Somatosensory changes may be present *(PIFP with somatosensory change)* or not present *(PIFP without somatosensory change)* on qualitative or quantitative somatosensory testing

BMS *(Termed Probable burning mouth syndrome if all diagnostic criteria but present for <3 mo)*	A. Oral pain fulfilling criteria B and C
	B. Recurring daily for >2 h/d for >3 mo
	C. Pain has both of the following characteristics:
	  i. Burning quality
	  ii. Felt superficially in the oral mucosa

(continued on next page)

Table 2 (continued)	
Diagnosis	**Diagnostic Criteria**
	D. Oral mucosa is of normal appearance, and local or systemic causes have been excluded
	Somatosensory changes may be present (*BMS with somatosensory change*) or not present (*BMS without somatosensory change*) on qualitative or quantitative somatosensory testing

Prevalence ranging from 0.3% to 2.1% is reported,[20–22] and women are more commonly affected than men, with increased incidence in middle-aged and older cohorts.[19,20] Presentation is more common in anterior, rather than posterior regions, with the maxilla being marginally more affected than the mandible.[20,23]

Pathogenesis

Diagnostic difficulty and late presentation following protracted patient journeys hamper understanding of the pathogenesis and etiology of PIDP.[20] Exact mechanisms have not yet been confirmed, however, it is likely that hyperalgesia and persistence are a result of peripheral and central sensitization of trigeminal nociceptive pathways alongside ectopic spontaneous activity of afferent neurons, with impaired function of the descending inhibitory pain pathway perpetuating the pain.[20,23,24] Poor localization, referral, and allodynia are likely to be a result of peripheral nerve sprouting at central nerve terminals.[20]

POSTTRAUMATIC TRIGEMINAL NEUROPATHIC PAIN

Historic alternative terminology: atypical odontalgia; phantom tooth pain deafferentation pain; and traumatic neuropathy.

Posttraumatic trigeminal neuropathic pain (PTTN) and PIDP, discussed in the previous section, were historically considered a single entity. As **Table 2** shows, these conditions differ in that, for PTTN, there is an identifiable traumatic event to the trigeminal nerve for example, tooth extraction in the 3 to 6-month period before onset of the pain.

Presentation

Presentation mirrors that of PIDP, the only difference being more localized presentation, with pain in PTTN tending to affect single teeth or the area around a single tooth. Prevalence rates for PTTN following endodontic treatment are reported as 3% to 6%, and of 3% following major facial trauma.[25,26]

Pathogenesis

PTTN is thought to be driven by peripheral afferent nerve damage, the resultant release of local inflammatory mediators and growth factors, which perpetuate increased afferent signaling (peripheral sensitization).[27] Induced changes in second-order and third-order neurons (central sensitization) are thought to lead to hyperexcitability, allodynia, and hyperalgesia.[27]

PERSISTENT IDIOPATHIC FACIAL PAIN

Historic alternative terminology: atypical facial pain

Persistent idiopathic facial pain (PIFP) is a poorly localized facial pain occurring for more than 2 hours per day for a period of at least 3 months, in the absence of any neurologic deficit.[1] The ambiguous nature of PIFP's presentation commonly leads to misdiagnosis.[28]

Presentation

Pain features mimic PIDP and PTTN, although for PIFP pain presents in the face and not the dentoalveolar region. Pain is poorly localized and most commonly unilateral with severe intensity.[28–30] Pain descriptors include aching, burning, throbbing, and stabbing.[28] Wide radiation patterns are common and the pain may present deep within the tissues or superficially.[28] PIFP predominantly affects middle-aged women.[29]

The lifetime prevalence of PIFP is currently thought to be around 0.03%, making the condition extremely rare.[31] However, presentation in specialist centers has been shown to be higher. For example, 21% to 27% of patients referred to a tertiary neurology team were diagnosed with PIFP, in orofacial pain clinics PIFP is thought to make up 10% to 21% of referrals.[28,30]

Pathogenesis

Mechanistically, PIFP demonstrates altered peripheral, central, and inhibitory nociceptive function, as described for PIDP and PTTN.[28,32,33] In addition, alterations in the nigrostriatal dopaminergic system have been observed.[34] Interestingly, qualitative sensory testing does not demonstrate a difference in individuals with confirmed unilateral PIFP when compared with both contralateral, unaffected sites, and control subjects, suggesting pain mechanisms in PIFP do not involve the trigeminal somatosensory system.[28,35]

DIAGNOSTIC CLUES (PERSISTENT IDIOPATHIC DENTOALVEOLAR PAIN DISORDER, POST TRAUMATIC TRIGEMINAL NEUROPATHIC PAIN, AND PERSISTENT IDIOPATHIC FACIAL PAIN)

Persistence of the pain beyond the usual timeframe of healing, repeated dental treatments that have failed to resolve the pain, and the fact that the patients sleep is unaffected by the pain would support a diagnosis of PIDP and PTTN rather than odontogenic pain. The persistence of pain after completion of a dental intervention by a well-intentioned dentist (eg, endodontic treatment or tooth extraction) may also help to refute an odontogenic condition as the cause of the painful symptoms. Indeed, patients presenting with PIDP, PTTN, and PIFP often report dental treatments, which have not in any way changed the pain, either for better or worse.

Stabbing pains in these conditions, if present, are not usually paroxysmal and lack a refractory period in contrast to trigeminal neuralgia. Furthermore, headache features such as aura, photo-sensitivity and phono-sensitivity, and other symptoms, such as nausea and emesis, would not usually be seen in PIDP, PTTN, or PIFP, helping to differentiate these conditions from migraine. Additionally, mean age of onset for PIDP, PTTN, and PIFP differs slightly, with initial presentation most common in the fourth decade of life, slightly later than usual onset for migraine, and earlier than usual onset of trigeminal neuralgia.

The dentoalveolar region should be thoroughly assessed, and oral pathology ruled out clinically and radiographically. In the neurology setting, this is likely to involve a general assessment of dentition and intraoral soft tissues under good lighting, and potentially radiographic imaging, as previously described, followed by formal referral to an oral or dental specialist for definitive assessment.

Digital pressure over the alveolar bone or tapping of the teeth in the region of pain has not been shown to be beneficial in the diagnosis of PIDP or PTTN.[19] In specialist orofacial clinics, somatosensory testing can be used to assess sensory changes in the affected dentoalveolar tissues.[19,36] Mechanical and thermal allodynia (sensory gain) has been demonstrated in PIDP and PTTN compared with control populations.[19,23,36]

FURTHER INVESTIGATIONS (PERSISTENT IDIOPATHIC DENTOALVEOLAR PAIN DISORDER, POST TRAUMATIC TRIGEMINAL NEUROPATHIC PAIN, AND PERSISTENT IDIOPATHIC FACIAL PAIN)

Neuronal function can be affected by several systemic conditions, and it is sensible to use a neuropathic blood panel to exclude potential causes of neuropathic pain and allow correction of abnormalities, as shown in **Table 3**. Detailed clinical and radiographic dental examination may be supplemented with three-dimensional imaging, such as cone beam computed tomography to definitively exclude causes of odontogenic pain. This is most appropriately facilitated by referral to a dental specialist.

Rarely, other pathologic conditions such as multiple sclerosis or neoplasms may cause symptoms similar to trigeminal neuropathies,[37,38] and depending on the presenting features, MRI may be justifiable to rule out central and/or peripheral pathologic condition, which could account for pain symptoms.

BURNING MOUTH SYNDROME

Historic alternative terminology: stomatodynia; glossodynia; stomatopyrosis; and primary/secondary burning mouth syndrome.

Burning mouth syndrome (BMS) is an idiopathic orofacial pain condition presenting with oral dysaesthesia, in the form of burning symptoms, in absence of any causative local, dental, mucosal, or systemic pathologic condition. Diagnostic criteria for BMS as defined in ICOP are shown in **Table 2**.

Presentation

Distribution is most commonly symmetric and bilateral, with the most affected site being the anterior two-thirds of the tongue, followed by dorsum and lateral borders of the tongue, anterior hard palate, and the mucosa of the lower lip.[1,39,40]

Table 3	
Blood investigations for PIDP, PTTN, PIFP, and BMS	
Diagnosis	**Further Investigations**
PIDP, PTTN, PIFP	**Full blood count**
BMS	**Urea and electrolytes**
	Thyroid profile
	HbA1c
	B_{12}
	Folate
	Ferritin
	Auto antibodies
	C-reactive protein
	Antinuclear antibody
BMS	Zinc
	Helicobacter pylori antibody[a]
	Vitamin B_1, B_2, and B_6

Tests in bold text are included in a neuropathic blood panel.
[a] If history indicates gastrointestinal disease.

Pain in BMS is usually constant, although its intensity can vary, demonstrating a tendency to worsen throughout the day, with one-third of patients reporting nocturnal pain.[39,40] There is often mechanical, thermal, and gustatory allodynia, with touching the mucosa aggravating pain symptoms, as well as hot, spicy, or acidic foods. Patients may report that symptoms are worse with stress or fatigue, and that they improve when distracted, or during oral intake, such as chewing gum. In addition to pain, patients commonly report dysgeusia in the form of a persistent bitter or metallic taste, changes in the intensity of taste perception, and xerostomia.[39,41]

Estimates of BMS prevalence in the United States, using strict diagnostic criteria, range from 0.1% to 0.4% with the highest prevalence in postmenopausal women (50–69 years of age).[40] Presentation is spontaneous in about 50% of individuals, and in others onset may be linked to urinary tract infections, dental procedures, antibiotic therapy, and traumatic life stressors.[39,42]

Pathogenesis

BMS is an oral pain diagnosis of exclusion; however, many other conditions and local or systemic factors can cause oral burning symptoms, as outlined in **Table 4**. Oral burning symptoms caused by other conditions were previously referred to as "secondary BMS"; however, this terminology is discouraged.[43] At present, the exact pathogenesis of BMS remains elusive; however, there is evidence of sensory dysfunction secondary to small and large fiber neuropathy,[41,44] centrally mediated pain through hypofunction of dopaminergic neurons in the basal ganglia,[45,46] central trigeminal neuropathy, and loss of central inhibition.[41,46]

Diagnostic Clues

The presentation of BMS localized to the oral soft tissues, and its usual symmetric and bilateral presentation means that BMS is less likely to be confused with other headache and orofacial pain disorders than some of the conditions discussed in this article. It is true, however, that patients presenting with oral burning symptoms are frequently underinvestigated for other local and systemic conditions, which cause oral burning symptoms (see **Table 4**), meaning that clinicians often miss an opportunity to provide effective treatment.

A diagnosis of BMS cannot be made until a thorough examination of the oral soft tissues, particularly in the region of painful symptoms, has been carried out to exclude a local cause. In the nondental setting, oral examination should be performed with good direct lighting to properly illuminate the oral cavity, allowing the assessment of the mucosal and gingival tissues for normal appearance, color, and texture. Examples of healthy mucosal and gingival tissues are shown in **Figs. 1** and **3**. If abnormalities of the oral soft or hard tissues are identified, referral to dental specialists would be appropriate.

Further Investigations

A comprehensive medical, drug, and social history should be taken, as well as an oral swab of the symptomatic area to assess for the presence of *Candida* and blood testing (see **Table 3**) to identify other systemic and local causes of oral burning symptoms, which should be treated promptly if identified. Diagnostic MRI is rarely necessary but may be appropriate in atypical presentations (young, male, unexpected additional symptoms, eg, neurosensory changes).[47] In such instances, MRI of the head and face, ensuring the image extends to the lower border of the mandible, is appropriate to exclude central or peripheral occult pathologic conditions mimicking BMS.

Table 4	
Conditions and factors known to cause symptoms of burning in the oral cavity (previously referred to as secondary BMS)	
Local Factors	**Systemic Factors**
Bacterial infection	**Endocrine**: Diabetes mellitus, hypothyroidism, menopause
Fungal infection (esp. candidiasis)	**Nutritional**: Ferritin, B_1, B_{12}, B_6, Folate, Zinc deficiencies
Viral infection	***H pylori* infection**
Dehydration, mouth breathing, and nasal obstruction	**Autoimmune**, eg, Sjögren syndrome
Xerostomia (34% patients with patients have xerostomia[58])	**Medications**: ACE inhibitors, angiotensin II reception blockers, antiretrovirals, psychotropics, anticholinergics, clonazepam, and chemotherapeutic agents
Mechanical trauma, eg, dentures or trauma from the dentition	**Conditions causing peripheral neuropathy:** HIV infection, sarcoidosis, multiple sclerosis, neuropathy in renal disease
Allergy	**Allergy**
Parafunctional habits, for example, tongue thrusting habit (predisposition to mechanical trauma)	**Gastro-oesophageal reflux disease** (51% of BMS patients have gastritis[59])
Dental prostheses, eg, decreased tongue space from a denture **Neoplasia** **Alcohol-based mouthwash** **Radiation induced stomatitis** **Vesiculobullous conditions**, for example, pemphigus vulgaris and mucous membrane pemphigoid **Aphthous stomatitis** **Oral lichen planus/oral lichenoid lesions/oral graft vs host disease** **Geographic tongue** (erythema migrans)	**Other neuropathies**: Inherited neuropathies, idiopathic small fiber sensory neuropathy, hereditary sensory amyloid polyneuropathy, postherpetic neuropathy, and posttraumatic peripheral sensory neuropathy

Table generated from in formation in refs.[39,42]

MANAGEMENT AND PROGNOSIS (PERSISTENT IDIOPATHIC DENTOALVEOLAR PAIN DISORDER, POST TRAUMATIC TRIGEMINAL NEUROPATHIC PAIN, PERSISTENT IDIOPATHIC FACIAL PAIN, AND BURNING MOUTH SYNDROME)

PIDP, PTTN, PIFP, and BMS are currently managed as neuropathic pain conditions. No treatment is absolutely effective, and unfortunately, the prognosis for these orofacial pain conditions is poor. In BMS for example, for individuals undergoing active management, longitudinal 5-year follow-up data demonstrate no change in symptoms for 49% of sufferers, worsening of symptoms in 10%, and remission of symptoms in just 3% of patients.[48]

As for all persistent pain conditions, cohesive biopsychosocial strategies to manage both the pain and its impact should be standard practice.[28,49] Pharmacologically, neuromodulatory agents in the form of antidepressant (eg, amitriptyline and duloxetine) and antiepileptic medications (eg, gabapentin and pregabalin) are routinely used, although robust evidence specific to trigeminal orofacial pain conditions is lacking,

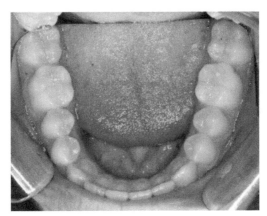

Fig. 3. Healthy oral mucosa including the gingival tissues and tongue dorsum. Note the uniform, noninflamed appearance of the gingival margins, and papillated appearance of the tongue dorsum.

meaning the certainty of their effect is low. Topical agents (eg, benzydamine, lidocaine, capsaicin, and clonazepam) seem to offer some temporary symptom reduction.[50,51] Despite lack of condition-specific data, the use of cognitive behavioral therapy and other active psychological therapies is encouraged due to their conservative nature and known benefit for other persistent pain conditions.[49,52,53] Nascent evidence exists for injectable treatments, such as botulinum toxin, and these could offer potential benefits to patients in the future.[54,55]

DISCUSSION

Just as headache disorders occasionally present to dental and orofacial pain clinics mimicking odontogenic or orofacial conditions, the converse is also true, with these conditions presenting to the nondental setting mimicking headache disorders.[56] The clinical presentations of odontogenic and orofacial pain conditions are usually straightforward to identify; however, this relies on an appropriate and comprehensive investigation strategy, which must involve a thorough examination of the oral cavity. For neuropathic disorders, such as BMS and the trigeminal neuropathies, exclusion of local or systemic factors, which would explain the patient's symptoms, is vital. This should include blood tests to identify relevant systemic conditions that may cause the presenting symptoms, and appropriate imaging where an occult pathology is suspected because of atypical symptoms or presentations.

Pain in the orofacial region is highly emotive,[57] and patients who present with these conditions may be highly distressed. It is therefore important that a multidisciplinary approach is taken to managing their condition from a biopsychosocial perspective. Where there is any question over the contribution of oral pathologies or pain originating from the orofacial region contributing to the patient's condition, then the assessing clinician should consider the early involvement of an oral or dental specialist in the patient's care as appropriate. Unfortunately, failure to consider this in a timely fashion may lead to inevitable harm to the patient due to inappropriate or ineffective treatments of their pain.

Clinicians in the neurology clinic or in general practice should be mindful of these conditions and keep such diagnoses in mind for patients who present with nontypical symptoms.

DISCLOSURE

The authors declare that there are no conflicts of interest. D. Edwards and J.R. Allison are supported by doctoral fellowship funding from the Wellcome Trust 4Ward North Clinical PhD Academy. All authors are supported by the NIHR Newcastle Biomedical Research Centre.

REFERENCES

1. International classification of orofacial pain, 1st edition (ICOP). Cephalalgia 2020; 40(2):129–221.
2. Headache Classification Committee of the International Headache Society (IHS). Classification and diagnostic criteria for Headache disorders, cranial neuralgias and facial pain. Cephalalgia 1988;8:1–96.
3. Headache Classification Subcommittee of the International Headache Society. 2nd edition. The international classification of headache disorders, 24. Cephalalgia; 2004. p. 1–160.
4. Headache Classification Subcommittee of the International Headache Society (IHS). 3rd edition. The international classification of headache disorders, 38. Cephalalgia; 2018. p. 1–211.
5. Lipton J, Ship J, Larach-Robinson D. Estimated prevalence and distribution of reported orofacial pain in the United States. JADA (J Am Dent Assoc) 1993; 124(10):115–21.
6. Office for National Statistics. Social survey division. information centre for health and social care. adult dental health survey. London: UK Data Service; 2012.
7. Edwards D, Rasaiah S, Hamzah Ahmed S, et al. The financial and quality of life impact of urgent dental presentations: A cross-sectional study. Int Endod J 2023; 56(6):697–709.
8. American Association of Endodontists. Endodontic diagnosis Online. . 2013; Available from: https://www.aae.org/specialty/wp-content/uploads/sites/2/2017/07/endodonticdiagnosisfall2013.pdf.
9. Trindade D, Carvalho R, Machado V, et al. Prevalence of periodontitis in dentate people between 2011 and 2020: A systematic review and meta-analysis of epidemiological studies. J Clin Periodontol 2023;50(5):604–26.
10. Dietrich T, Ower P, Tank M, et al. Periodontal diagnosis in the context of the 2017 classification system of periodontal diseases and conditions - implementation in clinical practice. Br Dent J 2019;226(1):16–22.
11. Byers MR, Wheeler EF, Bothwell M. Altered expression of NGF and P75 NGF-receptor by fibroblasts of injured teeth precedes sensory nerve sprouting. Growth Factors 1992;6(1):41–52.
12. Allison JR, Stone SJ, Pigg M. The painful tooth: mechanisms, presentation and differential diagnosis of odontogenic pain. Oral Surgery 2020;13(4):309–20.
13. Zhang X, Li L, McNaughton PA. Proinflammatory mediators modulate the heat-activated ion channel TRPV1 via the scaffolding protein AKAP79/150. Neuron 2008;59(3):450–61.
14. Lee C, Ramsey A, De Brito-Gariepy H, et al. Molecular, cellular and behavioral changes associated with pathological pain signaling occur after dental pulp injury. Mol Pain 2017;13. 1744806917715173.
15. Tsuboi Y, Iwata K, Dostrovsky JO, et al. Modulation of astroglial glutamine synthetase activity affects nociceptive behaviour and central sensitization of medullary dorsal horn nociceptive neurons in a rat model of chronic pulpitis. Eur J Neurosci 2011;34(2):292–302.

16. Siqueira JF Jr, Rôças IN. The microbiota of acute apical abscesses. J Dent Res 2009;88(1):61–5.

17. Heitz-Mayfield LJ. Systemic antibiotics in periodontal therapy. Aust Dent J 2009; 54(Suppl 1):S96–101.

18. Agnihotry A, Thompson W, Fedorowicz Z, et al. Antibiotic use for irreversible pulpitis. Cochrane Database Syst Rev 2019;(5).

19. Sanner F, Sonntag D, Hambrock N, et al. Patients with persistent idiopathic dentoalveolar pain in dental practice. Int Endod J 2022;55(3):231–9.

20. Coulter J, Nixdorf DR. A review of persistent idiopathic dentoalveolar pain (formerly PDAP/Atypical odontalgia). Oral Surgery 2020;13(4):371–8.

21. Ram S, Teruel A, Kumar SKS, et al. Clinical characteristics and diagnosis of atypical odontalgia: implications for dentists. J Am Dent Assoc 2009;140(2):223–8.

22. Nixdorf DR, Law AS, John MT, et al. Differential diagnoses for persistent pain after root canal treatment: a study in the national dental practice-based research network. J Endod 2015;41(4):457–63.

23. List T, Leijon G, Svensson P. Somatosensory abnormalities in atypical odontalgia: A case-control study. Pain 2008;139(2):333–41.

24. Costigan M, Scholz J, Woolf CJ. Neuropathic pain: a maladaptive response of the nervous system to damage. Annu Rev Neurosci 2009;32:1–32.

25. Al-Khudhairy MW, Albisher G, Alarfaj A, et al. Post-traumatic trigeminal neuropathy associated with endodontic therapy: a systematic review. Cureus 2022; 14(12):e32675.

26. Benoliel R, Birenboim R, Regev E, et al. Neurosensory changes in the infraorbital nerve following zygomatic fractures. Oral Surg Oral Med Oral Pathol Oral Radiol Endod 2005;99(6):657–65.

27. Korczeniewska OA, Kohli D, Benoliel R, et al. Pathophysiology of post-traumatic trigeminal neuropathic pain. Biomolecules 2022;12(12).

28. Benoliel R, Gaul C. Persistent idiopathic facial pain. Cephalalgia 2017;37(7): 680–91.

29. Maarbjerg S, Wolfram F, Heinskou TB, et al. Persistent idiopathic facial pain - a prospective systematic study of clinical characteristics and neuroanatomical findings at 3.0 Tesla MRI. Cephalalgia 2017;37(13):1231–40.

30. Zebenholzer K, Wöber C, Vigl M, et al. Facial pain in a neurological tertiary care centre–evaluation of the international classification of headache disorders. Cephalalgia 2005;25(9):689–99.

31. Mueller D, Obermann M, Yoon MS, et al. Prevalence of trigeminal neuralgia and persistent idiopathic facial pain: a population-based study. Cephalalgia 2011; 31(15):1542–8.

32. Forssell H, Tenovuo O, Silvoniemi P, et al. Differences and similarities between atypical facial pain and trigeminal neuropathic pain. Neurology 2007;69(14): 1451–9.

33. Derbyshire SW, Jones AK, Devani P, et al. Cerebral responses to pain in patients with atypical facial pain measured by positron emission tomography. J Neurol Neurosurg Psychiatry 1994;57(10):1166–72.

34. Hagelberg N, Forssell H, Aalto S, et al. Altered dopamine D2 receptor binding in atypical facial pain. Pain 2003;106(1–2):43–8.

35. Lang E, Kaltenhäuser M, Seidler S, et al. Persistent idiopathic facial pain exists independent of somatosensory input from the painful region: findings from quantitative sensory functions and somatotopy of the primary somatosensory cortex. Pain 2005;118(1–2):80–91.

36. Baad-Hansen L, Pigg M, Ivanovic SE, et al. Chairside intraoral qualitative somatosensory testing: reliability and comparison between patients with atypical odontalgia and healthy controls. J Orofac Pain 2013;27(2):165–70.
37. Moazzam AA, Habibian M. Patients appearing to dental professionals with orofacial pain arising from intracranial tumors: a literature review. Oral Surg Oral Med Oral Pathol Oral Radiol 2012;114(6):749–55.
38. Gupta K, Burchiel KJ. Atypical facial pain in multiple sclerosis caused by spinal cord seizures: a case report and review of the literature. J Med Case Rep 2016; 10:101.
39. Renton T. Burning mouth syndrome. Rev Pain 2011;5(4):12–7.
40. Kohorst JJ, Bruce AJ, Torgerson RR, et al. The prevalence of burning mouth syndrome: a population-based study. Br J Dermatol 2015;172(6):1654–6.
41. Ritchie A, Kramer JM. Recent advances in the etiology and treatment of burning mouth syndrome. J Dent Res 2018;97(11):1193–9.
42. The American Academy of Orofacial Pain. Orofacial pain: guidelines for assessment, diagnosis and management. 6th edition. Hanover Park, IL: Quintessence Publishing; 2018.
43. Currie CC, Ohrbach R, De Leeuw R, et al. Developing a research diagnostic criteria for burning mouth syndrome: Results from an international Delphi process. J Oral Rehabil 2021;48(3):308–31.
44. Forssell H, Jääskeläinen S, Tenovuo O, et al. Sensory dysfunction in burning mouth syndrome. Pain 2002;99(1–2):41–7.
45. Hagelberg N, Forssell H, Rinne JO, et al. Striatal dopamine D1 and D2 receptors in burning mouth syndrome. Pain 2003;101(1–2):149–54.
46. Lopez-Jornet P, Molino-Pagan D, Parra-Perez P, et al. Neuropathic pain in patients with burning mouth syndrome evaluated using painDETECT. Pain Med 2017;18(8):1528–33.
47. Suga T, Takenoshita M, Tu TTH, et al. A case of vestibular schwannoma mimicking burning mouth syndrome. Biopsychosoc Med 2021;15(1):7.
48. Sardella A, Lodi G, Demarosi F, et al. Burning mouth syndrome: a retrospective study investigating spontaneous remission and response to treatments. Oral Dis 2006;12(2):152–5.
49. Barker S, Urbanek M, Penlington C. Psychological interventions for persistent orofacial pain. Prim Dent J 2019;7(4):30–5.
50. Vickers ER, Cousins MJ, Walker S, et al. Analysis of 50 patients with atypical odontalgia. a preliminary report on pharmacological procedures for diagnosis and treatment. Oral Surg Oral Med Oral Pathol Oral Radiol Endod 1998;85(1): 24–32.
51. Rodríguez de Rivera Campillo E, López-López J, Chimenos-Küstner E. Response to topical clonazepam in patients with burning mouth syndrome: a clinical study. Bull Group Int Rech Sci Stomatol Odontol 2010;49(1):19–29.
52. Morley S, Eccleston C, Williams A. Systematic review and meta-analysis of randomized controlled trials of cognitive behaviour therapy and behaviour therapy for chronic pain in adults, excluding headache. Pain 1999;80(1–2):1–13.
53. Burns JW, Jensen MP, Thorn B, et al. Cognitive therapy, mindfulness-based stress reduction, and behavior therapy for the treatment of chronic pain: randomized controlled trial. Pain 2022;163(2):376–89.
54. Dawson A, Dawson J, Ernberg M. The effect of botulinum toxin A on patients with persistent idiopathic dentoalveolar pain—A systematic review. J Oral Rehabil 2020;47(9):1184–91.

55. Moreau N, Dieb W, Descroix V, et al. Topical review: potential use of botulinum toxin in the management of painful posttraumatic trigeminal neuropathy. J Oral Facial Pain Headache 2017;31(1):7–18.

56. Reyes AJ, Ramcharan K, Maharaj R. Chronic migraine headache and multiple dental pathologies causing cranial pain for 35 years: the neurodental nexus. BMJ Case Rep 2019;12(9):e230248.

57. Schmidt K, Forkmann K, Sinke C, et al. The differential effect of trigeminal vs. peripheral pain stimulation on visual processing and memory encoding is influenced by pain-related fear. Neuroimage 2016;134:386–95.

58. Klasser GD, Fischer DJ, Epstein JB. Burning mouth syndrome: recognition, understanding, and management. Oral Maxillofac Surg Clin 2008;20(2):255–71.

59. Brailo V, Vuéiaeeviae-Boras V, Alajbeg IZ, et al. Oral burning symptoms and burning mouth syndrome-significance of different variables in 150 patients. Med Oral, Patol Oral Cirugía Bucal 2006;11(3):252–5.

Moving?

Make sure your subscription moves with you!

To notify us of your new address, find your **Clinics Account Number** (located on your mailing label above your name), and contact customer service at:

Email: journalscustomerservice-usa@elsevier.com

800-654-2452 (subscribers in the U.S. & Canada)
314-447-8871 (subscribers outside of the U.S. & Canada)

Fax number: 314-447-8029

Elsevier Health Sciences Division
Subscription Customer Service
3251 Riverport Lane
Maryland Heights, MO 63043

Printed and bound by CPI Group (UK) Ltd, Croydon, CR0 4YY

03/10/2024

01040474-0013